The Science & Philosophy of Teaching Yoga and Yoga Therapy

A SUN YOGA BOOK

ISBN: 978-0-9556423-4-0

Printed in USA
Cover design: Workbridge

This book is dedicated to all the Sun Yoga teachers in the world who share our vision and walked our path.

May the long time sun shine upon you
SAT NAM

Also from Sun Yoga:

BOOKS

Simply Yogic. Food for the mind, body & soul

Live Patanjali! Yoga Wisdom for Everyday Living

Peaceful Warrior Handbook

DVD

YogaSense™ Master Sequence, Exercises and Routines

Groovy Creatures Yoga DVD (for children's yoga)

CD

Popular Yoga Mantra

Children's Yoga Music

YOGA CARDS

Fun With Sun Yoga.
Yoga Cards and Booklet for Children's Yoga

Yogasana flash cards

www.sunyoga.com

The Science & Philosophy of Teaching Yoga and Yoga Therapy

by Jacqueline Koay & Theodora Barenholtz

BOOK ONE:
THE SCIENCE & PHILOSOPHY OF TEACHING YOGA

BOOK TWO:
YOGA THERAPY

BOOK THREE:
YOGASENSE™ YOGA SEQUENCES

BOOK ONE: THE SCIENCE & PHILOSOPHY OF TEACHING YOGA

Chapter 1 Introduction: The Spirit of Yoga
1.1 "Experience, then believe" *(p3)*
1.2 The meaning of yoga *(p3)*
1.3 History, religion and key practices *(p4)*
1.4 The yoga tree *(p7)*
1.5 Seven historical yoga teachers *(p10)*
1.6 Seven influential yoga teachers *(p14)*
1.7 Seven contemporary yoga teachers *(p18)*
1.8 Related spiritual practices / schools *(p21)*
1.9 Six experiences of yoga *(p23)*

Chapter 2 Philosophy, Ethics & Lifestyle
2.1 Moving beyond the physical *(p27)*
2.2 *Shad Darshan*: the Six Philosophies of Life *(p31)*
2.3 The books of yoga *(p37)*
2.4 Yoga Sutra of Sri Patanjali *(p40)*
2.5 *Ashtanga yoga*: the eightfold path *(p51)*
2.6 Living life as a modern yogi *(p56)*

Chapter 3 Anatomy
3.1 Body mechanics *(p62)*
3.2 Parts of the skeletal system *(p68)*
3.3 Anatomical positions and planes of movement *(p72)*
3.4 The spine *(p74)*
3.5 The pelvis *(p78)*
3.6 The upper extremities *(p81)*
3.7 The lower extremities *(p83)*
3.8 The muscular system and *yogasana* *(p85)*
3.9 Muscles of the back *(p89)*
3.10 Abdominal muscles *(p95)*
3.11 Muscles of the lower extremities *(p98)*
3.12 Muscles of the upper extremities *(p107)*
3.13 Summary notes: muscles covered in this chapter *(p112)*
3.14 Treatment for overstretched/torn muscles *(p119)*

Chapter 4   Physiology
4.1 The basic concepts *(p121)*
4.2 Main systems of the body *(p123)*
4.3 Common ailments and symptoms *(p136)*
4.4 High risk categories *(p143)*
4.5 Important points for the yoga teacher *(p145)*

Chapter 5 The Brain and The Mind
5.1 The philosophical-physiological perspective *(p149)*
5.2 The brain: the Western perspective *(p149)*
5.3 Anatomy and physiology of the brain *(p150)*
5.4 Effects of yoga on the brain *(p155)*
5.5 The mind and science *(p159)*
5.6 The yogic mind *(p162)*
5.7 Yogic practices for a healthy brain and mind *(p173)*

Chapter 6 Yogic Anatomy & Ayurvĕda
6.1 Anatomy of light *(p178)*
6.2 Ayurvĕda *(p181)*
6.3 The three *dosha* *(p184)*
6.4 *Dhatu*, *ojas* and *tejas* *(p190)*
6.5 *Prana* and *agni* *(p193)*
6.6 Energy conduits of the body *(p198)*
6.7 The *chakra* system *(p202)*
6.8 The subtle bodies *(p204)*
6.9 The yogic way to good health *(p210)*

Chapter 7 Techniques
7.1 The yoga universe *(p214)*
7.2 Practicing *yogasana* *(p216)*
7.3 YogaSense™: The Seven Core Principles *(p218)*
7.4 *Drishti* *(p223)*
7.5 *Bandha* *(p223)*
7.6 Meditation *(p228)*
7.7 *Pranayama* *(p230)*
7.8 Relaxation and visualization *(p240)*
7.9 Sanskrit chants *(p241)*

Chapter 8 Teaching Methodology
8.1 Ethics of a yoga teacher *(p245)*
8.2 The teacher-student relationship *(p248)*
8.3 Teaching yoga as a yogi: the *yama* *(p251)*
8.4 Teaching *drishti* *(p253)*
8.5 Teaching *bandha* *(p255)*
8.6 Teaching meditation *(p259)*
8.7 Teaching *pranayama* *(p262)*
8.8 Teaching relaxation and visualization *(p266)*
8.9. Teaching YogaSense™ *(p267)*
8.10 Teaching *padmasana* *(p270)*
8.11 Teaching safely *(p272)*
8.12 Structuring a yoga class *(p274)*

BOOK TWO: YOGA THERAPY

Chapter 1 Introduction: The Spirit of Yoga Therapy

1.1 What is Yoga Therapy? *(p280)*
1.2 Key elements *(p280)*
1.3 Key yoga tools *(p282)*
1.4 Physical benefits of *yogasana* *(p285)*
1.5 Emotional benefits of *yogasana* *(p288)*
1.6 Scope of practice *(p289)*
1.7 Limitations *(p289)*
1.8 Yoga Props *(p290)*
1.9 Gong *(p291)*
1.10 Caregiver *(p292)*

Chapter 2 Neurology

2.1 Yoga for neurological conditions *(p294)*
2.2 Parkinson's Disease *(p296)*
2.3 Multiple Sclerosis *(p300)*
2.4 Cerebral Vascular Accident *(p302)*
2.5 Traumatic Brain Injury *(p304)*
2.6 Alzheimer's *(p305)*
2.7 Vestibular Disorder *(p306)*
2.8 Peripheral Neuropathy *(p308)*

Chapter 3 Medical

3.1 Introduction *(p312)*
3.2 Diabetes *(p314)*
3.3 Obesity *(p315)*
3.4 Irritable Bowel Syndrome and Gastroesophageal Reflux *(p316)*
3.5 Coronary Artery Disease *(p317)*
3.6 Pulmonary Disease *(p318)*
3.7 Cancer *(p321)*
3.8 Infectious Diseases: HIV/AIDS *(p322)*

Chapter 4 Orthopedic

4.1 Introduction *(p326)*
4.2 Spinal alignment and pathology *(p327)*
4.3 Scoliosis *(p331)*
4.4 Osteoporosis *(p332)*
4.5 Arthritis *(p334)*
4.6 Lower back *(p335)*
4.7 Neck *(p337)*
4.8 Upper extremities *(p339)*
4.9 Lower extremities *(p341)*
4.10 Hyperextended joints *(p343)*

BOOK THREE: YOGASENSE® SEQUENCES

The YogaSense™ Roadmap *(p345)*
Sun breath sequence *(p346)*
Brain organizing & grounding meditation *(p347)*
Vestibular rebalancing exercise *(p348)*
Posture awareness exercise *(p349)*
Balance sequence *(p350)*
Spinal alignment exercise *(p352)*
Core strengthening exercise *(p354)*
Supported strengthening sequence *(p356)*
Wheelchair / chair yoga *(p357)*
Hip and hamstring opening exercise *(p358)*
Shoulder opening exercise *(p359)*
Lower back routine *(p360)*
Pelvic floor routine *(p361)*
Restorative yoga *(p362)*
Foot care routine *(p363)*
Pawanmuktasana sequence *(p364)*
Gastrointestinal (GI) sequence *(p364)*
Guided relaxation *(p365)*
Tantra yoga *(p366)*

BOOK ONE: THE SCIENCE & PHILOSOPHY OF TEACHING YOGA

Chapter 1   Introduction: The Spirit of Yoga

1.1 "Experience, then believe"..3

    1.1.1. Live your yoga 3

1.2 The meaning of yoga 3

    1.2.1. Origin of the word yoga 3

1.3 History, religion and key practices..4

    1.3.1. History..4

    1.3.2. Religion 5

        svadhyayat ista-devata samprayogah [Yoga Sutra 44, II]...............5

        yatha abhimata dhyanat va [Yoga Sutra 39, I] 5

    1.3.3. Key Practices 6

1.4 The yoga tree...7

    1.4.1. The Hatha Yoga branch 7

    1.4.2. The Raja Yoga branch 7

    1.4.3. Bhakti Yoga..8

    1.4.4. Jnâna yoga..8

    1.4.5. Naad Yoga 8

    1.4.6. Laya Yoga 9

    1.4.7. Karma Yoga 9

    1.4.8. Contemporary Branches of Yoga...9

1.5 Seven historical yoga teachers 10

    1.5.1. Swami Sivananda Saraswati (*1887 - 1963*) 10

    1.5.2. Krishnamacharya (*1888–1989*) 11

    1.5.3. Sri K Pattabhi Jois (*1915 - 2009*) 12

    1.5.4. BKS Iyengar (*1918 - *)...12

    1.5.5. Indra Devi (*1899 - 2002*) 12

    1.5.6. Harbajan Singh Khalsa / Yogi Bhajan (*1929 - 2004*)............13

    1.5.7. Sri Swami Satchidananda (*1914 - 2002*) 14

1.6 Seven influential yoga teachers...14

    1.6.1. Vanda Scaravelli (*1908 - 1999*)...14

    1.6.2. Yogi Amrit Desai (*1932 - *) 15

    1.6.3. Gurmukh Kaur Khalsa (*1943 - *) 15

    1.6.4. TKV Desikachar (*1938 - *) 16

    1.6.5. John Scott (*1957 - *) 16

    1.6.6. Deepak Chopra (*1947 - *) 17

    1.6.7. Doug and David Swenson (*1950's - *) 17

1.7 Seven contemporary yoga teachers 18

    1.7.1. Joseph Michael Levry / Gurunam...18

    1.7.2. Bikram Choudhury 19

    1.7.3. Sharath Rangaswamy 19

1.7.4. Baron Baptiste 19

1.7.5. Shiva Rea 20

1.7.6. Seane Corn 21

1.7.7. Rodney Yee 21

1.8 Related spiritual practices / schools 21

1.8.1. Art of Living (AOL) 21

1.8.2. Transcendental Meditation (TM) 21

1.8.3. Brahma Kumaris 22

1.8.4. Osho (*1931 – 1990*) 22

1.8.5. *Kirtan* 22

1.9 Six experiences of yoga 23

1.9.1. Living in the moment 23

1.9.2. Journaling 23

1.9.3. Mindful Eating 24

1.9.4. Spiritual fire 24

1.9.5. Commitment 24

1.9.6. Letting go 24

References 25

Chapter 2   Philosophy, Ethics & Lifestyle

2.1 Moving beyond the physical 27

2.1.1. The deeper meaning of yoga 27

2.1.2. Self-study / studying the scriptures (*svadhyaya*) 27

yogahcittavrittinirodhah [Yoga Sutra 2, I] 27

2.1.3. The five sheaths (*kosha*) 28

2.2 *Shad Darshan*: the Six Philosophies of Life 31

2.2.1. Introduction 31

2.2.2. The Universe according to Samkhya..32

2.2.3. Samkhya and Yoga...33

2.2.4. Vaisheshika and Nyaya 34

2.2.5. Mimamsa and Vedanta..36

svadhyayat ista devata samprayogah [Yoga Sutra 40, II] 36

2.3 The books of yoga..37

2.3.1. Yoga Sutra of Sri Patanjali 37

2.3.2. Vedas 37

2.3.3. Upanishad 38

2.3.4. Mahābhārata and Rāmāyana 38

2.3.5. Bhagavad Gita 38

2.3.6. Hatha Yoga Pradipika...39

2.4 Yoga Sutra of Sri Patanjali 40

2.4.1. Introduction to the Yoga Sutra...40

2.4.2. How to study the Yoga Sutra..41

2.4.3. The framework 41

2.4.4. Chapter 1: Samadhi Pada 42

    yogaschittavritti nirodhah [Yoga Sutra 2, I]...43

    vrttayah pancatayyah klista aklistah [Yoga Sutra 5, I]...............................44

    pramana viparyaya vikalpa nidra smrtayah [Yoga Sutra 6, I] 44

    pratyaksa anumana agamah pramanani [Yoga Sutra 7, I] 45

    abhyasa vairagyabhyam tan-nirodhah [Yoga Sutra 12, I]..........................45

    vitarka vicara ananda asmita rupa nugamat samprajnata [Yoga Sutra 17, I] 46

2.4.5. Chapter 2: Sadhana Pada 47

    Tapah-svadhyayesvara-pranidhananikriya-yogah [Yoga Sutra 1, II] 47

    kayendriya-siddhir asuddhi-ksayat tapasah [Yoga Sutra 43, II]...................48

    samadhi-bhavanarthah klesa-tanu-karanarthas ca [Yoga Sutra 2, II] 48

    avidyasmita-raga-dvesabhinivesah klesha [Yoga Sutra 3, II] 49

    sukhanusayi ragah [Yoga Sutra 7, II] 49

    anityasuci-duhkhanatmasunitya-suci-sukhatmakhyatir avidya [Yoga Sutra 5, II].........50

    te pratiprasava-heyah suksmah [Yoga Sutra 10, II] 50

    dhyana-heyas tad-vrttayah [Yoga Sutra 11, II] 50

    Heyam duhkham anagatam [Yoga Sutra 16, II].......................................50

2.5 *Ashtanga yoga*: the eightfold path...51

2.5.1. The eightfold path 51

    Yama niyama asana pranayama pratyhara dharana dhyana samadhyo astavangani [Yoga Sutra 29, II] 51

2.5.2. <u>*Yama*</u> 52

    ahimsa satya asteya brahmacharya aparigraha yamah [Yoga Sutra 30, II] 52

    jati desa kala samaya annavachinnah sarva-bhaumah maha-vratam [Yoga Sutra 31, II] 53

2.5.3. <u>*Niyama*</u> 53

    sauca santosa tapah svadhyaya Isvara-pranidhanani niyamah [Yoga Sutra 32, II] 54

    santosat anuttamah sukha labhah [Yoga Sutra 42, II].............................54

2.5.4. <u>*Asana*</u> 54

2.5.5. <u>*Pranayama*</u> 55

2.5.6. <u>*Pratyhara*</u> 55

2.5.7. <u>*Dharana and dhyana*</u> 55

2.5.8. <u>*Samadhi*</u> 55

    tada drastuh svarupe avasthanam [Yoga Sutra 3, I]................................55

    tatra sthitau yatnah abhyasa [Yoga Sutra 13, I].....................................55

    abhyasa vairagyabhyam tan-nirodhah [Yoga Sutra 12, I]..........................56

    visoka va jyotismati [Yoga Sutra 36, I]...56

2.6 Living life as a modern yogi...56

2.6.1. Renaissance of yoga 56

2.6.2. Living a yogic life...57

    Jati-desa-kala-samaya-annavachinnah sarva-bhauma maha-vratam [Yoga Sutra 31, II] 57

yoga-anga-anusthanad asuddhi-ksye jnana-diptir a viveka-khyateh [Yoga Sutra 28, II] 57

2.6.3. Starting on the path...58

References 60

Chapter 3   Anatomy

3.1 Body mechanics...62

3.1.1. Strength and flexibility of the body 62

3.1.2. Internal scaffolding of the body 62

3.1.3. Construction of the spine..63

3.1.4. Vulnerability of the spinal column 64

3.1.5. Other vulnerable parts of the body 66

3.2 Parts of the skeletal system 68

3.2.1. Bones 68

3.2.2. Joints...70

3.2.3. Ligaments..70

3.2.4. Tendons 71

3.2.5. Muscle contraction 71

3.2.6. Fascia 71

3.3 Anatomical position and planes of movement 72

3.3.1. Anatomical position..72

3.3.2. Anatomical planes (diagram 3.3)..72

3.3.3. Planes of movement (diagram 3.3) 72

3.3.4. Anatomical descriptions (diagram 3.3)...73

3.4 The spine..74

3.4.1. Function of the spine..74

3.4.2. Bones of the spine (diagram 3.2) 74

3.4.3. Vertebrae (diagram 3.2) 74

3.4.4. Intervertebral discs (diagram 3.2) 75

3.4.5. Curves of the spine 75

3.4.6. Understanding the internal movement of the spine...76

3.4.7. Special considerations for the neck..77

3.5 The pelvis 78

3.5.1. Pelvic bones 78

3.5.2. Ligaments..79

3.5.3. Muscles and movement..80

3.5.4. Alignment..80

3.6 The upper extremities..81

3.6.1. Bones of the upper extremities...81

3.6.2. Joints...81

3.6.3. Muscles and movement..82

3.6.4. Alignment..83

3.7 The lower extremities 83

    3.7.1. Bones of the lower extremities 83

    3.7.2. Joints 84

    3.7.3. Muscles and movement 84

    3.7.4. Alignment 85

3.8 The muscular system and *yogasana* 85

    3.8.1. Introduction 85

    3.8.2. Workings of the muscles 86

    3.8.3. Studying muscles 87

    3.8.4. Notes on the following sections 88

3.9 Muscles of the back 89

    3.9.1. Trapezius (diagram 3.8) 89

    3.9.2. Latissimus dorsi (diagram 3.8) 90

    3.9.3. Rhomboids (diagram 3.9) 91

    3.9.4. Levator scapulae (diagram 3.10) 92

    3.9.5. Serratus posterior (diagram 3.9) 93

    3.9.6. Erector spinae 94

    3.9.7. Transversospinalis muscles 94

3.10 Abdominal muscles 95

    3.10.1. Rectus abdominis 95

    3.10.2. Internal and External Obliques 95

    3.10.3. Transverse abdominals 96

    3.10.4. Breathing and the abdominals 96

    3.10.5. Diaphragm 97

3.11 Muscles of the lower extremities 98

    3.11.1. Quadratus lumborum 98

    3.11.2. Psoas muscles (psoas major and iliacus) 98

    3.11.3. Tensor fascia lata 99

    3.11.4. HIP ABDUCTORS 99

    3.11.5. THE EXTERNAL HIP ROTATORS 101

    3.11.6. THE ADDUCTORS 102

    3.11.7. Quadriceps 103

    3.11.8. Hamstrings 104

    3.11.9. Gastrocnemius, soleus and tibialis posterior 105

    3.11.10. Sartorius 105

    3.11.11. MUSCLES OF THE FOOT 106

3.12 Muscles of the upper extremities 107

    3.12.1. Deltoids 107

    3.12.2. Scapula region 107

    3.12.3. ARMS 108

    3.12.4. Sternocleidomastoid 110

    3.12.5. PECTORAL REGION (front of body) 110

    3.12.6. THORAX 111

3.13 Summary notes: muscles covered in this chapter 112

3.14 Treatment for overstretched/torn muscles 119

Chapter 4   Physiology

4.1 The basic concepts...121

    4.1.1. Physiology 121

    4.1.2. Organization of the human body 121

    4.1.3. Main cellular structures 121

4.2 Main systems of the body...123

    4.2.1. Introduction 123

    4.2.2. The nervous system..125

    4.2.3. The immune system 131

    4.2.4. The lymphatic system 132

    4.2.5. The endocrine system..132

    4.2.6. The digestive system 133

    4.2.7. The circulatory system...134

    4.2.8. The respiratory system..134

    4.2.9. The urinary system 135

    4.2.10. The genital system...135

    4.2.11. The integumentary system 136

4.3 Common ailments and symptoms...136

    4.3.1. The parameters of *yogasana* 136

    4.3.2. Fever...137

    4.3.3. Stress 137

    4.3.4. Hypertension..138

    4.3.5. Persistent headaches..139

    4.3.6. Depression 140

    4.3.7. Migraine..141

    4.3.8. Frequent sore throats, fevers, coughs and colds 142

    4.3.9. Influenza ('flu') 142

    4.3.10. When it is not appropriate to attend yoga 142

4.4 High risk categories...143

    4.4.1. Diabetes 143

    4.4.2. Cancer...143

    4.4.3. Recovery from surgery (including caesarean births).......................................143

    4.4.4. Slipped disc and other trauma of the spine..144

    4.4.5. Senior citizens 144

    4.4.6. Pregnancy...145

4.5 Important points for the yoga teacher 145

    4.5.1. Managing your practitioners' expectations 145

    4.5.2. Yoga is not the cure for everything 146

    4.5.3. Yoga is not suitable for everybody 146

4.5.4. You are a yoga teacher, not a doctor 146

References 147

Chapter 5   The Brain and The Mind

5.1 The philosophical-physiological perspective 149

    5.1.1. Dualism 149

    5.1.2. The yogic perspective 149

5.2 The brain: the Western perspective 149

    5.2.1. The scope 149

    5.2.2. Brain biology 150

5.3 Anatomy and physiology of the brain..150

    5.3.1. Major internal parts of the brain..150

    5.3.2. The surface of the cerebrum (cerebral cortex) 152

    5.3.3. Cerebral cortex lobes..153

    5.3.4. Beneath the cerebral cortex 153

    5.3.5. The limbic system 154

5.4 Effects of yoga on the brain 155

    5.4.1. Accepted benefits of yoga 155

    5.4.2. Emotional management 156

    5.4.3. Improving basic vital life functions...156

    5.4.4. Changing perspectives on life 157

    5.4.5. Physical coordination..157

    5.4.6. Right-left hemisphere balancing 158

5.5 The mind and science 159

    5.5.1. Introduction 159

    5.5.2. Psychology 160

    5.5.3. Psychiatry...161

    5.5.4. Application of psychology and psychiatry 161

5.6 The yogic mind 162

    5.6.1. The mind according to the Yoga Sutra of Sri Patanjali 162

        yogaschittavritti nirodhah [Yoga Sutra 2,I]....................................162

        pramanaviparyayavikalpanidrasmrtayah [Yoga Sutra 6, I].........162

        tada drashtuh svarupe avasthanam [Yoga Sutra 3,I]....................162

    5.6.2. Anatomy of the mind...162

    5.6.3. States of consciousness 163

    5.6.4. Moving through the states of consciousness....................................165

    5.6.5. Birth of the mind 166

    5.6.6. From mind to matter 167

    5.6.7. Manifestations of the mind...170

    5.6.8. Pathology of the ego...171

5.7 Yogic practices for a healthy brain and mind..173

5.7.1. How yoga works 173

5.7.2. The practices 173

References 176

Chapter 6　　Yogic Anatomy & Ayurvĕda

6.1 Anatomy of light 178

    6.1.1. Introduction 178

    6.1.2. Advent of modern Western medicine 178

    6.1.3. Foundations of holistic medical sciences..180

    6.1.4. Branches of the holistic medical sciences 181

6.2 Ayurvĕda 181

    6.2.1. An introduction 181

    6.2.2. Origins of Ayurvĕda 182

    6.2.3. Ayurvĕda in the Western world 182

6.3 The three *dosha*...184

    6.3.1. The foundations 184

    6.3.2. *Dosha* and their attributes 185

    6.3.3. *Doshic* signature 186

    6.3.4. Characteristics of *vata* 187

    6.3.5. Characteristics of *pitta* 188

    6.3.6. Characteristics of *kapha* 189

6.4 *Dhatu, ojas* and *tejas* 190

    6.4.1. *Dhatu* 190

    6.4.2. *Ojas* 192

    6.4.3. *Tejas* 192

6.5 *Prana* and *agni* 193

    6.5.1. *Prana* and *agni* 193

    6.5.2. The five *prana* 193

    6.5.3. Experiencing the five *prana* 196

6.6 Energy conduits of the body 198

    6.6.1. Movement of energy in the body...198

    6.6.2. *Merudanda* and *sushumna* 198

    6.6.3. *Nadi* 198

    6.6.4. *Ida* and *Pingala*...199

    6.6.5. *Chakra* 200

6.7 The *chakra* system...202

    6.7.1. *Mooladhara*: the earth *chakra* (dark red)..202

    6.7.2. *Svadisthana*: the creative *chakra* (deep orange) 202

    6.7.3. *Manipura*: the feelings *chakra* (bright yellow)....................................202

    6.7.4. *Anahata*: the love *chakra* (intense green)...203

    6.7.5. *Visuddha*: the truth *chakra* (cool blue)..203

    6.7.6. *Ajna*: the knowing *chakra* (midnight blue) 204

6.7.7. *Sahasrara*: the angel *chakra* (violet) 204

6.8 The subtle bodies 204

    6.8.1. The five *kosha* 205

    6.8.2. The Ten Bodies 207

6.9 The yogic way to good health 210

    6.9.1. Do everything in balance 210

    6.9.2. Eat a balanced diet 210

    6.9.3. Live a balanced life 210

    6.9.4. Cultivate balanced relationships (stay away from destructive ones)........211

    6.9.5. The Ayurvĕdic way..211

References 212

Chapter 7   Techniques

7.1 The yoga universe...214

    7.1.1. Introduction 214

    7.1.2. The main schools of yoga...214

7.2 Practicing *yogasana* 216

    7.2.1. Introduction to *yogasana* 216

    7.2.2. Scope of this book 216

    7.2.3. How many postures are there? 217

7.3 YogaSense™: The Seven Core Principles...218

    7.3.1. Respect your body 218

    7.3.2. Starting the fire 219

    7.3.3. Optimal alignment...220

    7.3.4. Balancing opposing forces 221

    7.3.5. Opening like a flower 221

    7.3.6. Nurturing...222

    7.3.7. Live it! 222

7.4 *Drishti*...223

    7.4.1. Focus, clarity and alignment 223

7.5 *Bandha* 223

    7.5.1. Sending the energy upwards..223

    7.5.2. *Moolabandha* 224

    7.5.3. *Uddiyanabandha* 226

    7.5.4. *Jalandharabandha* 227

    7.5.5. *Mahabandha* 227

7.6 Meditation..228

    7.6.1. Meditation: a simple explanation 228

    7.6.2. The Yoga Sutra and meditation..228

        desa bandhas cittasya dharana [Sutra 1, Pada III]....................229

        tatra pratyaya-ekatanata dhyanam [Sutra 2, Pada III]..............229

        trayam ekatra samyamah [Sutra 4, Pada III]...........................229

      taj-jayat prajna-alokah [Sutra 5, Pada III] 229

7.7 *Pranayama* 230

   7.7.1. Spirit of *pranayama* 231

   7.7.2. Definition of *pranayama* 231

   7.7.3. Benefits of *pranayama* 231

   7.7.4. Key features of *pranayama* 232

   7.7.5. Anatomy of *pranayama*: Western view 233

   7.7.6. Yogic anatomy of *pranayama* 233

      udana-jayat-jala-panka-kantaka-adishuasanga utkrantis-ca [Sutra 40, Pada III].......234

      samana-jayaj jvalanam [Sutra 41, Pada III] 234

   7.7.7. Learning *Pranayama* 236

   7.7.8. Summary of basic *pranayama* techniques 236

   7.7.9. *Pranayama* and the Yoga Sutra 239

      sthira sukham asanam [Sutra 46, Pada II] 239

      prayatna saithilya ananta samapattibhyam [Sutra 47, Pada II] 239

      tatah dvanda anabhighatah [Sutra 48, Pada II] 239

      tasmin sati svasa-prasvasayor gati-vicchedah pranayamah [Sutra 49, Pada II] 239

   7.7.10. Living *Pranayama* 239

7.8 Relaxation and visualization 240

   7.8.1. Go within and heal 240

7.9 Sanskrit chants 241

   7.9.1. AUM (OM) 241

   7.9.2. Gâyatrî Mantra 242

   7.9.3. Asatho Maa 242

   7.9.4. Mantra of Ashtanga Vinyasa Yoga 242

References 243

Chapter 8   *Teaching Methodology*

8.1 Ethics of a yoga teacher 245

   8.1.1. "Sat Nam" – teach truthfully 245

   8.1.2. Be firmly rooted in your practice 245

   8.1.3. Teach with integrity 246

   8.1.4. Be a <u>real</u> teacher, not a false prophet 246

   8.1.5. "I am a teacher" 247

   8.1.6. Let your students go with grace 247

   8.1.7. Teach an empty class 248

8.2 The teacher-student relationship 248

   8.2.1. Stay within your scope of practice 248

   8.2.2. Sexual misconduct 249

   8.2.3. Respect boundaries 249

   8.2.4. Respect your students' rights 251

   8.2.5. Socializing with students 251

8.3 Teaching yoga as a yogi: the *yama* 251

    8.3.1. *Ahimsa* – non-violence 251

    8.3.2. *Satya* – truthfulness...252

    8.3.3. *Asteya* – non-stealing 252

    8.3.4. *Brahmacharya* – focused and committed 253

    8.3.5. *Aparigraha* – non-grasping 253

8.4 Teaching *drishti* 253

    8.4.1. Focus and adjustment from within 253

    8.4.2. The yoga eye exercise...254

    8.4.3. Using the mind's eye: disappearing objects (beginner) 255

    8.4.4. Using the mind's eye: mountain and rock (intermediate)............255

8.5 Teaching *bandha* 255

    8.5.1. Getting in touch with the energy locks....................................255

    8.5.2. *Moolabandha* – root lock..256

    8.5.3. *Uddiyanabandha* 257

    8.5.4. *Jalandharabandha* 257

    8.5.5. *Mahabandha* 258

8.6 Teaching meditation 259

    8.6.1. Meditation via concentration 259

    8.6.2. Some common types of meditation 259

    8.6.3. Methods for leading meditation 260

    8.6.4. Moving meditation 261

    8.6.5. Meditation in motion 262

8.7 Teaching *pranayama* 262

    8.7.1. Explaining *pranayama* 262

    8.7.2. *Pranayama* within a class setting..262

    8.7.3. The technical points...263

    8.7.4. *Pranayama* basics...263

    8.7.5. Teaching *pranayama* 264

    8.7.6. Developing your students' breath capacity 265

    8.7.7. Teaching *pranayama* 265

8.8 Teaching relaxation and visualization...266

    8.8.1. How to teach 266

8.9. Teaching YogaSense™ 267

    8.9.1. Finding your own way *YogaSense™ Guiding Principle #7: Live it!*...............267

    8.9.2. Foundations of teaching asana 268

8.10 Teaching *padmasana* 270

    8.10.1. Why the lotus? 270

    8.10.2. Preparing for *padmasana* 271

8.11 Teaching safely 272

    8.11.1. Before you start..272

    8.11.2. Importance of warming up 273

8.12 Structuring a yoga class...274

8.12.1. What to teach? 274

8.12.2. Components of a yoga class 274

8.12.3. Designing a *vinyasa* 275

8.12.4. Tuning-in 275

8.12.5. Duration of a yoga class 276

8.12.6 "How many times a week?" 276

BOOK TWO: YOGA THERAPY

Chapter 1   Introduction: The Spirit of Yoga Therapy

1.1 What is Yoga Therapy? 280

   1.1.1. The art and science of self-healing 280

   1.1.2. Holistic approach 280

1.2 Key elements 280

   1.2.1. Essential principles 280

   1.2.2. Mindfulness 281

1.3 Key yoga tools 282

   1.3.1. *Yogasana* 282

   1.3.2. Restorative Yoga 282

   1.3.3. Yoga Nidra 282

   1.3.4. *Pranayama* 283

   1.3.5. Meditation 283

   1.3.6. Positive Affirmation 284

   1.3.7. Guided Relaxation 284

1.4 Physical benefits of *yogasana* 285

   1.4.1. Flexibility 285

   1.4.2. Strength 285

   1.4.3. Posture 285

   1.4.4. Balance 286

   1.4.5. Cardiovascular system 286

   1.4.6. Pulmonary function 286

   1.4.7. Nervous system 287

   1.4.8. Immune system 287

   1.4.9. Sensory system 288

1.5 Emotional benefits of *yogasana* 288

   1.5.1. Inner strength 288

   1.5.2. Inner peace 288

1.6 Scope of practice 289

   1.6.1. Credentials 289

1.7 Limitations 289

1.7.1. Not a miracle cure 289

1.7.2. Adjunct to Medical Care 289

1.8 Yoga Props 290

1.8.1. Blankets 290

1.8.2. Blocks, stools and chairs 290

1.8.3. Straps or ties 290

1.8.4. Chairs or table or bed 290

1.8.5. Beanbags, cushions and bolsters 291

1.8.6. Wall, counter or desk 291

1.8.7. Ball 291

1.9 Gong 291

1.9.1. Gong and vibration 291

1.10 Caregiver 292

1.10.1. Taking care of the caregivers 292

Chapter 2   Neurology

2.1 Yoga for neurological conditions 294

2.1.1. Nervous system 294

2.1.2. Muscle tone 295

2.1.3. Sensation 295

2.1.4. Postural control, balance reactions, protective reactions 296

2.2 Parkinson's Disease 296

2.2.1. Description and pathology 296

2.2.2. Presentation 297

2.2.3. Yoga intention 297

2.2.4. Key problems and recommended *yogasana* 297

2.2.5. Common muscle imbalances 299

2.2.6. Safety and special consideration 299

2.3 Multiple Sclerosis..300

2.3.1. Description and pathology 300

2.3.2. Presentation 300

2.3.3. Yoga intention 300

2.3.4. Muscle imbalances 300

2.3.5. Key problems and recommended *yogasana* 301

2.3.6. Safety and special commentary 301

2.4 Cerebral Vascular Accident 302

2.4.1. Description and pathology 302

2.4.2. Presentation 302

2.4.3. Yoga intention 302

2.4.4. Key problems and recommended *yogasana* 303

2.4.5. Safety and special commentary 303

2.5 Traumatic Brain Injury 304

2.5.1. Description and pathology..304

2.5.2. Presentation..304

2.5.3. Yoga Intention..304

2.5.4. Key problems and recommended *yogasana* 304

2.5.5. Safety and special commentary..304

2.6 Alzheimer's...305

2.6.1. Description and Pathology...305

2.6.2. Presentation..305

2.6.3. Yoga Intention..305

2.6.4. Key problems and recommended *yogasana* 305

2.6.5. Muscle imbalances...306

2.6.6. Safety and special commentary..306

2.7 Vestibular Disorder...306

2.7.1. Description and pathology...306

2.7.2. Presentation..307

2.7.3. Yoga Intention..307

2.7.4. Key problems and recommended *yogasana* 307

2.7.5. Muscle imbalances...307

2.7.6 Safety and special commentary...307

2.8 Peripheral Neuropathy 308

2.8.1. Description and pathology...308

2.8.2. Causes of neuropathy..308

2.8.3. Common nerves involved in neuropathy...309

2.8.4. Presentation..309

2.8.5. Yoga intention 309

2.8.6. Key Problems and recommended *yogasana* 310

2.8.7. Safety and special commentary..310

Chapter 3   *Medical*

3.1 Introduction 312

3.1.1. Benefit of yoga for medical conditions..312

3.1.2. Systems and Organs 312

3.2 Diabetes 314

3.2.1. Description and pathology...314

3.2.2. Key problems and recommended *yogasana* 314

3.2.3. Safety and special commentary..315

3.3 Obesity 315

3.3.1. Description and pathology...315

3.3.2. Key problems and recommended *yogasana* 316

3.3.3. Safety and special commentary..316

3.4 Irritable Bowel Syndrome and Gastroesophageal Reflux 316

3.4.1. Description and pathology...316

3.4.2. Key problems and recommended *yogasana* 317

3.4.3. Safety and special commentary 317

3.5 Coronary Artery Disease 317

3.5.1. Description and pathology 317

3.5.2. Key problems/risk factors and recommended *yogasana* 318

3.5.3. Safety and special commentary 318

3.6 Pulmonary Disease 318

3.6.1. Description and pathology 318

3.6.2. Key problems and recommended *yogasana* (common for both restrictive and
obstructive lung disease) 319

3.6.3. Safety and special commentary 321

3.7 Cancer 321

3.7.1. Description and pathology 321

3.7.2 Yoga intention (applicable to all medical conditions) 321

3.7.3. Key problems and recommended *yogasana* 322

3.7.4. Safety and special commentary 322

3.8 Infectious Diseases: HIV/AIDS 322

3.8.1. Description and pathology 322

3.8.2. Key problems and recommended *yogasana* 323

3.8.3. Safety and special commentary 323

Chapter 4   Orthopedic

4.1 Introduction 326

4.1.1. Yoga and modern orthopedic medicine 326

4.1.2. Acute and chronic traumatic injury 326

4.1.3. YogaSense™ Effectiveness 327

4.2 Spinal alignment and pathology 327

4.2.1. Abnormal posture and alignment of the spine 327

4.2.2. Pathologies of the spine 328

4.2.3. Yoga intention 329

4.2.4. Key problems and recommended *yogasana* 329

4.2.5. Safety and special commentary 330

4.3 Scoliosis 331

4.3.1. Description and pathology 331

4.3.2. Presentation 331

4.3.3. Yoga intention 331

4.3.4. Key problems and recommended *yogasana* 332

4.3.5 Safety and special commentary 332

4.4 Osteoporosis 332

4.4.1. Description and pathology 332

4.4.2. Presentation 333

4.4.3 Yoga intention 333

4.4.4. Key problems and recommended *yogasana* 333

4.4.5. Safety and special commentary 334

4.5 Arthritis 334

4.5.1. Description and Pathology 334

4.5.2. Presentation 334

4.5.3. Yoga Intention 334

4.5.4. Key problems and recommended *yogasana* 335

4.5.5. Safety and special commentary 335

4.6 Lower back 335

4.6.1. Description and pathology 335

4.6.2. Presentation 336

4.6.3. Yoga intention 336

3.6.4. Key problems and recommended *yogasana* 336

3.6.5. Safety and special commentary 337

4.7 Neck 337

4.7.1. Description and pathology 337

4.7.2. Presentation 338

4.7.3. Yoga Intention 338

4.7.4. Key problems and recommended *yogasana* 338

4.7.5. Safety and special commentary 338

4.8 Upper extremities 339

4.8.1. Abnormal alignment of the upper extremities 339

4.8.2. Common pathologies and injuries 339

4.8.3. Yoga intention 340

4.8.4. Key Problems and recommended *yogasana* 340

4.9 Lower extremities 341

4.9.1. Abnormal alignment of the lower extremities 341

4.9.2. Common pathologies and injuries 341

4.9.3. Yoga intention 342

4.9.4. Key Problems and recommended *yogasana* 342

4.9.5 Safety and special commentary 343

4.10 Hyperextended joints 343

BOOK THREE: YOGASENSE® SEQUENCES

The YogaSense™ Roadmap 345

Sun breath sequence 346

Brain organizing & grounding meditation 347

Vestibular rebalancing exercise 348

Posture awareness exercise 349

Balance sequence 350

Spinal alignment exercise 352

Core strengthening exercise 354

Supported strengthening sequence 356

Wheelchair / chair yoga...357

Hip and hamstring opening exercise 358

Shoulder opening exercise...359

Lower back routine..360

Pelvic floor routine 361

Restorative yoga..362

Foot care routine...363

Pawanmuktasana sequence 364

Gastrointestinal (GI) sequence..364

Guided relaxation 365

Tantra yoga 366

Diagrams and Tables Index

Diagram 2.1. The five *kosha*..28

Diagram 2.2. *Shad Darshan*: the Six Visions of Life 31

Diagram 2.3. *Shad Darshan* and self-enlightenment 32

Diagram 3.1. Construction of the S-curve of the spine from the stacking of vertebral discs. 64

Diagram 3.2. Main bones of the human body 69

Diagram 3.3. Planes of the body 73

Diagram 3.4. Bones of the pelvis..78

Diagram 3.5. The shoulder girdle 82

Diagram 3.6. Hyperextension of the elbows..83

Diagram 3.7. Keeping the eyes of the elbows facing forward with a slight bend to the arms 83

Diagram 3.8. External muscles of the back..89

Diagram 3.9. Muscles of the upper back (after the trapezius and a segment of the
         rhomboideus minor had been removed)...92

Diagram 3.10. Levator scapulae 93

Diagram 3.11. External musculature of the abdominal wall 97

Diagram 3.12. Psoas major and iliacus 98

Diagram 3.13. Tensor fascia latae and iliotibial tract 99

Diagram 3.14. External hip rotators (left) and with quadratus femoris (right) 101

Diagram 3.15. The adductor muscles 102

Diagram 3.16. The quadriceps muscles 103

Diagram 3.17. The hamstrings (back view of the lower leg)........................104

Diagram 3.18. Muscles of the calf 105

Diagram 3.19. Biceps and triceps of the right arm...................................108

Diagram 3.20. Sternocleidomastoid muscle 110

Diagram 3.21. Main muscles of the body in action during *yogasana* 118

Diagram 4.1. A typical cell..122

Diagram 4.2. Neuron 126

Diagram 4.3. Organization of the nervous system 126

Diagram 4.4. Depiction of the body's sympathetic NS and parasympathetic NS. 129

Diagram 4.5. The transformation effects of *pranayama* on the autonomic NS 130

Diagram 5.1. Main regions of the brain and their functions (midsaggital plane) 151

Diagram 5.2. Transverse slice of the brain 152

Diagram 5.3. Cerebral cortex lobes and their functions......................................153

Diagram 5.4. Transverse slice showing gray and white matters of the brain..............................153

Diagram 5.5. Location of the basal ganglia, thalamus and hypothalamus 154

Diagram 5.6. Main components of the limbic system.......................................155

Diagram 5.7. Effects of yoga on the brain 159

Diagram 5.8. The three stages of consciousness 164

Diagram 5.9. Realms of the conscious states..166

Diagram 5.10. *Tamas* and sensory perceptions 168

Diagram 5.11. The energetic properties of the three *gunas* 168

Diagram 5.12. The creation of the organic universe 169

Diagram 5.13. The creation of the inorganic universe 169

Diagram 5.14. *Ahamkara*, *buddhi* and *manas* 170

Diagram 5.15. *Asmita* 171

Diagram 5.16. Yogic practices for a healthy brain and mind 175

Diagram 6.1. "Anatomy Lesson of Dr. Nicolaes Tulp" by Rembrandt van Rijn, 1632..................178

Diagram 6.2. Microscopic section through one year old ash (Fraxinus) wood. Drawing of Antonie van Leeuwenhoek..179

Diagram 6.3. Image from Koehler's Medicinal-Plants 1887 183

Diagram 6.4. Creation of the gross, causative elements.................................184

Diagram 6.5. The three *dosha* from the five *bhuta*....................................185

Diagram 6.6. Dosha and their attributes 185

Diagram 6.7. Yogin with seven chakras. Painting. Kangra school. Late 18th century A.D...........200

Diagram 6.8. The main *chakra* and the endocrine system 201

Diagram 6.9. The five *kosha*...205

Diagram 7.1. Stages of the mind...228

Diagram 7.2. The five *prana* of the body 235

Diagram 8.1. Yoga eye exercise...254

Table 4.1: Summary of the main functions of the body's systems 124

Table 5.1. The three universal qualities...167

Table 6.1. *Chakra*, location, correspondence with the endocrine plexus and organs innervated 201

Table 6.2. The Ten Bodies...208

Table 7.1. *Ashtanga yoga*: the eight limbs of yoga 215

Table 7.2. Weaknesses of the body..219

Table 8.1. Surya Namaskar meditation 261

Namaste from the authors, Jacqueline Koay and Teddi Barenholtz

Acknowledging the many pathways in life, the authors hope to inspire and enlighten the readers on the positive benefits of yoga. Whether you are a teacher, health professional or completely new to yoga, this book will take you on a wondrous journey.

Jacqueline, a mother of five children, has found yoga to be a pathway for the modern family. Yoga philosophy reinforces healthy family living by cultivating exercise, healthy nutrition and a peaceful state of mind as part of daily life.

Teddi as a health professional, has found that yoga brings a deeper level to therapy by fostering active participation and self-healing. This book thus demonstrates how yoga therapy complements western medicine.

We hope this book will deepen your practice and enrich your life.

Love, peace, light,
Jacqueline & Teddi
Connecticut, July 2009

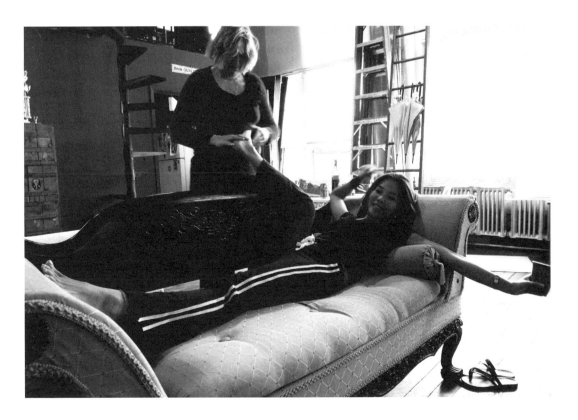

Book 1
The Science & Philosophy of Teaching Yoga

CHAPTER ONE

Introduction: The Spirit of Yoga

OVERVIEW OF THE CHAPTER

1.1	"Experience, then believe"
1.2	The meaning of yoga
1.3	History, religion and key practices
1.4	The yoga tree
1.5	Seven historical yoga teachers
1.6	Seven influential yoga teachers
1.7	Seven contemporary yoga teachers
1.8	Related spiritual practices / schools
1.9	Six experiences of yoga

1.1. "Experience, then believe"

1.1.1. Live your yoga

Yoga is multi-faceted like a diamond: it means different things to different practitioners. For some, it is merely a system of physical exercise, weight management or stress relief. For others, it is a spiritual path handed down for centuries to help us make sense of the world today. And for some practitioners, yoga is simply a way of life.

As a teacher, your task is to lead your students to their inner teacher, so that they may find their own yoga. You are merely a facilitator, passing down the centuries-old teaching like a conduit, but you are never the master. The innate knowledge and inner wisdom already lie within each and every one of us. Your job is to guide your students to this space. But of course, you have to experience your own yoga before you can teach it with integrity. You have to believe in it, and that belief can only come with direct experience.

"Experience, then believe" *Yogi Bhajan, Master of Kundalini Yoga*

The experience of yoga cannot be bought from books or assimilated from the most expensive teacher training course: it has to come from a desire within you to find your yoga, to live your yoga. And you can do this simply by practicing.

"99% practice, 1% theory" *Sri K Pattabhi Jois, Ashtanga Yoga*

1.2. The meaning of yoga

1.2.1. Origin of the word yoga

The language of yoga is Sanskrit (*section 2.6*). It is believed that the word yoga is derived from the Sanskrit root word, *yuj*, which is translated to mean "yoke", "tying together" and "to unite".

The most common interpretation of the word yoga is the yoking together of mind, body and spirit. This is achieved in practice when practitioners are totally absorbed in their yoga, resulting in the mind, body and spirit merging into one entity.

A less common interpretation of the word *yuj* is the unification of the individual consciousness (*citta*) with the universal consciousness (*Cit*). A practitioner finds enlightenment when the boundaries surrounding her individual consciousness (ego) are melted away, freeing her to reach her limitless potential (Creative Source).

1.3. History, religion and key practices

1.3.1. History

Nobody really knows when yoga began. If we define yoga as the practice for attaining spiritual enlightenment and expanding consciousness, then yoga is probably as old as mankind. It has been said[1] that Dead Sea scrolls pointed to yoga being practiced as far back as the time of the Sat Yurg era ('Civilization of Light') thousands of years ago. More conservative estimates place yoga's origin to between four and eight thousand years ago. It is also believed by some scholars that yoga predates the Vedic times, from detailed descriptions of its practices in ancient Hindu texts, the Vedic *shastra*. The practice of yoga can also be traced back to the Rig Veda, the oldest Hindu text, which mentioned the yoking of the human mind with the Sun of Truth.

The first physical evidence that yoga was practiced in ancient times is in the form of a seal excavated from Mohenjo-Daro, an ancient city located in modern-day Pakistan. The city of Mohenjo-Daro flourished between 2600 BCE and 1900 BCE, although the first signs of settlement in the area have been dated to the period of 3500 BCE (Kenoyer, 1998). The Mohenjo-Daro seal, measuring less than a couple of inches on each side, depicted a 'yogi' sitting on a meditation chair in a traditional cross-legged yoga pose with his hands resting on his knees The meditation chairs of today still bear the same ancient design. This artifact points to the practice of some form of spiritual-physical science during the times of the Harappan Culture (Indus

---

[1] Yogi Bhajan, Master of Kundalini Yoga

Valley civilization). Yoga also flourished in ancient civilizations of South America and along the Indo-China border, though it took strongest root in India.

1.3.2. Religion

Yoga predates most of the main modern religions. Ancient yogis were men who denounced their world in pursuit of enlightenment. It was widely believed in those days that enlightenment came after years of austere living in distant mountain caves and river valleys, living a harsh, simple life dedicated to contemplation, meditation, breathing exercises and the physical practice of postures. These yogis were sometimes nomadic and itinerant. They would meet up in forest clearings and remote caves to study under a teacher. The tradition then was to study at the feet of the teacher, sitting near, and learning was transmitted orally. This is called *upanishad*.

Yoga is intricately woven into Buddhist and Jain philosophies. The similarities found in yoga and certain Buddhist teachings, practices and words come from the intersection between the two at some point in history: there is evidence to suggest that Buddha was part of several *Upanishad* in his time: learning, sharing and teaching spiritual knowledge with his peers. Though there are some influences of religion in yoga (for example, Hinduism in Hatha Yoga; Sikhism in Kundalini Yoga), yoga does not preach a jealous god. In yoga, there are no rituals, dogmas or ceremonies associated with most religions. Indeed, the teachings of yoga, according to the Yoga Sutra, exhort practitioners to find their own God according to their own beliefs.

> *svadhyayat ista-devata samprayogah* [Yoga Sutra 44, II]
> Self-study leads towards the realization of one's own God.

> *yatha abhimata dhyanat va* [Yoga Sutra 39, I]
> Or serenity can come by the way of meditation in harmony with one's own religious heritage
> *ista* = personal choice
> *yatha abhimata* = as desired (according to one's own religious heritage)

Yoga is an unaffiliated spiritual practice rather than a religious one, with self-enlightenment and creating a better world as its central themes. Its aim is to guide practitioners to find a quiet place to sit within themselves, to commune with their own God, rather than converting practitioners into worshipping Hindu deities. But for millions of practitioners worldwide, yoga is no more than a system of physical exercise and relaxation.

1.3.3. Key Practices

<u>The Eight Limbs of Yoga (*ashtanga yoga*)</u>
True practitioners of yoga should practice the eight limbs of yoga, as outlined in the Yoga Sutra (*sections 2.4, 8.3*). Designed to lead practitioners to self-realization ultimately, and consist of both external and internal limbs:

I.   *Yama*: The Great Universal Vows (actions onto others)
II.   *Niyama*: Personal Observances (actions onto self)
III. *Asana*: Sitting comfortably (often translated as posture practice)
IV.   *Pranayama*: Conscious breathing
V.   *Pratyhara*: Withdrawal of the senses
VI.   *Dharana*: One-pointed concentration
VII. *Dhyana*: Meditation
VIII. *Samadhi*: Self-realization, bliss, enlightenment.

According to Sri K. Pattabhi Jois, the physical body must be made strong through *asana* and *pranayama* practices before the internal limbs can be mastered successfully.

<u>Vegetarianism</u>
One of the fundamental principles of yoga is *ahimsa*, which is non-harming and non-violence. Eating meat, which can only be the result of *himsa* (harm and violence), can never be justified if this principle is to be embraced in its entirety. Yogic diet is discussed briefly in *section 2.6.3* and comprehensively in The Kundalini Yoga Cookbook (Koay, 2006).

<u>Purification (*kriya yoga*)</u>
To increase the effectiveness of one's yoga practice, the body needs to be purified first. There are various yogic purification techniques of Ayurvĕda and personal observances such as vegetarianism and *tapas* (generating and conserving spiritual fire to burn off the impurities).

<u>Committed practice (*sadhana*)</u>
The fruits of yoga can only be found at the end of a long road of committed, daily, spiritual practice of the eight limbs.

1.4. **The yoga tree**

1.4.1. **The Hatha Yoga branch**

Hatha (pronounced *ha-ta*) yoga is probably the most popular form of yoga practiced in the West. It was introduced by Swami Swatmarama, a 15th century Indian sage and the compiler of the text on Hatha yoga, *Hatha Yoga Pradipika.*

Classical translations of Hatha yoga include:
i.   *Ha* = sun; *tha* = moon (balancing the opposing forces)
ii.   'Forceful' yoga

For the Hatha yogis, enlightenment is realized through the physical body. Hatha yoga involves combining physical postures with breathing, energy locks and meditation techniques to purify and strengthen both the physical and esoteric bodies. According to *Hatha Yoga Pradipika,* Hatha yoga is the preparation for the practice of Raja Yoga (*section 1.4.2*).

Amongst the schools of yoga in this branch are:
i.   Ashtanga Vinyasa Yoga (Sri K Pattabhi Jois)
ii.   Iyengar Yoga (BKS Iyengar)
iii.   Sivananda Yoga (Swami Sivananda)

1.4.2. **The Raja Yoga branch**

The word Raja means 'royal' in Sanskrit. This is the royal road to reintegrating unit consciousness (*citta*) with universal consciousness (*Cit*). Its way to self-realization is through meditation, referring specifically to Sri Patanjali's system that is described in the Yoga Sutra.

Popular schools of Raja yoga include:
i.   Sahaja Yoga (Nirmala Srivastava)
ii.   Ananda Marga Yoga (Sri Sri Anandamurti)

1.4.3. Bhakti Yoga

Bhakti yoga is the yoga of devotion; practitioners' spiritual practice involves cultivating loving devotion, selfless love and pure giving to God. This is described as a religious form in the Bhagavad Gita. This is expressed through prayers and chants (*japa*) and service to humanity (often in the form of free canteens open to the public).

Perhaps one of the most well-known faces of Bhakti yoga is the International Society for Krishna Consciousness (commonly known as 'the Hare Krishnas').

1.4.4. Jnâna yoga

In Sanskrit, *jnâna* means 'knowledge'; therefore, Jnâna Yoga is the path of knowledge. It draws the mind away from delusions generated by false perceptions and emotions, to clear the path to liberation and self-realization.

Jnâna Yoga is mentioned in the Bhagavad Gita. In one reference, Krishna said that *jnâna* is about understanding the body and the soul, and the difference between both. The practice of Jnâna Yoga is about learning the four means of salvation, namely discrimination, detachment, the virtues and cultivating an intense desire for liberation (*moksha*).

1.4.5. Naad Yoga

Naad Yoga is the yoga of sounds, as *naad* is the essence of all sounds. The practice of Naad Yoga therefore centers around conscious communication and chanting.

With Naad Yoga, practitioners learn how to use mantra, scripture, harmonious communication and musical sounds that elevate, heal, and balance. With each repetition (*jap*), the illusory layers of ego are gradually removed so that the True Self can be experienced.

1.4.6. Laya Yoga

Kundalini Yoga is a form of Laya Yoga[2]. Laya means the melting away of obstacles and old layers of karma by working on the *chakra* and focusing on raising the *kundalini* energy that lies dormant at the base of the spine. The practice of Laya Yoga would include *asana*, *pranayama*, mantra, visualization and meditation. These techniques mend, heal and strengthen the *chakra* and to awaken and raise the *kundalini*.

1.4.7. Karma Yoga

Karma Yoga is the yoga of action; it is the selfless service for the benefit of the community. The word *karma* is a Sanskrit word meaning action or deed. Karma also means the result of an action. This is rather like the laws of physics: for every action, there is a resultant reaction. This law of Karma is also a fundamental doctrine in Hinduism, Buddhism and Jainism.

A Karma yogi performs his duty selflessly, devoting all the fruits of his action to the Lord. He should have no attachment to the results. Giving with no attachment purifies the heart, preparing it for knowledge of the True Self and frees one from the endless cycle of birth-death-rebirth.

1.4.8. Contemporary Branches of Yoga

The yoga renaissance of the 20th century spawned new branches of yoga from the classical schools, each with its distinct philosophies, methodology and following. These schools' practices are often a contemporary take on the ancient subject, tailored to the needs of a modern client base.

Examples of contemporary branches are:

Kripalu
Founder: Yogi Amrit Desai, inspired by Swami Kripalvananda
Focuses on proper alignment, breathwork and meditation to encourage inward focus and spiritual attunement. The gentle Hatha yoga practice in the Kripalu tradition fosters compassion for the body, thus facilitating physical healing and spiritual transformation.

---

[2] Kundalini Yoga also embodies elements of Hatha, Raja and Karma Yoga.

Jivamukti
Founders: David Life and Sharon Gannon
The emphasis is on teaching yoga as a spiritual practice, and is delivered through vigorously physical and intellectually stimulating yoga, which incorporates breathwork, scriptures and mantra.

Anusara
Founder: John Friend
Hatha-based system that incorporates yoga positions that flow from the heart based on alignment principles, 'Universal Principles of Alignment™'.

Bikram
Founder: Bikram Choudhury
Set series of 26 yoga poses, including two *pranayama* exercises, practiced in a heated room. The aim of this is to promote sweating to rid the body of toxins; the elevated temperature also makes the body very warm, and therefore increases its flexibility.

Sun Yoga
Founder: Jacqueline Koay
Moving towards spiritual and physical liberation through *vinyasa*, *pranayama*, mantra and meditation practices. Heavily influenced by the scriptures, Ashtanga yoga, medical sciences and dance. Emphasis on living the yoga philosophy in everyday life.

1.5. Seven historical yoga teachers

1.5.1. Swami Sivananda Saraswati *(1887 - 1963)*

Swami Sivananda Saraswati is the founder of The Divine Life Society and the Sivananda Ashram. A spiritual teacher, yoga master and Vedanta proponent, Swami Sivananda was a medical doctor for ten years in Malaysia (then Malaya) before returning to India to embrace monasticism in 1923.

Swami Sivananda was initiated by his spiritual teacher, Swami Vishwananda Saraswati, in Rishikesh, where he remained to immerse himself in his spiritual practices as well as helping the sick.

Swami Sivananda then travelled widely throughout India, seeking and sharing spiritual knowledge. He was the author of many books on a wide variety of subjects, and through his writing (initially short articles), his fame grew. The Sivananda Ashram proliferates around the world today.

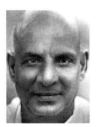

"Truth is to be perceived intuitively or realized"

- Sri Swami Sivananda

1.5.2. **Krishnamacharya** *(1888–1989)*

Sri Tirumala Krishnamacharya is known as the Father of Modern Yoga. His students include the well-known teachers of our time, namely Sri K. Pattabhi Jois, Sri BKS Iyengar, the late Indra Devi and Krishnamacharya's own sons T.K.V. Desikachar and T.K. Sribhashyam.

Krishnamacharya's foundations were in classical Indian philosophy. He studied logic and Sanskrit at the University of Benares, followed by stints at Queens College and Patna University. Krishnamacharya was a great scholar who had been awarded many titles.

Krishnamacharya's education in yoga came from Yogeshwara Ramamohan Brahmachari, who lived in a cave in the foothills of Mount Kailash. Under the patronage of the Maharajah of Mysore, Krishnamacharya taught yoga and wrote books on the subject. He was also a trained Ayurvedic physician and practiced as a healer in later life (often incorporating healing into yoga).

1.5.3. Sri K. Pattabhi Jois *(1915 - 2009)*

Sri K. Pattabhi Jois is the founder of the Ashtanga Yoga Research Institute, and is widely credited as the originator of the highly popular form of yoga, Ashtanga Vinyasa Yoga ('Ashtanga Yoga').

After attending a lecture by Sri Tirumala Krishnamacharya (*section 1.5.2*), the twelve year old Pattabhi Jois was so impressed that he became a student of Krishnamacharya for the next twenty five years.

Pattabhi Jois established his Ashtanga Yoga Research Institute in Mysore (it receives thousands of international visitors each year) and at the time of writing, he still teaches at the Institute with his daughter Saraswati and his grandson Sharath. Ashtanga Yoga is one of the most widely practiced schools of yoga today, and its form has remained unchanged over the decades.

1.5.4. B.K.S. Iyengar *(1918 -)*

B.K.S. Iyengar is known for his unique form of yoga, where meticulous details are paid to the alignment of the body for therapeutic benefits. As a child, Iyengar was weak and sickly, and his road to health was paved for him when he fortuitously went to live with his brother-in-law, Sri Tirumala Krishnamacharya (*section 1.5.2*), who taught him the practice of *yogasana*. With the encouragement of his guru, Iyengar developed his own system of practice, which is now known simply as Iyengar Yoga.

B.K.S. Iyengar has been practicing and teaching yoga for more than 75 years, and has gathered millions of disciples from all over the world.

1.5.5. Indra Devi *(1899 - 2002)*

Indra Devi is one of the most influential female yogis of her time. Born to Russian nobility as Eugenia Peterson, she trained as an actress and dancer. In 1927, she moved to India to embrace the culture and spirituality. She was influenced by the philosopher, J. Krishnamurthi, and studied yoga under Sri Tirumala Krishnamacharya (*section 1.5.2*) with the specific purpose of healing her cardiac illness.

Indra Devi then took yoga worldwide. She returned to the Soviet Union in 1960 and became known as the woman who brought yoga to the Kremlin. She conducted a meditation in Vietnam in 1966. She traveled frequently to India. During one of her trips, she met and became a follower of Satya Sai Baba.

In 1985, she moved to Argentina, where she taught yoga to thousands and set up the Indra Devi Foundation. She spread yoga throughout South America, along with holding seminars and classes in the U.S. and Europe. Over the years she published a number of books, including Forever Young, Forever Healthy, Yoga for Americans, and Sai Yoga, Renew Your life Through Yoga.

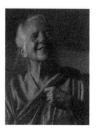

"In yoga, relaxation is taught as an art, breathing as a science and mental control of the body as a means of harmonizing the body, mind and spirit"

– Indra Devi

1.5.6. Harbajan Singh Khalsa / Yogi Bhajan *(1929 - 2004)*

Yogi Bhajan was the Master of Kundalini Yoga and the leader of the Sikhs in the Western world until his death; he brought Kundalini Yoga and Sikhism to the United States in 1968 with his migration from India by the way of Canada. And it is the confluence of Yogi Bhajan's two pillars of faith that made Kundalini Yoga unique: it bears influences of Sikhism instead of Hinduism.

Yogi Bhajan sought knowledge and wisdom from reclusive hermits, yogis and holy men of India. His principal teacher was Sant Hazara Singh, who declared Yogi Bhajan a Master of Kundalini Yoga at the age of sixteen. Yogi Bhajan also held a Masters degree in Economics and a doctorate in the Psychology of Communication.

His legacies are his foundation, 3HO (Healthy, Happy, Holy Organization), Miri Piri Academy and the technology of Kundalini Yoga which has brought much healing and meaning to countless practitioners in the world.

1.5.7. **Sri Swami Satchidananda** *(1914 - 2002)*

Sri Swami Satchidananda is the founder of Integral Yoga. Born as C. K. Ramaswamy Gounder, he led a comparatively unyogic life until the death of his wife when he was 28. Swami Satchidananda then went on a long spiritual quest, where he subsequently met Swami Sivananda (*section 1.5.1*) who ordained him into the Sannyasa order. This is the stage of life where a Hindu renounces all in pursuit of spiritual contemplation.

As a *sannyasin*, Swami Satchidananda taught at his spiritual teacher's ashram in Sri Lanka, where he modernized the ancient practices. His philosophies were then integrated into his brand of yoga, Integral Yoga, which he propagated when he migrated to the United States in 1966. Integral Yoga rapidly became established in the United States and the world by the time of Swami Satchidananda's death and continues to grow worldwide.

1.6. Seven influential yoga teachers

1.6.1. **Vanda Scaravelli** *(1908 - 1999)*

One of the most inspiring teachings of *yogasana* is to be found in the works of Vanda Scaravelli, who exhorted her students never to let gravity kill a posture.

B.K.S. Iyengar (*section 1.5.4*) was her teacher, and the full life that Scaravelli had led before coming to yoga in her forties shone through in her teachings. Yoga for Scaravelli was *allegrezza*, or the intelligent heart: "You become intelligent and at the same time you are happy".

Scaravelli published one beautiful book on yoga with the title, *Awakening The Spine*, and since her death in 1991, several teachers continue keeping her teachings alive.

1.6.2. Yogi Amrit Desai *(1932 -)*

A disciple of Swami Kripalvanandji, Yogi Amrit Desai came to the United States as an art student in 1960. With his deepening practice of yoga, he discovered a beautiful form of meditation in movement, which he called Kripalu Yoga, named in honor of his spiritual teacher.

In his own words, Yogi Amrit Desai described Kripalu Yoga's origins as *"during my routine practice of hatha yoga postures I found my body moving spontaneously and effortlessly while at the same time I was being drawn into the deepest meditation I had ever experienced"*.

Yogi Amrit Desai established his first ashram in 1970, and a second one in 1975. The Kripalu Center for Yoga and Health was established in 1983, with branches in North America, Europe and India. Yogi Amrit Desai served as Director until 1994. He currently teaches at Amrit Yoga Institute in Florida, USA.

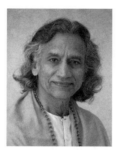

"Find freedom by living in the moment."

– Yogi Amrit Desai

1.6.3. Gurmukh Kaur Khalsa *(1943 -)*

A direct student of Yogi Bhajan *(section 1.5.6)*, Gurmukh Kaur Khalsa has been a committed practitioner and teacher of Kundalini Yoga as taught by Yogi Bhajan since first embracing the path in 1971.

Gurmukh has travelled far from her place of birth (Chicago). Her travelling found its purpose when she met Yogi Bhajan in 1971 in an ashram in Arizona. Together with other Kundalini Yoga pioneers, Gurmukh threw herself whole-heartedly into her practice, and was given the name Gurmukh by Yogi Bhajan which means 'one who takes thousands across the world ocean'.

Gurmukh is the co-founder of Golden Bridge Yoga, which offers Kundalini Yoga classes as well as fostering the yogic lifestyle and wellness.

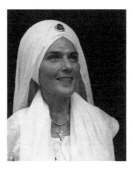

"When we gather to do yoga in a group, there is a healing wisdom that benefits everyone who participates"

- Gurmukh

1.6.4. T.K.V. Desikachar *(1938 -)*

T.K.V. Desikachar is the son and student of Sri Tirumala Krishnamacharya (*section 1.5.2*). An engineer by training, he lived and studied with his father until his father's death in 1989, sharing the belief that *yogasana* practice should be individualized, taking account of health, energy, physique, gender, place and age. Desikachar's contribution to yoga is through his book, *The Heart of Yoga*. Here, one finds the integration of *yogasana* with an uplifting translation of the Yoga Sutra.

Desikachar currently teaches at the school founded in his father's memory in Madras, as well as in Europe, the United States, Australia, and New Zealand.

1.6.5. John Scott *(1957 -)*

John Scott has studied extensively with Sri K. Pattabhi Jois (*section 1.5.3*). He is currently one of the most popular Ashtanga Yoga teachers in the world today.

His first experience of yoga was with Derek Ireland, who inspired him to take his practice further. Experienced and creative, John Scott takes his practitioners far with his clean, concise interpretation of Ashtanga Yoga, which he studied intensively with Sri K Pattabhi Jois.

John and his wife Lucy Scott run Stillpoint Ashtanga Yoga Center in New Zealand, and both travel extensively to teach.

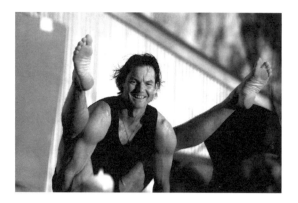

"Lead with the heart, follow with the head" – *John Scott*

1.6.6. Deepak Chopra *(1947 -)*

Deepak Chopra is a best-selling author who brought yoga to millions through his books. He is an Indian-American medical doctor and has written widely about mind-body medicine. From his literary success in 1996, he established The Chopra Center for Wellbeing in California, which practices his system of integrating the best of Western medicine with natural healing traditions.

One of Deepak Chopra's most well-known books is the *Seven Spiritual Laws of Yoga,* which he co-authored with David Simon.

1.6.7. Doug and David Swenson (*1950's -)*

Brothers Doug and David Swenson began their yoga practice early in their lives. Doug introduced David to Hatha Yoga, which they both learned from books. In 1973, David began Ashtanga Yoga which he then introduced to Doug. Both studied with some of the well-known teachers, notably Sri K. Pattabhi Jois (*section 1.5.3*) who was their primary yoga influence.

The Swensons' teachings are joyous and thoughtful, instilling softness into the otherwise austere discipline of Ashtanga Yoga. Humor is always close at hand to bring humanity and humility to their teachings, ""There is a difference between doing yoga or just making an *asana* of ourselves"!

Perhaps the clearest insight into the Swenson brothers' desire to share their love of yoga comes from David's comment, "It is very easy to make things difficult and very difficult to make things easy".

David Swenson

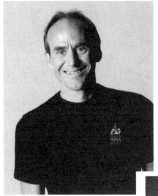

"There are fears that keep us alive and fears that keep us from living. Wisdom is understanding the difference."

- David Swenson

Doug Swenson

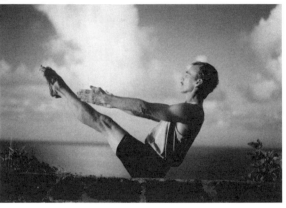

1.7. Seven contemporary yoga teachers

1.7.1. Joseph Michael Levry / Gurunam

Gurunam is a renowned Kundalini and Kabbalah teacher and the developer of Harmonyum, a transcendental healing system born out of Universal Kabbalah. By combining his three systems, Gurunam creates a practice which is both healing and uplifting, and one which can be integrated into everyday life.

Trained as an industrial engineer, Gurunam began his study into the esoteric arts when he was 12. He is the author of many books on Kabbalah and he lectures far and wide on the subject. He often lectures on the symbols of Kabbalah, secrets within the doctrines of Judaism.

Gurunam is the founder of Universal Force Yoga Center in New York City, and he teaches internationally several months a year.

1.7.2. Bikram Choudhury

Bikram Choudhury is famed for creating a system of yoga that consists of 26 postures practiced in a heated room. As a boy, Bikram studied under Bishnu Ghosh at the College of Physical Education in Calcutta, and had won the National India Yoga Championships several times.

Though often maligned for his much-publicized love of gold Rolls Royces, Speedo swimming trunks and sunglasses, Bikram's system of yoga (named after him) has nonetheless reached thousands of new practitioners searching for innovative and effective ways of losing weight and increasing their flexibility.

1.7.3. Sharath Rangaswamy

Sharath Rangaswamy is the grandson of Sri K. Pattabhi Jois (*section 1.5.3*), and began his *yogasana* practice at the age of seven. He spent most of his teen years focusing on academic education, but returned inevitably to his grandfather's Ashtanga Yoga when he was 19. He established a strict routine of getting up at 3.30 a.m. to begin his personal practice (though it is reputed that Sharath starts his practice at 2.00 a.m. these days).

He teaches at Ashtanga Yoga Research Institute (AYRI), where he also serves as its Assistant Director.

1.7.4. Baron Baptiste

Baron Baptiste's Power Vinyasa Yoga is a powerful and intense yet accessible form of vinyasa flow yoga that leaves practitioners energized, exhilarated and empowered. The practice contains elements of Ashtanga, Bikram & Iyengar yoga, but has evolved during the 30 years that Baptiste has been a teacher to also include elements of modern fitness. Although often branded as sensationalism, Baptiste's yoga has real 'wow' appeal and promises honest results.

Baron began practicing yoga at the age of seven, and that journey has continued to the present day. He teaches students from all walks of life in classes, workshops and yoga bootcamps. His books, DVDs and CDs have been translated into numerous languages.

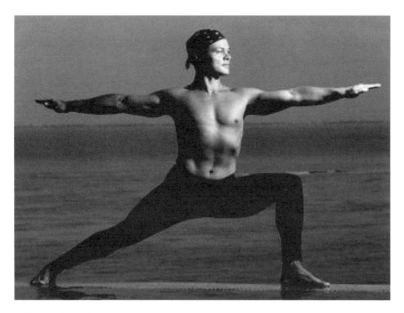

Baron Baptiste

1.7.5. Shiva Rea

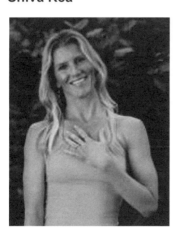

Shiva Rea was named by her artist father. Inspired by her Indian name, Shiva embarked on an exploration of yoga at the age of 14. Her influences are wide and varied, ranging from dance to *kalaripayyatu* (an ancient Indian martial art). Her philosophy stems from Sri Tirumala Krishnamacharya (*section 1.5.2*) lineage.

Shiva's classes are beautiful, flowing and inspirational, as are her dancelike *vinyasa* which has made her a household name in yoga circles. Perhaps the most captivating aspect of Shiva's transformational *vinyasa* (or commonly known as 'flow') is her warmth, humor and artistry that shine through in her yoga.

1.7.6. Seane Corn

Seane Corn's yoga is unapologetically spiritual, and from this spirituality emerges something very beautiful: "your connection to spirit is what that's really important in this practice, beyond the physical expression". She puts a lot of emphasis on connecting with the breath and the Inner Self through the natural movements of the body.

1.7.7. Rodney Yee

Rodney Yee was a gymnast and a ballet dancer trained in the Iyengar style. Deep, slow and conscious repetition leading to mindful practice is Yee's *yogasana* signature. He is reputed to be a good teacher with a grasp on modern issues such as fat burn, abs reshaping and muscle density.

1.8. Related spiritual practices / schools

1.8.1. Art of Living (AOL)

Founded by Sri Sri Ravi Shankar (*1956 -*), AOL's philosophy is creating a violence-free world by eliminating stress. At the heart of AOL is the *sudarshan kriya,* a powerful practice that leads to transformation. Meditation and other techniques are also utilized to make the mind calm and focused, so that challenges can be met gracefully.

AOL preaches wisdom and service as a way to a better world, spreading its word through the Art of Living Foundation and its many followers. It has been estimated that more than 100 million people have gone through AOL workshops globally, and the Foundation undertakes charitable projects in many parts of the world.

1.8.2. Transcendental Meditation (TM)

TM is a form of meditation (name trademarked) introduced by the Maharishi Mahesh Yogi (*1917 – 2008*). Maharishi Mahesh Yogi is probably best known as the spiritual guru to The Beatles and other celebrities.

TM is a technique for quieting the mind. It requires dedicated self-practice (20 minutes twice a day) after being inducted into the program by a set procedure. During the 20 minute period of TM, practitioners use a sacred sound (*mantra*) to draw their attention inwards into the mind, experiencing its deeper levels and gradually bringing them into the conscious realms. TM survives despite controversies surrounding its practice, and there is some scientific evidence pointing to the effectiveness of TM for various medical conditions.

1.8.3. Brahma Kumaris

The Brahma Kumaris is a spiritual organization built on the belief that self-realization can be achieved based on meditation and positive thinking. It falls in the Raja Yoga branch of yoga (*section 1.4.2*), whereby meditation is used to clear the mind and calm the heart. Contemplation on God is also a Brahma Kumaris way of turning the focus inwards to reach the inner self and to work on achieving balance between the inner and outer worlds. All Brahma Kumaris courses and seminars are offered free of charge, providing an entree for those seeking higher answers on God, life, spirituality and the external world.

1.8.4. Osho *(1931 – 1990)*

Osho was an Indian mystic and a spiritual teacher who garnered much controversy in his life. His beliefs on sexuality, institutionalized religion and other topical issues gave him a certain degree of notoriety. His legacy is his ashram, the Osho International Meditation Resort in India, and his teachings based on love, awareness, meditation, creativity and joy have won him many followers in the West, especially after his death.

1.8.5. *Kirtan*

Kirtan is an Indian tradition of devotional songs, which can be practiced as a personal spiritual practice (*japa*) or with much merriment, dancing and musical instruments. For those who do not find meditation easy, *kirtan* is a good option.

Because *kirtan* is based on call-and-response, it is accessible to all. *Kirtan* is a participatory event, and one would discover through *kirtan* that chanting can heal the heart. In the West, the proliferation of *kirtan* is driven by the International Society for Krishna Consciousness (ISKCON) and popular singers such as Jai Uttal and Krishna Das.

1.9. Six experiences of yoga

1.9.1. Living in the moment

One of the most profound teachings of yoga is the belief that "there is only now". It is a call to every one of us to live each moment of our life to the full and to our best ability, because for the yogi, the past is dead and the future is but imaginary.

Experiencing this key belief – written about and marketed by many spiritual teachers and psychologists – can be as simple as spending a few moments each day sitting comfortably in a quiet place, breathing deeply and slowly.

1.9.2. Journaling

Self-inquiry is one of the tenets contained within the Yoga Sutra. The physical body is but a sheath which sometimes misleads and distracts us from the path of truth. Noisy background chatter also serves to distract us from the true purpose of life.

Journaling is simply sitting down with a notebook and a pen, and letting your inner self flow through from your heart to your arm to your hand holding the pen. There is no right or wrong when it comes to journaling. And more importantly, there should be no judgment or criticism of what flows freely from within, for this is the reflection of your true self. You are who you are.

1.9.3. Mindful Eating

In the rush of our daily lives, we often forget to give thanks. Although vegetarianism is one of the teachings of yoga and a principle that all yogis should strive to achieve, the practice of giving thanks for our food should be easy enough to embrace.

Take a few seconds out before each meal to say a silent thank you to the sun, earth, seas, winds and animals that made the meal possible. And perhaps devote one day a week to silent dining to deepen the practice.

1.9.4. Spiritual fire

Spiritual fire is not necessarily confined to the ubiquitous definition of 'heat generated from the physical practice of *yogasana'*.

By turning our focus inward, we redirect our energy to fuel the spiritual fire and not waste our resources on negative words, vicious thoughts and harmful actions. This practice is simply one of "think no evil, say no evil and do no evil".

1.9.5. Commitment

Commitment to practice and to a spiritual path is the key to one's success in yoga. For a Hatha yogi, the commitment entails *yogasana* practice six days a week and living the Yoga Sutra through his actions in every waking hour.

A simple lesson in commitment begins with choosing a spiritual practice (for example meditation, journaling or observing the breath) for three minutes each day, and ensuring that this practice is not broken whatever the circumstances for a minimum of 21 days.

1.9.6. Letting go

Though a yogi must be committed to her practice, she must not be attached to the fruits of her practice. According to the Yoga Sutra, the illusion of possession and ownership is the cause of suffering. Life is transient, and it should be lived and let go of.

To experience this aspect of yoga, try unloading the rocks in your heart by forgiving those you carry a grudge against. This simple practice can save a lifetime of needless suffering.

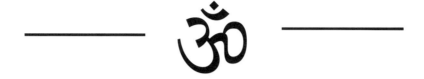

References

Kenoyer, J. M. (1998) *Ancient Cities of the Indus Valley Civilization*. Karachi, Oxford University Press.

Koay, J. (2006). *The Kundalini Yoga Cookbook*. London, UK: Gaia Octopus.

CHAPTER TWO

Philosophy, Ethics & Lifestyle

OVERVIEW OF THE CHAPTER

2.1   Moving beyond the physical
2.2   *Shad Darshan*: the Six Philosophies of Life
2.3   The books of yoga
2.4   Yoga Sutra of Sri Patanjali
2.5   *Ashtanga yoga*: the eightfold path
2.6   Living life as a modern yogi

2.1. Moving beyond the physical

2.1.1. The deeper meaning of yoga

The origins of yoga have never been accurately established by historians and scholars (*section 1.3.1*), but it is widely agreed that yoga is an ancient practice leading to self-enlightenment.

However, a huge proportion of the yoga that is practiced today by the masses is mat-based. *How does jumping on the mat lead one to self-enlightenment?*

Over the passage of time, yoga has evolved into so many guises, some barely recognizable from its origins. But if taught honoring its rich philosophies, traditions and history, yoga has much to offer its practitioners in terms of 'inner benefits'. Increasingly, it has been found to provide an alternative or as a complement to allopathic (modern Western) medicine, thus beginning the renaissance in this ancient science in recent decades.

With *yogasana*, the muscles and ligaments are stretched open from the outside. With conscious breathing practice (*pranayama*), the body is stretched from the inside so that it unfurls like a flower. With the opening of the body, the mind will become less rigid and more embracing.

2.1.2. Self-study / studying the scriptures (*svadhyaya*)

The yoga path, though unknown to many practitioners, is one of introspection, or *svadhyaya*. With the *Svadhyaya* path the Teacher, the Universal Wisdom and the Ultimate Truth are to be found within oneself. The classic mistake many yogis make is relying solely on their external senses (eyes and ears) for information which often gets jumbled up because of faulty cognitive processes, coloring from their ego and the distraction of continuous background noises. The first lesson is therefore silence (and patience to absorb the silence). Yoga is about silencing the chattering of the mind.

yogahcittavrittinirodhah [Yoga Sutra 2, I]

Withdrawal of the senses from the distractions of the external world, concentration and meditation take one deeper within oneself for an

27

encounter with one's True Self, in which Eternal Bliss resides. This is, in a nutshell, the basis of many philosophies on self-enlightenment.

The next step (or one that should be taken concurrently) is studying appropriate texts to guide oneself into an understanding of the obstacles and how they can be overcome through diligent practice to reach the light within. Thus, combining the physical practices of yoga (*asana* and *pranayama*) with philosophy, ethics and lifestyle makes yoga a powerful system for living a beautiful, bountiful and blissful life.

2.1.3. The five sheaths (*kosha*)

Many people's yoga journey starts with physical practice, *asana*, for one very simple reason: according to yogic anatomy, we have five layers of being which are arranged rather like the layers of an onion (*diagram 2.1*):

1. *Annamaya kosha* - physical
2. *Pranamaya kosha* – breath/energy
3. *Manomaya kosha* – mental
4. *Vijnamaya kosha* – wisdom
5. *Anandamaya kosha* - bliss

***Diagram 2.1.* The five kosha**

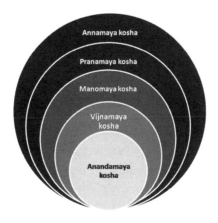

(Further description of the *kosha* is given in *section 6.8.1*)

Annamaya kosha

A Hatha-based yoga practice starts with the outermost layer, namely, the physical body. The physical body is a mass of bones, flesh, muscles, organs, cells. Appropriate practice of *yogasana* and *kriya* will keep the body healthy and functioning optimally. This would include, in Western speak, healthy internal functions (such as digestion and excretion), good cardiovascular health, supple joints, the right amount of body fat and good muscle tone.

But physical practice alone is not enough, even for the physical body. The physical body is nourished by the food we eat. According to the words of Yogi Bhajan, Master of Kundalini Yoga, "when we eat, we are building our future selves" (Koay, 2006). Therefore, though it is not common practice, the yoga teacher should advise his students on their diet, and move them towards a more appropriate diet if they are intent on the yogic path. "You are what you eat" is a common Western saying. If you put dirty fuel into an engine, there is no way the engine will run smoothly. There is not much point in practicing yoga, even for a good-looking body, if you continue to feed the wrong food into your body.

Another important aspect of keeping the physical body healthy is relaxation. The body needs time to rest, rejuvenate and repair itself. By continuously bombarding the body with rigorous demands without rest periods in between would harm it. As you can see, even on the first sheath alone, to embrace yoga wholly would involve a change in lifestyle, namely moving towards a more appropriate diet and honoring your body by giving it the rest it needs.

Pranamaya kosha

The *pranamaya kosha* is the next sheath inwards that brings us closer to the Self. This layer is accessed through the breath, utilizing *pranayama*. But *pranayama* is more than correct breathing, though correct breathing is vital to harness this energetic force. We need pranayama for the mind, too. I am always saying to my students, "Your breath is your emotional signature". A stressed out person breathes shallowly, forcing the breath into the body by aggressive, grasping movements – this will have long-lasting detrimental impacts on the overall health (*section 4.2.2*).

As human beings, we tend to accumulate our life's experiences in the form of *klesha*, poisionous mental states, either from ignorance or fear of death. Our consciousness starts revolving around these experiences and memories, spurred on by ego. When stored in the inner mind, these become *samskara*, or impressions. With *pranayama*, we learn to eliminate or transform the *samskara*, and this is one of the key goals of *pranayama*.

Manomaya kosha

The practice of *pratyhara*, the fourth limb of ashtanga yoga, leads us to *manomaya kosha*. *Manomaya kosha* is at the level of the *mana*, or mind. By harmonizing the *pranamaya kosha*, we are accessing the *manomaya kosha:* when we are at peace with ourselves, we have a clearer, more impartial insight through this *kosha*. This level, and the other two deeper ones, namely, the *vijnamaya* kosha and the *anandamaya* kosha, are the skeletons of our being, on which *annamaya kosha* and *pranamaya kosha* are built upon: if the skeleton is bent and crooked, so too will our being be.

Vijnamaya kosha and Anandamaya kosha

Traditional yoga practices work on righting and strengthening the three deeper levels of *kosha*, and indeed, this is the way of Raja Yoga.

But how many yogis actually reach into these deeper layers, distracted by the perennial preoccupation with the physical body? We might have sculpted our body to its ideal dimensions on the outside, but if the inner structures are unstable, then this perfection is only superficial. There is form but without substance. It's like an apple that has been grown in commercial situations with genetic modifications and fed on an abundance of pesticides – it might look good, but what does it contribute to you when you eat it?

Similarly, what does a physically perfect looking person contribute to the world if his/her core is diseased and rotten? A yogi is not someone with a toned body and a black heart. Obsession with appearance is fool's gold, because it does not last long, whereas the soul is eternal. Hence, the practice of yoga should be inward-looking, namely one of coming home.

2.2.   *Shad Darshan*: the six philosophies of life

2.2.1.   Introduction

Darshan is the Sanskrit word for philosophy (from the root word *drsh*, which means to contemplate and to see by divine intuition), and yoga is one of the six main *darshana*, or schools of classical Indian philosophy and cosmology (*diagram 2.2*):

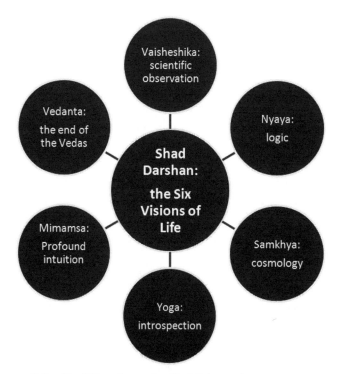

Diagram 2.2. **Shad Darshan: the Six Visions of Life**

Samkhya, Vaisheshika and Nyaya explore the physical world, whereas Mimamsa, Vedanta and Yoga are about delving into the inner reality as a means to understanding outer reality.

For the contextualization of yoga, the two most important philosophies are Samkhya and Vedanta.   Samkhya, on which the medical science of Ayurvĕda (Chapter 6) is based upon, strongly influenced the writings of Sri Patanjali, who formulated Yoga.

Diagram 2.3. **Shad Darshan and self-enlightenment**

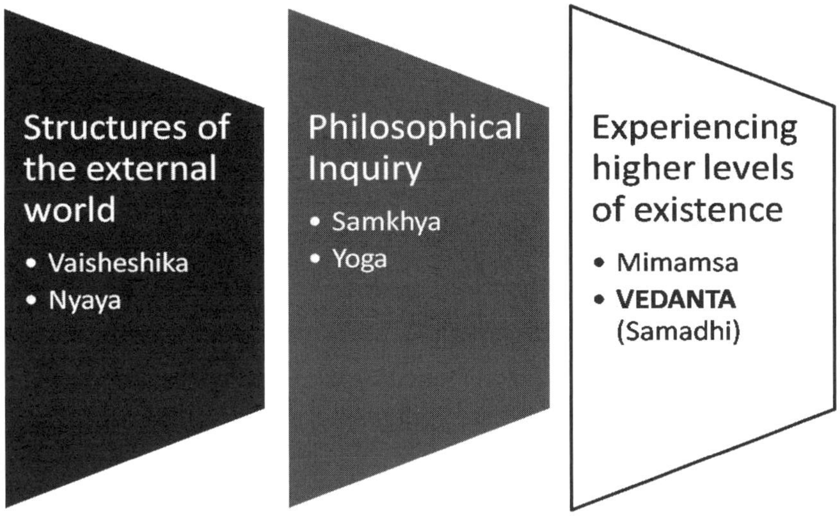

Structures of the external world
- Vaisheshika
- Nyaya

Philosophical Inquiry
- Samkhya
- Yoga

Experiencing higher levels of existence
- Mimamsa
- **VEDANTA** (Samadhi)

Vaisheshika (scientific observation)
formulated by Kanada:
building the Universe from nine causative substances, *nava karma dravya*

Nyaya (logic)
formulated by Gotama:
reasoning and logic leading to proof of truth

Samkhya (cosmology)
formulated by Kapila:
understanding the truth of life

Yoga (introspection)
formulated by Sri Patanjali:
the eightfold path to experiencing the Inner Self

Mimamsa (profound intuition)
formulated by Jaimini:
of God, deities and truth

Vedanta (the end of the Vedas)
formulated by Badarayana:
knowledge to end all knowledge

2.2.2. The Universe according to Samkhya

[REFER TO *section 5.6.5*]

Purusha is the unmanifested matter – quiet, formless, shapeless and with no attributes. It is passive and plays no part in creation. It is an observer, a witness, the potential energy that is sleeping.

Prakriti is the first of the 24 principles of creation. Prakriti is the womb from which the Universe was born. It is the Divine Mother. Without *purusha*, there can be no *prakriti.* However*, purusha* can exist without *prakriti* (Note: think about this). The unmanifested state of *purusha* and *prakriti* is called Brahma, or Pure Consciousness. Coming together gives physical expression (*vyakata*) to the unmanifested matter. This is the process of creation, which gives birth to consciousness.

The first expression of this creation is *Mahad*, the supreme intelligence. From *Mahad* comes *Ahamkara*, the ego. *Ahamkara*, the ego, introduces "I" into the scenario. The separateness creates *Buddhi* (individual awareness) from *Mahad* (universal awareness). Consciousness and all matter in the Universe come from *Hiranyagarbha*, or the Golden Egg. Pulsations of cosmic *prana* (or life force) caused the Egg to split into three universal qualities, *sattva, rajas* and *tamas*. *Sattva* is the quality of light and purity. *Rajas* is fiery and transformational. *Tamas* is heaviness and inaction. All matter is made up of these three qualities, in different proportions. However, there are some objects that arise solely from *sattva.*

Rajas, the transformation energy, moves *sattva* to create the world of sensory perception:
- The Five Senses (hear, see, touch, taste and smell)
- The Five Actions (speech, procreation, walking, grasping, elimination)
- The Mind

Similarly, *rajas* moves *tamas* to create the five elements of Ether or Space (*Akasha*), Air (*Vayu*), Fire (*Agni*), Water (*Apas*) and Earth (*Prthivi*), which contain qualities of *sattva* and *rajas*. These five elements are also known as the *maha bhutas*, the gross causative elements.

2.2.3. Samkhya and Yoga

Samkhya and Yoga are the divine pairing of *jnâna* (knowledge) and *karma* (action). Through dedicated practice of Yoga, the practitioner moves from experiencing the gross states to the subtle elements, moving inwards to experience the cosmology described by Samkhya. To reach this verdant inner universe where Reality exists, one has to detach oneself from the external world through the practices given in the Yoga Sutra by Sri Patanjali.

2.2.4. Vaisheshika and Nyaya

To understand Samkhya and Yoga, the pairing of Nyaya and Vaisheshika may be used to create structures of the external world from which philosophical inquiry can be contemplated.

Nyaya and Vaisheshika are ancestors of modern scientific methodology. They are about the process of establishing proof by methodical investigative means to elevate a conjecture to truth.

Vaisheshika is very similar to the Atomic Theory. According to the Atomic Theory, the world is made up of indivisible units called atoms. Each atom has its individual characteristics, and they combine with other atoms to form larger entities called molecules. These are the building blocks to all objects that exist.

According to Vaisheshika, there are nine causative substances of the Universe (*nava karma dravya*):

1. Ether/Space (*Akasha*)
2. Air (*Vayu*)
3. Fire (*Agni*)
4. Water (*Apas*)
5. Earth (*Prthivi*)
6. Soul (*Atman*)
7. Mind (*Manas*)
8. Time (*Kala*)
9. Direction (*Dig*)

Ether, Air, Fire, Water and Earth are the equivalent of atoms. Under the will of the Supreme Being, they combine to form other matters; they separate and annihilate as they form in this eternal dance of life. The soul in Vaisheshika philosophy is part of Consciousness. The soul is therefore the Self, something that does not need body or mind to exist. It is the aim of life to move the mind from *mudha* (lowest state – unbalanced) to *mukta* (highest state – enlightened) through a series of observances and practices.

In the state of *mudha*, the individual is focused on power, wealth, sex, prestige and other empty benchmarks to the exclusion of everything else. Indeed, much of Sri Patanjali's Yoga Sutra and other meditation practices are about transforming the mind; for example, taming the *kspita* (chattering mind) to the state of *ekagra* (one-pointed focus) and finally leading to *mukta*.

Time is a flow. In today's world, time is commonly measured with clocks and watches. In ancient times, it was the observation of seasons, the positions of the sun and other celestial entities and other natural means that gave man a measure of change and movement. In the yogic world view, time is measured in terms of prana. One *prana* is one breath (one cycle of inhalation and exhalation). Life is measured in the number of breaths taken; therefore, pranayama (or breathing consciously) is about longevity.

The final causative substance in the Vaisheshika philosophy is direction. One of the uses of direction is in positioning one's dwelling in such a way that the occupants receive the blessings from the elements. This practice, known as *vashtu shastra*, is similar to *feng shui*.

Nyaya provides the reasoning and logic to make sense of the theories of Vaisheshika. In the Nyaya philosophy, there are four sources of valid knowledge, or methodology of proof, which can be applied to rationalize everything:

1. Perception (*Pratyaksha*)
2. Inference (*Anumana*)
3. Comparison (*Upamana*)
4. Testimony (*Shabda*)

Perception is the rudimentary Ayurvĕdic diagnostic tool, and perception in this context is based on accurate input received from the five senses (*laukika*) and from the more intangible senses (*alaukika*): pain, pleasure, soul, memories, etc. Inference is drawn from past experience and knowledge, and is useful where *laukika* is not possible. The next – third – step in Nyaya's methodology of proof is the process of comparison. Finally, testimony from the patient or from other diagnostic methods, are held as sacred truth and play an important role in Ayurvĕdic medicine.

2.2.5. Mimamsa and Vedanta

Once the steps of Vaisheshika and Nyaya have been taken with the conscious mind to experience the world of Samkhya through the practices of yoga, the practitioner is ready to embrace spiritual technologies of Mimamsa to reach Vedanta. The realization of the Vedanta is equivalent to samadhi in the context of Sri Patanjali's Yoga Sutra. There are parallels between Mimamsa and Chapter 3 of Sri Patanjali's Yoga Sutra. This is why many new practitioners are put off by this chapter, or at worst, they regard the Yoga Sutra as a religious treatise rather than a technique for self-enlightenment. In fact, Sri Patanjali clearly exhorts practitioners to find their own God in accordance with their own beliefs:

> **svadhyayat ista devata samprayogah** [Yoga Sutra 40, II]
> *svadhyayat* = self-study; study of scriptures
> *ista* = personal choice, beloved
> *devata* = deity
> *samprayogah* = communion

The basis of Mimamsa is that there is an ultimate creator, who is God. This God is not a God that is distant and separate from us, but One who is reflected in each and every one of us. This belief resonates strongly with the words of Yogi Bhajan, Master of Kundalini Yoga: "If you can't see God in all, you can't see God at all". Apart from God, believers of Mimamsa believe in deities who contribute to our well-being and that of our world. And apart from God and deities, there is also Ultimate Truth, which can be found through selfless service in *dharma*. Based on the teachings of the Vedas, Mimamsa is highly ritualistic, with fasting, *puja* and sacrifices among its practices. In Ayurvĕda, only few of these rituals are adopted for healing purposes.

In Vedanta, there is only Consciousness. God is this Consciousness, or Brahma. The study of Vedanta involves surrendering the pursuit of knowledge after a certain level to walk in the path of faith, under the guidance of an enlightened teacher. This is Upanishad, which means sitting near a teacher or master, and absorbing his light with a totally open heart. Vedanta is the end of knowledge, because in the journey of life, the most important book to read is one's self. It is from here that we realize life, to see life without our vision being fettered, and ultimately, to coalesce our lower self into the higher Self.

36

2.3. **The books of yoga**

2.3.1. **Yoga Sutra of Sri Patanjali**

[REFER TO *section 2.4*]

2.3.2. **Vedas**

The Sanskrit word *véda* means knowledge or wisdom, and is derived from the root *vid-* which means 'to know'. The Vedas are therefore the book of knowledge. Knowledge in the Vedic era was passed down via oral transmission (known as Śrauta), recited like poetry with complex text, pronunciations and accents. This is considered the oldest unbroken oral tradition. The chant Om (*section 7.9.1*) is found throughout the Vedas, and the popular Gayatri mantra (*section 7.9.2*) is Rig Vedic by origin.

The Vedas are the oldest Sanskrit text in existence. The contents are mostly ritualistic. There are several books which are collectively known as the Vedas, of which the Rig Veda is probably the best known. The oldest Vedas, Samhitas, date back to 1500 - 1000 BC (though various estimates exist). The Vedas are widely studied as befitting their position as the oldest Sanskrit text in existence. Different schools have different interpretations of the Vedas. Moreover, the parameters of what constitutes as Vedic literature are not clearly defined. Other closely related texts include:

1. Upanishad (*section 2.3.3*)
2. Bhagavad Gita (*section 2.3.5*)

2.3.3. **Upanishad**

The Upanishad chronicles the Vedanta. Vedanta is a spiritual tradition not unlike Yoga, where the ultimate aim is self-realization, namely to know Brahman (or Ultimate Consciousness). While the Vedas are mostly about rituals, the Upanishad is about philosophies and practices (in particular, the forms of meditation) leading to self-realization.

The Vedanta Sutra, composed after the Vedic period, is known as 'knowledge to end all knowledge' (*véda* = 'knowledge'; *anta* = 'end'). The vast universe of Vedic ideas was collated into one treatise by the scribe Bandarayana, who was also known as Vyāsa.

Vedanta forms one half of Mimamsa, namely the Uttara Mimamsa. The other half of Mimamsa is Pūrva Mimamsa. These are the process of inquiry and rituals discussed in *section 2.2.5.*

2.3.4. Mahābhārata and Rāmāyana

These are the texts of Hindu mythology. Written in Sanskrit, the epic stories of Mahābhārata and Rāmāyana span the centuries, and exist today as modern cartoon books and children's DVD, selling the age-old values of duty and purpose. When performed correctly and with pure intent, they ultimately lead to liberation and escape from the karmic cycle.

The earliest portion of the Mahābhārata was probably composed in the late Vedic period. Like the Vedanta, the Mahābhārata is attributed to Bandarayana (Vyāsa). This epic has about 1.8 million words in total!

The Mahābhārata is about the lives of two families, the Kauravas and the Pandavas, who fought each other in the Kurukshetra War. Parallels on moral values from the thoughts and deeds of the main characters are drawn from this epic and applied to daily life. Its spin-off, the Bhagavad Gita (*section 2.3.5*), makes an easier reading.

The Rāmāyana shares its place in history with the Mahābhārata. Compiled by the sage Valmiki, it is no less unwieldy with 24,000 verses contained in seven books. In brief, the Rāmāyana, or 'Rama's Journey', is about Rama (an incarnation of Vishnu), whose wife Sita is abducted by Ravana, the demon king of Lanka. Rama's faithful servant, the monkey god Hanuman, helps Rama find Sita. The story emphasizes the omnipresent concepts of right action and selfless service (which still form the backbone of Hindu society today).

2.3.5. Bhagavad Gita

Bhagavad Gita means the 'Song of God'. A derivative of the Mahābhārata, it has only 700 verses. The story revolves around the conversation between Krishna, the incarnation of the Lord, and Arjuna the archer. It takes place in the battlefield of Kurukshetra, as Arjuna is about to take up arms against his own family.

Through Arjuna's confusion and moral dilemma, parallels are drawn with those encountered in daily life. The ever-patient and wise teacher Krishna guides Arjuna through his turmoil, and Krishna's timeless lessons are still used as moral compass today by many Hindus. The wisdom espoused in the Bhagavad Gita shares many common themes with Yoga philosophy, namely stilling the chattering of the mind, freeing it from desires (the root of suffering), and surrendering to the Lord. It is built around Bhakti Yoga (*section 1.4.3*), Jnâna Yoga (*section 1.4.4*) and Karma Yoga (*section 1.4.7*).

2.3.6. Hatha Yoga Pradipika

Hatha Yoga Pradipika, the seminal text for the practice of Hatha Yoga, was ascribed to the sage Svatmarama, and is believed to have been written in the 15th century CE.

The word *pradipika* comes from the Sanskrit verb, 'to flame forth'. Thus, the text is the light on yoga. For the physical practice of yoga, Svatmarama connects life, breath, *prana, nadi, chakra* and the mind. He further describes the practice of breathing exercises and *mudra* (energy seals created with fingers). Parallel to the Yoga Sutra, Swatmarama also describes *samadhi* in Hatha Yoga Pradipika.

Although it is a classic, many students of yoga are disappointed by the small number of *asana* presented in this book. Most of the *asana* to be found here are those that work towards enabling the practitioner to sit for long periods in meditation, rather than a compilation of the *asana* of Hatha Yoga. However, it presents another not too dissimilar take on Sri Patanjali's Yoga Sutra, for example:

- Yoga perishes by these six: overeating, overexertion, talking too much, performing needless austerities, socializing and restlessness.

- Yoga succeeds by these six: enthusiasm, openness, courage, knowledge of the truth, determination and solitude.

2.4. Yoga Sutra of Sri Patanjali

2.4.1. Introduction to the Yoga Sutra

When talking about yoga philosophy, we are invariably referring to Sri Patanjali's Yoga Sutra. This is where we find *yama, niyama, pranayama, asana, pratyhara, dharana, dhyana, samadhi* and a whole host of yogic practices. As a yoga practitioner and /or a yoga teacher, this book is as important to you as the yoga mat.

There are over 50 translations in English of the original work by Sri Patanjali. Yoga in its earliest inception was an oral tradition (*section 2.3.1*), with nothing written down but passed directly from master to disciples in a living energetic *yantra* made up of gestures, gazes, sounds (such as mantras and chants), as well as other methods of non-verbal energetic transmission. This wisdom came from the sages and wise men in deep meditation. It became knowledge – the Universal Truth - when tempered with the fire of time. Sri Patanjali was the scribe who documented this corpus of information. He was not the 'inventor' of yoga: yoga was the collective wisdom from sages and wise men of that time.

According to lore, Sri Patanjali was the incarnation of the serpent Ananta, whom Lord Vishnu, the Lord of Creation, rested upon. Sri Patanjali came to being when he fell in the form of a little snake into the cupped hands of the maiden Gonika, who was offering water to the sun. We do not know much about Sri Patanjali, other than he was a scholar who was also a yogi.

It is difficult to estimate when yoga practices began, with estimates ranging from 10,000 years to as recent as four thousand years ago. In the ancient literature, the principles of yoga are mentioned in the four Vedas (*section 2.3.2*). One of the earliest relics that bore evidence to yoga's existence in prehistoric times is the Mohenjo-Daro seal that some archaeologists believe represents a yogi sitting in meditation posture (*section 1.3.1*).

Based on style, language, literary technique, historians place Sri Patanjali's Yoga Sutra as approximately 2,000 years old. Sutra is the Sanskrit word for thread. Sri Patanjali wrote in the form of aphorism, which is a shorthand way of writing, and his writing is steeped in Samkhya philosophy of the time (*section 2.2*). All in all, Sri Patanjali's Yoga Sutra has only 196 verses, and from hearsay, was contained in 10 pages of large texts. These verses are in four chapters (called *pada*), though many argue that the fourth chapter is incomplete and more have been added on posthumously.

2.4.2. How to study the Yoga Sutra

Translation of Sri Patanjali's original words would require knowledge of Sanskrit, yoga, philosophy, historical context of the time the Sutra was written and an appreciation of today's thinking. But in this world where anyone can be an 'expert', there are many books translating Patanjali's words. Invest in one from a reputable scholar and work through this book slowly. It could take you several years. (Note: Koay (2008) had written a simple, readable version of this book which provides a suitable entree to the subject).

However, the best version of Patanjali's Yoga Sutra is yours, your own version. Reason: Patanjali's Yoga Sutra is not a textbook. It is a laboratory practical book – you have to do the experiments to understand it. Patanjali's words are merely the signposts that you cannot understand by intellect and rationale. You need to study with the guidance of a teacher, and to meditate on those words, to live with a few of those words on a daily basis. Word-for-word translations are meaningless, because the most profound teachings come from the silences and spaces between the words. So don't get bogged down trying to memorize all the Sanskrit words in a short time; focus instead on what each Sutra is trying to say to you each day.

But you have to live the Yoga Sutra and not only study the aphorisms. Sri Patanjali tells us that we must be anchored in our own experiences, no matter how authoritative the pre-conceived beliefs are. Therefore, the only way to know the Yoga Sutra is to experience it for yourself. Success in yoga is through practice and practice only. In the words of Sri K Pattabhi Jois, "Do your practice, and all is coming".

2.4.3. The framework

The Yoga Sutra belongs to the school of Raja Yoga (*section 1.4.2*), and as such, *samadhi* is approached principally through the meditation route. Hindrances to meditation (and hence, to achieving *samadhi*) are in the forms of *klesha, samskara, vasana, vrtti* and *karma*. These are the result of *avidya* (ignorance) and /or where you are in your karmic cycle. Apart from meditation, remedies to these obstacles include *ashtanga yoga* and *kriya yoga*.

Even with *karma* permitting, the only way you can hope to reach *samadhi* is by doing, namely through showing commitment to your *sadhana*. You cannot understand Patanjali's Yoga Sutra by reading a book hoping to glimpse self-enlightenment through the written word. Reading involves mental machinations (such as power of analysis, conceptual thoughts, philosophical extrapolation, the study of semantics, memorization of facts, etc), which are all *vritti*. *Vritti* can be imagined as a whirlpool going round and round on its own momentum. And the aim of yoga, of course, is to stop the chattering of the mind so that we can sit in silence and experience the Self, the Ultimate Reality.

Sri Patanjali did not write a prescriptive text, advocating one method over the other. You cannot follow his recipe to *samadhi*, because he has not given us the recipe. In the Yoga Sutra, he used the word *va*, which means 'or', instead of *ca* (and) when describing methods. Therefore, you need to experience for yourself, to find your path.

Note: only chapters 1 and 2 are covered in this book, because the author does not have sufficient mastery to disseminate the final two chapters.

2.4.4. Chapter 1: Samadhi Pada

Samadhi Pada gives us an overview of Raja Yoga. The Ultimate Reality, Source of Consciousness (called *Cit*) and the Divine is obscured by the fog of our mind (*citta-vrtti*). This disconnection or spiritual estrangement, put there by ignorance (called *avidya*) is the cause of suffering (*dukha*). Yoga is the practice of bringing together the Creator and the Creation, the yoking together of mind, body and soul with the Universal. This is the state of *samadhi*.

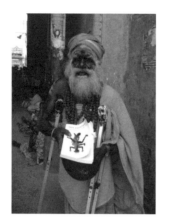

Disconnection from True Reality: explains why some people, despite wealth, status and other blessings remain discontent and unhappy, while others with very little live each day in bliss and serenity. Ending this spiritual estrangement to attain *samadhi* is the only way to true and everlasting happiness.

Remedies for spiritual estrangement (*pratishedha*) include: *vairagya, nirodha, virama-pratyaya, Isvara pranidhana, dhyana, eka-tattvabhyasa, japa, shradda, virya, prajna, maîtri, karuna, upeksanam, mudita, bhava, rtam prajna*. Note: Look up the meaning of these words, and practice living with one or two each day.

Deep inside, we are already familiar with the *samadhi* that yoga is taking us to, because in our original true nature (*svarupa*), we were already there. The fluctuations of the mind, *vritti*, and the trappings of individual consciousness (*cit*) in this mental state (*citta-vritti*) can be annulled (*nirodhah*) by yogic practices that facilitate the connection with our true nature.

Cit/citta is pure and clear consciousness (*sattva*), but is colored by other influences (*rajas* and *tamas*). It can be purified by yogic practices such as *pranayama* and *kriya yoga*. Yoga is thus the application and techniques (*sadhana*) for the purpose of annulling (*nirodhah*) the imprisonment of consciousness (*cit*) by the machinations of the mind (*vritti*) so that we can return to our true state (*svarupa*) to achieve bliss, self-realization and spiritual liberation (*samadhi*).

yogaschittavritti nirodhah [Yoga Sutra 2, I]

The goal of yoga is to still the chattering of the monkey mind. This sutra also goes on to say that this chattering, or fluctuation, distorts or limits the field of consciousness (*citta-vritti*) [Sutra 3-4, I]. A good way to illustrate this is to put a coin at the bottom of a glass of water – if we shake the glass so that the water swirls, it is difficult to see the coin clearly through the swirling water. In this analogy, the coin is Ultimate Reality, Truth and the Inner Self, while the water is the fluctuations of our mind. We have to cease identifying with these fluctuations in order to attain the state of Yoga.

Patanjali went on to describe the fluctuations of the mind and methods of controlling them [Yoga Sutra 5-16, I] so that we may experience that moment of clarity to know the Ultimate Reality.

vrttayah pancatayyah klista aklistah [Yoga Sutra 5, I]
pramana viparyaya vikalpa nidra smrtayah [Yoga Sutra 6, I]

There are five types of fluctuations (*vritti*), which can be difficult and even painful, and they are:
1. *pramana* – comprehension, or right knowledge
2. *viparyaya* – miscomprehension, or wrong knowledge
3. *vikalpa* – imagination
4. *nidra* – deep sleep
5. *smrtayah* – memory

Pramana is awareness of the real situation, and comes from:
• Inference or *anumana*
• Direct perception or *pratyaksha*
• Verbal testimony or *shabda pramana*

Viparyaya is obstruction to the Truth:
• Egoism or *asmita*
• Hatred or *dvesa*
• The sense of self-preservation or *abhinivesa*
• Ignorance or *avidya*
• Attachment or *raga*

In *nidra* or deep sleep, there is no mental activity present in the brain as it sinks into heaviness. Memory is the retention of all our past experiences – when we have experienced something in the past with our five senses, we build an entry of that experience in our image bank, which we subconsciously retrieve when faced with a situation in the present moment.

When we meditate, we are in effect witnessing the rise and fall of the *vritti*. By getting to know our *vritti*, we gain power over them so that they lose their ability to mislead us.

Vritti produce *klesha*, which are mental and emotional afflictions. We experience *klesha* when feelings of anger, rage and jealousy raise their ugly heads. This is when we act out of ignorance, spurred on by negative conditioning, past programming and old habits. These *klesha* come to you from your past life through the law of cause and effect (*karma*), though you may know (*drsta*) or may not know (*drsta-adrsta*) their origins. It's a downward spiral – negative *karma* feeds these *klesha*, and actions arising from these *klesha* induce a bigger negative *karma*. Therefore, we can see *klesha* as the root cause of the continuation of negative *karma*. When you begin on the yoga or any other spiritual path, you are making a conscious decision to break free from this spiral.

pratyaksa anumana agamah pramanani [Yoga Sutra 7, I]

pramana - comprehension, or right knowledge

agamah – testimony from those who know(parents, teachers etc) who can testify *pramana*

anumana – inference: logical, deductive activity of the mind

pratyaksa – direct perception

Comprehension (or right knowledge) implies a belief system. When meditating, we have to let go of *pramana*, which is a vritti. Letting go of *pramana* is difficult, as it is the belief system from which we build the foundations of 'I'. The other three components which form *pramana*, too, have to be let go. The *pratyaksa* we are letting go of is not wisdom, but a dualistic belief that we understand the external world. Instead, to attain *nirbija samadhi*, we need to find a different kind of wisdom, namely *jnâna*. The key is that yoga is a direct experience through *sadhana*, not based on intellect, instructions or 'proof'.

abhyasa vairagyabhyam tan-nirodhah [Yoga Sutra 12, I]

The significance of this sutra is that it tells us yoga is a process-oriented process, not goal-directed, i.e. we must practice non-attachment to the results of our practice. Just because you are faithfully doing your *sadhana* every morning does not guarantee you *samadhi*. Thus, we should practice yoga out of love and devotion, not a profit-minded, goal-oriented exercise. Yoga does not owe you anything, and Sri Patanjali promises nothing.

Sadhana should therefore be approached with:
- *abhyasa* – continuous practice
- *vairagyabhyam* – freedom from attachment.

Sutra 17 onward deals with different types of *samadhi*. It is more abstract, requiring a leap of faith, since few of us have personally experienced *samadhi*. (Note that there is no consensus among scholars about the segmentation of *samadhi*). But as previously mentioned, Sri Patanjali meant for the Yoga Sutra to be experiential, so this argument is theoretical until you are experiencing *samadhi* yourself.

vitarka vicara ananda asmita rupa nugamat samprajnata

[Yoga Sutra 17, I]

samprajnatah – *samadhi* with seeds

anugamat – followed by

rupa – form

asmita – sense of being, I-ness

ananda – rejoicing

vicara – reflecting

vitarka – reasoning

Patanjali distinguished two broad categories of *samadhi, samprajnatah* and *asamprajnatah*. *Samprajnata samadhi* is further divided into *vitarka* (reasoning), *vicara* (reflecting), *ananda* (rejoicing) and *asmita* (pure I-am-ness) [Sutra 17, I]. *Vitarka samadhi* and *vicara samadhi* are in turn further divided into two: *savitarka samadhi* (when the mind is focused on the name, form, appearance of the object) and *nirvitarka samadhi* (when the name, form and appearance of the object fall away so that duality breaks down). Then consciousness moves to: *savichara samadhi* (contemplating the subtle layers of the object, contemplating the layers that are beyond the grasp of our senses) and *nirvichara samadhi* (where our Inner self illuminates brightly).

The final stages of *samprajnatah samadhi* are *ananda* (rejoicing, with pure bliss) and *sasmita* (sense of pure being). Up to here (*samprajnatah samadhi*) we have seeds, which are the *samskara* (impressions). We have to get rid of the seeds (links to the physical world) and the *citta-vritti* before we can move on to *nirbija samadhi*: *tasyapi nirodhe sarva nirodhat nirbijah samadhih* [Sutra 51, I].

Samadhi Pada:
Yoga is about moving our awareness
from *asmita* (ego-centric world-view) and *vitarka* (material)
to the more subtle (*vicara*)
to beyond even the most subtle (*nirvicara*)
to *nirguna* (devoid of the *guna*)
to *arupa* (formless)
to *nirvikalpa* (transconceptual)

to *nirodhah, asamprajnatah* (non-dual)
and eventually…
to *nirbija samadhi* (which is the last step).

2.4.5. Chapter 2: Sadhana Pada

Sadhana Pada is the chapter detailing the journey from *sadhana* to *samadhi* (a state of awakening) and on to the final *samadhi* (*nirbija samadhi* – 'seedless samadhi'), where even the future seeds of vritti have been annulled (*nirodhah*).

The 'do' part of this chapter is *sadhana*, starting off with *kriya* (pre-requisite purification) followed by yogic practices (*tapas, svadhyaya*, and *Isvara pranidhanani*). Samadhi Pada introduces *ashtanga yoga*, going into detail of the first five limbs. It finishes off with *svadhyaya, tapas* and *Isvara pranidhanani*.

The most important point about *sadhana* is your attitude – it should not be seen as a discipline, hard work, something you have to do to get to *samadhi*. *Sadhana* should be approached with joy, and it should be seen as an honor to be able to perform *sadhana*. Selfless giving in *sadhana* is where your practice of *vairagya* (renunciation, letting go) solidifies. In the end, when *samadhi* is achieved, we surrender even the practice.

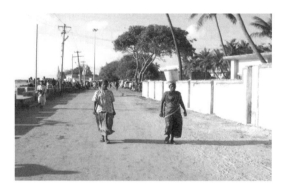

<u>Just do it</u>. Surrender, let go, love and embrace your practice with joy. That's the road to *samadhi*.

Tapah-svadhyayesvara-pranidhananikriya-yogah
[Yoga Sutra 1, II]

To get to the state of yoga (connection between Self and *samadhi*), these are the actions for purification (*kriya yoga*):
1. Renouncing distracting activities so that you can channel your energies inwards to start the spiritual fire (*tapas*);
2. Self-study to understand your Self (*svadhyaya*);

3. Surrendering to God, the light behind Consciousness, whatever you believe (*Isvara pranidhanani*).

.

Basically, you are not practicing yoga if you are just jumping on the mat, but still think (and worse still, speak) ill of other people, if you do not try to understand what's really in your heart, and if you have no faith.

Experiencing *tapas*

You can put these all into practice in a simple meditation session – sit tall and straight in *padmasana*, bring awareness to your breath. Create a steady flow of prana through your body with proper breathing techniques (and holding *bandha* – body locks to hold pranic energy).

In meditation, do not fight whatever that is going through your mind. Just sit quietly and witness your passing thoughts. When those thoughts silence, delve into your memory and think of one person you do not like. Turn what you perceive that is negative about that person into a positive thought – we waste too much energy on hatred. Find something in that person that you admire. Let go of the negative thought associated with that person forever: from this point thence, this person is bathed in the positive light you create.

Work through this, and then just sit quietly and BE. There is no goal, no aim, to this practice. It is a few moments of nothingness in your busy day. Learn to see it this way, rather than as a 'discipline', an 'exercise', a 'sacrifice'.

kayendriya-siddhir asuddhi-ksayat tapasah
[Yoga Sutra 43, II]

The sense organs are purified through the destruction of the impurities by *tapas*, the fire of your practice. With hard work and discipline you burn the impurities from your body/mind whether using a meditation to "let go of attachments" or practicing a challenging *yogasana*.

samadhi-bhavanarthah klesa-tanu-karanarthas ca
[Yoga Sutra 2, II]

Samadhi doesn't occur instantaneously (unless you are in a particular stage of your karmic cycle). In fact, it is a step-wise process as we grow in our practice (*bhavana*). It starts first with the burning off of the negative afflictions (*klesha*) that traps us in *dukha* (sorrow), so that the purpose of our practice or intention (*artah*) becomes clear. With the lessening (*tanu*) of the *klesha*, our intentions become clear and the path to *samadhi* becomes more attainable. If our intention is to attain *samadhi* (*samadhi-bhavanarthah*), we should practice *tapas* not only during a yoga class, but in our everyday life. "If you want to find God, feed the world".

avidyasmita-raga-dvesabhinivesah klesha
[Yoga Sutra 3, II]

This is about the afflictions that we are trying to destroy. As mentioned in the previous Sutra, we need to destroy *klesha* so that we can cultivate *samadhi* (*samadhi bhavanarthah*). The major *klesha* is ignorance (*avidya*). Ignorance of our True Self gives birth to *asmita* (ego-driven, arrogance, conceit, focus on the 'I, me, myself'), *raga* (excessive attachment, desire), *dvesa* (repulsion, aversion, hatred, fear), and, *abhinivesa* (the fear of death when there is no need to because of the eternity of the Self).

Raga is contemplated on again in:

sukhanusayi ragah [Yoga Sutra 7, II]
anusayi = clinging

When we talk about pleasure (*sukha*), it is not merely pleasure of the flesh but of the mind, such as (perceived) freedom from fear, desire and temporary satiation of the mind's needs (often ego and greed). This is not to be confused with *santosa* (true contentment) and *ananda* (bliss), which is a natural state of being when we surrender and become One with our True Self. Excessive attachment and clinging as characterized by *raga* is a waste of time – it's like trying to find the pot of gold at the foot of the rainbow.

Raga also fills a void that exists in us when there is no True Love in our life. But with love for our true Self, we will know that we are all part of everything, that we are complete, that there is no need for 'more'. In ourselves, we are whole, because we are all part of a Universal Whole. With the realization that we each are a little river flowing into the ocean, the fear of death (*abhinivesa*) is unnecessary. There is no need to cling to life.

In everyday terms, *abhinivesa* is manifested in clinging to the present in the mistaken belief that what that gives us security, peace, happiness, will go on forever. *Abhinivesa* is the greatest source of some of the most corrosive emotions, such as desire, fear and materialism. We are fearful of change, and in that fear we cling on to what we currently have – but have you tried clinging to a handful of sand? The harder your grasp, the more the sand flows out of your hands. So the lesson with *abhinivesa* is simply to relax and enjoy what you have, and simply to BE.

anityasuci-duhkhanatmasunitya-suci-sukhatmakhyatir avidya
[Yoga Sutra 5, II]

Pleasures that so many human beings sacrifice and destroy their lives for are transient, temporary, and an illusion (think of it as scratching an itch – isn't it better not to scratch, despite the fact that it gives you pleasure when you scratch? Scratching an itch can cause damage to you!).

But because of *avidya*, we blindly run after pleasure and similar things (success, bigger house, fame, status) which will inevitably plunge us into suffering (*dukha*). When we are on this path of self-destruction, we confuse the non-self (*anatama*) with the True Self (*atman*), resulting in *asmita* (false identification). We also confuse the pure (*suci*) with the impure (*asuci*), and the mistaken belief that the ever-changing world (*anitya*) is static and permanent (*nitya*).

The following Sutra is actually revisiting *tapas*:

> ### *te pratiprasava-heyah suksmah* [Yoga Sutra 10, II]
> *suksma* = small, subtle
> *heya* = destroy
> *pratiprasava* = sending back to the Source

One interpretation is that we get rid of even the smallest of *klesha* by returning it to its Origin. How do we do this? Through meditation, of course:

dhyana-heyas tad-vrttayah [Yoga Sutra 11, II]

When you meditate, you just sit there and wait for your *klesha* to appear. It could be something as deep as buried childhood anger, as frivolous as anticipated pleasure or as mundane as wanting a drink. By not reacting to the klesha but merely witnessing them, you are dissipating their energy and potency, and they melt away. It is through trying to fight them or trying to analyze them that we begin a hide-and-seek game where we end up being tortured by our monkey-mind.

Heyam duhkham anagatam [Yoga Sutra 16, II]

With meditation, we can eliminate (*heya*) sorrows that are in the future (*anagatam*). 'You think, therefore you are'. How often have you tortured yourself with imagining the worst? Intellect and analytical prowess is very different from discriminatory awareness; the former are the products of the thinking mind while the latter comes from wisdom.

What is discriminatory awareness? Basically, even though yoga philosophy expounds 'oneness' (with oneself, with the society, with the whole Universe, with our Creator), there also exists 'differentness' (which is not to be confused with ego) such as *purusha/prakriti*, Shiva/Bhakti, etc. By merely being aware is not enough – we need the awareness of awareness (*viveka*). It is the light within the light, and it is this that brings upon wisdom (*prajna*), and with the dawning of wisdom, *avidya* falls away, and as *avidya* falls away, more wisdom shines through. To cultivate that discriminatory awareness, or differentiated consciousness, Sri Patanjali recommends *ashtanga yoga*, the eight limbs which come in seven stages:

1. *yama* and *niyama*
2. *niyama* and *asana*
3. *asana* and *pranayama*
4. *pranayama* and *pratyhara*
5. *pratyhara* and *dharana*
6. *dharana* and *dhyana*
7. *dhyana* and *samadhi*

2.5. *Ashtanga yoga*: the eightfold path

2.5.1. The eightfold path

Yama niyama asana pranayama pratyhara dharana dhyana samadhyo astavangani [Yoga Sutra 29, II]

yama = The Great Universal Vows (actions onto others)
niyama = Personal Observances (actions onto self)
asana = Sitting comfortably (often translated as posture practice)
pranayama = Conscious breathing
pratyhara = Withdrawal of the senses
dharana = One-pointed concentration

51

dhyana = Meditation

samadhyo = Self-realization, bliss, enlightenment

astavangani = eight limbs

2.5.2. <u>Yama</u>

Yama is *mahavratam*, or the Great Universal Vows.   There are five instructions contained within *yama*:

ahimsa satya asteya brahmacharya aparigraha yamah

[Yoga Sutra 30, II]

ahimsa = non-violence

satya = truthfulness

asteya = non-stealing

brahmacharya = focus on the Divine, continence

aparigraha = non-grasping, freedom from greed

yamah = The Great Universal Vows (actions onto others)

The five *yama* are the self-restraints that all yogis are exhorted to practice in their relationship with others, including animals and the environment. The first *yama*, *ahimsa*, relates to acts, words and thoughts that should be non-injurious onto others. Plotting the downfall of others and thinking ill of people are the more subtle acts of *himsa* that contravene the first *yama*.

Satya is truth, and that includes truth to oneself. A common non-truth that some yogis fall into is trying to 'accelerate' their practice instead of being devoted to it simply out of love for what they do. These yogis miss the real spirit of yoga: yoga is where you are at this moment in time and how you live your life, not what you can do with your body (Koay, 2008).

Asteya involves non-stealing, and this includes the non-stealing of intangibles, such as ideas, intellectual properties and goodwill. *Asteya* links with *aparigraha*, non-grasping. It is only by accepting that all life is impermanent that one can truly let go of one's desire to accumulate and to cling.   Running around attending endless number of yoga workshops simply for the sake of certificates or in the hope of accelerated learning are going against the grain of *aparigraha*.

Brahmacharya is popularly taken to mean sexual continence. It ties in with the history and tradition of yoga, where the ancient yogis were celibate.

However, in the wider context, *brahmacharya* means being focused (*acharya* = religious teacher) on the Divine (*brahma*). A simple way of walking the path of *brahmacharya* is simply not to waste one's time doing pointless activities like pursuing fool's gold, gossiping or thinking fruitless thoughts.

The practice of *yama* for yoga teachers is discussed in detail in *section 8.3*. Sri Patanjali adds another dimension to the practice of *yama*, where he exhorts that these universal great vows (*sarva-bhaumah maha-vratam*) are to be practiced on everyone, irrespective of status (*jati*), in all places (*desa*) and at every single time (*kala*), unlimitedly and unconditionally (*annavachinnah*):

> *jati desa kala samaya annavachinnah sarva-bhaumah*
> *maha-vratam* [Yoga Sutra 31, II]

It is only when we absorb in totality the principles of *yama* and extend the practice to all facets of our lives that we begin to make the world a better place. Swami Shyam (2001) phrases this elegantly: "...*Yam* (*yama*) reaches its peak when one becomes so established in it that he always acts and thinks for the universe as a whole. Then he thinks beyond the bounds of any kind of species and beyond any space, nation, or time. This yam (*yama*) is known by the word *maha vratam,* greatest observance."

2.5.3. *Niyama*

The *niyama* are actually a deeper level of *yama*, where the practices are taken deeper and applied to one's own self. While the *yama* form a list of 'do not dos', the *niyama* are the seeds of actions and attitudes that Sri Patanjali asks us to cultivate in our consciousness.

Niyama are important because they are about the practices that keep us on track to self-realization. The five practices are:
1.   both internal and external purity (*sauca*)
2.   contentment (*santosa*)
3.   purification (*tapas*)
4.   self-study / study of scriptures (*svadhyaya*)
5.   surrender to the Lord (*Isvara-pranidhanani*)

> *sauca santosa tapah svadhyaya Isvara-pranidhanani niyamah*
> [Yoga Sutra 32, II]

Purity in the Yoga Sutra sense extends beyond wearing clean clothes and bathing five times a day. It encompasses thinking pure thoughts (thoughts which are free from malice), eating a *sattvic* diet (*section 2.6*), buying things that do not involve child labor, and other observances that do not cause harm down the line.

Contentment (*santosa*) helps one to stay on the path of self-realization, because with contentment, one negates the need to steal and to grasp (the two *yama,* namely *asteya* and *aparigraha*). This *niyama* has nothing to do with the external world: some of the greediest people are also the richest. Wealth has never been the foundation that happiness is built upon: it is only from contentment that one knows real happiness:

santosat anuttamah sukha labhah [Yoga Sutra 42, II]

Santosa can be realized through *yogasana*: when consciousness flows with the breath, energy and light surge through every cell in our body, bathing our whole being with *santosa*. Many practitioners define *tapas* as austerity, but really, *tapas* is about the spiritual fire that burns the mental and physical impurities away. It helps to keep our mind and body pure (*sauca*). Self-study or the study of scriptures - *Svadhyaya* (*section 2.1.2*) – helps us to define our path. It *is* our path, as we need time out from the bustling, noisy external world to know where we are going.

But knowing where we are going is not enough. At the end of every intellectual or contemplative journey, we ultimately need to surrender to God or the Divine (or whatever you believe in) to be truly free. Ultimately, we need to unconditionally surrender the fruits of our practice to reach this highest point.

2.5.4. *Asana*

[REFER TO *section 7.2*]

2.5.5. _Pranayama_

[REFER TO _section 7.7_]

2.5.6. _Pratyhara_

The external world exists to set us free, because it is only through mastering our senses that we can be free of their machinations and experience ultimate freedom and bliss. With _pratyhara_, we withdraw from the tendency to cling to the emptiness of the external world so that the energy can be channeled towards building a relationship with the Inner Self. With _pratyhara_, too, we free ourselves from being slaves to the ego. _Pratyhara_ can be experienced through these two simple practices:

1. not adding additional flavorings (such as sugar and salt) to food and
2. practicing _mouna_, or social silence for any length of time.

2.5.7. _Dharana_ and _dhyana_

[REFER TO _section 7.6_]

2.5.8. _Samadhi_

The supreme goal of yoga is _nirbija_ (seedless) _samadhi_. Many other Eastern spiritual practices, share the same goal. According to the Yoga Sutra, the True Self (_svarupe_) is realized when the vacillations of the mind ceases:

tada drastuh svarupe avasthanam [Yoga Sutra 3, I]

The way of getting to this point, according to the Yoga Sutra, is by practicing the eight limbs (_section 2.5_) steadily (_sthitau_), continuously (_yatnah_) and repeatedly (_abhyasa_):

tatra sthitau yatnah abhyasa [Yoga Sutra 13, I]

but without attachment to the fruits of the practice:

abhyasa vairagyabhyam tan-nirodhah [Yoga Sutra 12, I]

These practices serve to still the mind and purify the body, so that the lens through which we view our True Self is no longer distorted by vacillations of the mind and impurities. When we reach the innermost core of our being, a serenity or shining light will be experienced:

visoka va jyotismati [Yoga Sutra 36, I]

2.6.   Living life as a modern yogi

2.6.1. Renaissance of yoga

The Hatha yogi should live in a secluded hut free of stones, fire, and dampness to a distance of four cubits in a country that is properly governed, virtuous, prosperous and peaceful.
Hatha Yoga Pradipika

Historically, yogis live austere and celibate lives in remote mountain caves and riverbeds, studying in small groups under the guidance of a teacher and practicing in solitude. This is the tradition of yoga. Hatha Yoga Pradipika stated that Hatha Yoga should be practiced in secret to maintain its potency.

With the renaissance of yoga, we now see yogis in designer lycra with yoga mats swinging on their toned shoulders emerging from sleek yoga studios in downtown Los Angeles, Beijing and Perth. Yoga has become the new 'in' thing: easily accessible, cool, sexy and beneficial to health. It has also proven to be effective as an antidote against the ills of modern living, such as stress, anxiety attacks, insomnia, obesity and high blood pressure, to name but a few.

In a 2008 survey by Yoga Journal, it is estimated that in America alone, there are 15.8 million people practicing yoga.

2.6.2. Living a yogic life

Practicing yoga as an exercise is not the same as living a yogic life (though it is a start). Living a yogic lifestyle is about living in awareness and living consciously. It is practicing *brahmacharya* (in the sense of devotion) by consciously moving from *vitarka* to *nirvitarka* and from *vicara* to *nirvicara* until our vibrations and awareness are raised and we are moved only by the Pure Love within. This is the stage that all *sadakh* aspire to. But yoga practice, and indeed, the yogic lifestyle, is not one that is ruled by fear and promises:

Jati-desa-kala-samaya-annavachinnah sarva-bhauma maha-vratam

[Yoga Sutra 31, II]

This Sutra was introduced in *section 2.5.2* and introduces us to the concept *mahavratam*, or the Universal Vow. As mentioned in the previous section, the yogic path is not one of having an external set of rules that one is compelled to obey, lest he/she gets punished for disobeying or for committing a sin. Rather, the *sadakh* undertakes a vow to act in the light of the *yama*, solely out of love, not of fear of punishment or hope of a reward.

In the challenging environs of modern life, it is of course difficult to stay on the course of righteousness. For example, for a typical working person, it requires a lot of commitment and dedication to devote an hour or two every day to *yogasana*. Yet we need to practice the eight limbs – which includes *asana* – to know our Self. Yoga is a slow process, and there is no other way of getting there other than practice, practice, practice. Note that this differentiates Patanjali's system from others – in the path of *ashtanga yoga*, we do not gather knowledge externally, but instead begin a journey inward to the inner wisdom that resides there, and for that we need patience.

In today's quick-fix world, patience is an outdated concept. People prefer to take vitamins instead of the inconvenience of eating a healthy diet, to cram academic studying in as efficiently as possible instead of enjoying the learning, seeking shortcuts all the time. Yoga is the contrary to this rushing, grasping, snatching, me, me, me modality:

yoga-anga-anusthanad asuddhi-ksye jnana-diptir a viveka-khyateh

[Yoga Sutra 28, II]

Diptir is a word meaning shining, radiant light. Through the devoted and committed practice of the eightfold-path, the impurities (*asuddhi*) which cloud the light of wisdom (*jnâna diptir*) are annihilated. This process is also enhanced by cultivating that discriminatory awareness. As Swami Rama stated, "Yoga is *samadhi*". *Ashtanga yoga* is the container that holds the light: through a long period of dedicated practice with the right attitude, the *sadakh* becomes the container holding the light.

2.6.3. Starting on the path

Start with experiencing off-the-mat yoga (*section 1.9*).

Take your time to immerse yourself in the experience. If you jump into the river, your body reacts, whereas if the change is more gradual, your body adapts. Adaptations are long lasting and permanent, whereas reactionary changes are temporary, and at worst, damaging. So if you are making any changes to your lifestyle, make sure you make the changes gradually, and that you are able to sustain those changes permanently.

Embrace your yoga practice with total commitment. If you are a yoga teacher, make sure that you have a strong and consistent practice (*sadhana*). It is all too easy to be too busy teaching yoga to practice your own yoga. Remember, you should not be teaching yoga if you do not have a personal practice: these are the principles of *satya* and *asteya*.

<u>Time management</u>
Make a point of going to sleep an hour earlier, and rising an hour earlier. If you are not getting enough sleep, then aim to go to sleep two hours earlier every night.

Eliminate unnecessary activities that eat up your time. Cut down on your journeys to the shops by planning efficiently and spending less time in front of the television.

With that one extra hour you have every morning, do your *yogasana* practice. Do this every day, except on moon days. If you are unable to commit to one hour a day, start with 20 minutes, and gradually build that up over the months. Never start with one hour, then slump off to ten minutes, then zero.

Moving towards a yogic diet

Try to avoid eating after sundown.

If you are a meat eater, try to cultivate a love for fruits and vegetables. Incorporate more fruits and vegetables into your meals every day, and introduce new varieties into your repertoire. Seek out exciting fruits – passion fruits, pomegranates, lychees, mangosteens, to name but a few. Buy a vegetarian cookbook, get together with one or two friends, and make one day of the week a vegetarian day. Koay (2006) presented ideas for food cooked according to the Kundalini Yoga traditions.

Cooking the yogic way

Eliminate artificial flavorings (such as monosodium glutamate), salt and sugar from your cooking. This is *pratyhara*.

Cook for less time, so that your food retains its minerals (and remains in *sattvic* form). If possible, invest in a steamer and steam your vegetables. And when you cook, infuse your task with love and blessings, so that the food you make will be enriched.

Drink enough water

Start the day with warm water laced with squeezed lemon. Carry bottled water with you at all times, and make sure you drink at least the equivalent of eight glasses a day.

Gradually phase out caffeine, carbonated drinks and alcohol from your life. Opt instead for natural, freshly squeezed fruit juices and more water!

The yogic formulation is to eat until you are 1/3 full of food, 1/3 full of water and 1/3 full of air.

Open your mind

Buy a copy of the Yoga Sutra of Patanjali and devote one day to one Sutra. Whenever you have a spare moment in the day, contemplate the day's Sutra. (You might also like to invest in a copy of Bhagavad Gita).

Spend some time with yourself everyday

Allocate 15 minutes before bedtime every night for yourself. Find a quiet place where you will not be disturbed to meditate, or just sit in silence.

Contribute to the world

Live consciously. Take time to appreciate the people and the world around us. Help someone who needs a helping hand, make an effort to think environmentally, wake up each day asking, "How can I serve today?"

Sow good world-seeds

Look at your life and the people in your life with new eyes. Turn negative thoughts into positive thoughts, and try to find good in all.

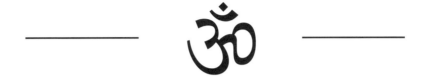

References

Koay, J. (2006). *The Kundalini Yoga Cookbook*. London, UK: Gaia Octopus.

Koay, J. (2008). *Live Patanjali! Yoga Wisdom for Everyday Living*. London, UK: Sun Yoga.

Swami Shyam (2001). *Patanjali Yoga Darshan*. India: International Meditation Institute, 3rd. Edition.

CHAPTER THREE
Anatomy

OVERVIEW OF THE CHAPTER

3.1   Body mechanics

3.2   Parts of the skeletal system

3.3   Anatomical positions and planes of movement

3.4   The spine

3.5   The pelvis

3.6   The upper extremities

3.7   The lower extremities

3.8   The muscular system and *yogasana*

3.9   Muscles of the back

3.10   Abdominal muscles

3.11   Muscles of the lower extremities

3.12   Muscles of the upper extremities

3.13   Summary notes: muscles covered in this chapter

3.14   Treatment for overstretched/torn muscles

3.1. **Body mechanics**

3.1.1. **Strength and flexibility of the body**

Strength and flexibility are two sides of a coin. Excessive strength (as seen in the bodies of weightlifters) or excessive flexibility (as seen in the bodies of gymnasts) can be detrimental to the overall functioning of the body, especially in the long run. In *yogasana*, we strive for balance between strength and flexibility so that the body can function optimally, gracefully, throughout a lifetime.

The pelvis is the core of our stability. The pelvis is the attachment point of the legs to the spine. This attachment forms a major joint that allows for forward and back bending. The pelvic structure is made up of several bones: two symmetrical ilium bones that are joined to form a bowl: the sacrum and coccyx. The extremities are joined with the pelvis by soft tissues. The muscles, connective tissues and tendons create the connection at the hip joint.

The pelvis is the bowl (pelvis means 'basin' in Latin) holding the visceral content of the abdomen. In *yogasana*, one should treat the pelvis like a bowl containing the sacred water of the Ganges. That is to say, pelvic stability must be maintained while holding postures so as not to spill the sacred water.

3.1.2. **Internal scaffolding of the body**

From the spine, the bones of the ribs emanate frontwards to the sternum to form the ribcage of the trunk. The trunk forms the connection between the upper and lower extremities. It also forms the cage protecting the soft internal organs.

The spine gives the body its length, but it is the muscles and soft tissues that hold it in place and attach the trunk to the extremities, thus making the body one cohesive unit. Without the action of the back and core muscles, the ribs will collapse all the way down to the pelvis under gravity. Thus, a large part of the purpose of *yogasana* is to build strong and supple back and core muscles to support the upward lift of the body.

3.1.3. Construction of the spine

Certain parts of the body are more prone to injury than others. Apart from the spine (including the neck), these are the areas for concern when practicing *yogasana*. The spine, being long, is one of the most vulnerable parts of the body.

The spine supports the weight of the upper body and houses the spinal nerves and the spinal cord, adding to its vulnerability and importance to the body as a whole.

The curvature of the spine is created by the stacking of individual vertebral units (*diagram 3.1*) in a sigmoid curve to give the body optimal function. The loss of the natural curvature of the spine is one of its greatest threats. This may come from trauma, disease, a lifetime of bad posture or inadequate muscular strength to offset the effects of gravity.

Spinal misalignment occurs when one or more vertebrae slip out of alignment within the stacking system and excessive curvature occurs, thus creating a compression on the concave side of that vertebra. This results in the narrowing of the spinal canal, causing nerve damage and pain.

As the spinal column houses a dense network of nerves, misalignment of the spine may cause pain and injury elsewhere in the body. For example, misalignment of the cervical vertebrae may affect the flow of blood to the brain, resulting in neurological problems. Spines with osteoarthritic vertebrae and herniated intervertebral discs are particularly prone to injury.

To facilitate deeper twists and bends in *yogasana*, lift the spine up first to create more space between adjacent vertebra, thereby allowing for a larger range of motion.

Always remember to create the lift first. Indeed, one of the principles aims of *yogasana* is to lengthen the spine. In twists, learn to twist from the belly and rib cage rather than the spine itself. The spine remains passive and relaxed.

Diagram 3.1. **Construction of the S-curve of the spine from the stacking of vertebral discs.**

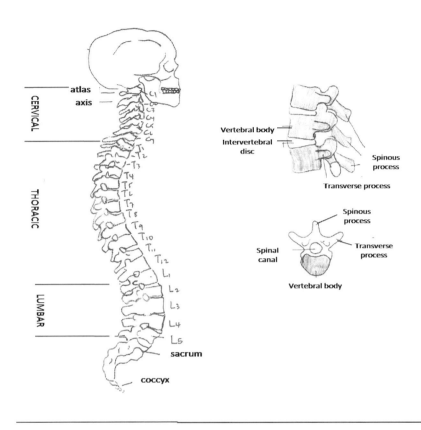

3.1.4. Vulnerability of the spinal column

A strong spine is one that is mechanically strong as well as flexible. *Yogasana* is good for spinal health because it patiently works on the individual vertebra as opposed to the spine as a whole. In Kundalini Yoga's Spinal Strengthening Kriya as taught by Yogi Bhajan, for example, each segment of the spine is exercised on, and light and awareness is brought to each region.

Weakness in the spine
Back pain that is not caused by pinched nerve is often caused by muscle imbalance and less-than-optimal spinal mechanics. To address this general weakness in the spine, the recommended *yogasana* are those strengthening the weak muscles of the back and abdomen, and stretching the tight muscles such as the hamstrings and hip flexors.

Weakness in the neck

A muscle imbalance in the neck, especially weak anterior neck muscles, tends to produce postures that reinforce the imbalance. When the neck muscles are weak, the neck tends to straighten, shifting the head forward, thus putting additional strain on the muscles of the upper back and those at the back of the neck.

The recommended *yogasana* are those that increase spinal cervical extension and the upper back, as well as stretching the front (chest openers).

Weakness in the lower back

When the lower back is weak, it tends to arch forward. This puts pressure and strain on the joints in that region. Good *yogasana* are those that involve stretching the overly tight muscles and building up the weak ones.

Abnormal curvature of the spine

Not everyone has a perfect spinal curvature. The main causes of abnormal spinal curvature include: trauma, genetics and a lifetime of poor posture. However, deviation from the optimal spinal curvature is greater in some people, resulting in:

- Hyper-lordosis (*page 84*)
- Hyper-kyphosis (*page 84*)
- Scoliosis

Disc degeneration and disc herniation

Due to compression, intervertebral discs may suffer degenerative changes, and nerves may be impinged causing pain.

Disc herniation is a common occurrence when the disc between the two vertebrae pushes outward. The disc may push outward anteriorly as when doing a back bend or posteriorly as when doing a forward bend. Wedging of the vertebrae occurs on the concave side of the spinal curvature. The increased pressure to the vertebrae can cause crumbling of the bone. Disc herniation generally occurs opposite of the wedging as the pressure from the wedging pushes the disc out.

Nerve impingement

When the vertebral canal shrinks, nerves may get impinged, giving rise to pain or weakness. Impingement can occur anywhere along the spine when the nerve is trapped or squeezed, interfering with nerve conduction. The goal of *yogasana* is to restore the normal alignment by lengthening the spine, opening the space between the vertebrae and correcting any muscle imbalance that is causing the impingement. In cases where there is ongoing nerve damage, surgery may be required to release the impingement before permanent damage occurs.

3.1.5. Other vulnerable parts of the body

<u>Knees</u>
The knee is another vulnerable area of the body. Knee injury is common to amongst athletes who do repetitive exercises or movements. One of the most effective ways of protecting the knee is by strengthening the quadriceps, hamstrings, calf muscles and the ankles.

The kneecap must be aligned: the front knee should never be over-extended (hyper-extended) in *yogasana* such as *parsvakonasana*, *virabhadrasana I* and *II*. Rather, the thigh, the knee and the foot must form a clean 90 degree angle, that is to say, when weight is put on the front leg, the knee should be directly aligned over the ankle.

Knees are particularly vulnerable to injury if they are weight-bearing in a seated position with the knees twisted back such as in *supta virasana* and *kapotanasana*. Even in straight-forward, weight-bearing position such as *utkatanasana*, proper alignment should be ensured to prevent injury. For those with knee problems, the knees should be hip-width apart in *utkatanasana*.

Forcing the legs onto *padmasana* before the muscles are ready is another common cause of avoidable knee injury. One of the most common causes of damage to the knees is jumping from one posture to another when the body is not ready: practitioners who do not have sufficient muscle power in the overall body should not be jumping in and out of *yogasana*.

> Knees must be:
> - **aligned** (not hyper-extended);
> - **stabilized**;
> - **protected** by not subjecting them to high-impact activities, and
> - **treated with respect** (i.e. not being forced into extreme contortions if the body is not ready).

Shoulder injury

It is advisable that preparatory poses or modifications should be offered to beginners until sufficient strength is gained to be able to execute weight-bearing *yogasana* such as *chaturanga dandasana* without compromising the shoulders.

Preparatory pose: standing press-ups against a wall.

Modification: caterpillar pose (knees, chest and chin on the floor).

If one is predisposed to shoulder injury, extra care should be taken to ensure that the shoulder joints are stabilized during *yogasana*. The shoulder is the most mobile joint of the body, and with increased mobility, there is a decrease in stability. Primary shoulder injuries are the rotator cuff injury, over-used syndrome and tendonitis.

In some of the *yogasana*, especially the weight-bearing ones, core strength is needed to assist the muscles of the arms in holding up the body weight. It is common to observe the concaving of the spine when beginners are attempting *chaturanga dandasana*, which puts strain on the spine (especially the weaker regions) and on the shoulder joints.

The shoulder joints are put at greater risk when weight-bearing *yogasana* such as *chaturanga dandasana* forms part of a dynamic sequence: the practitioner needs to have control of his weight throughout the entire range, especially the shortened range (i.e. lowering down from *chaturanga dandasana* to *bhujangasana / urdhva mukha svanasana* in *Surya Namaskar*). Without strength and stability, the whole body weight may come crashing down on the shoulder joints during the transition from the weight-bearing *yogasana* to the next one, causing a pull, tear or other injury.

Wrists

Vulnerable wrists must be thoroughly stretched and gently introduced to weight-bearing *yogasana*.

If wrists have been weakened through arthritis or other injuries such as carpal tunnel syndrome, they may be over-stressed by full weight-bearing *yogasana* such as *ardho mukha svanasana*. Strength should be built into the wrists beforehand with preparatory poses such as *bidalasana* (or the dynamic cat-cow).

3.2. **Parts of the skeletal system**

3.2.1. **Bones**

There are 206 bones in the adult skeleton (*diagram 3.2*). When the skeleton first develops, it begins as cartilage, and within a few weeks of conception, the bones develop. The bones which form the skeleton of the body protect the soft organs of the body and facilitate locomotion (working in tandem with the muscular system).

Bones are living entities. The soft bone marrow inside the long bones is the site of manufacturing of many components of the blood, such as red blood cells, white blood cells and platelets. Bones also store calcium, the mineral that makes bones hard.

Bone density decreases with age. With decreasing bone density, one of the most common injuries is osteoporosis, which women are particularly vulnerable to, especially post menopause (men are at risk from this, too). It has been estimated that about 1 of every 2 women and 1 in 8 men over 50 will have an osteoporosis-related fracture in their lifetimes (National Institutes of Health, 2002).

Bone density is affected by heredity factors, sex hormones, physical activity, diet, lifestyle choices (such as smoking and lack of exercise), and the use of certain medications. Weight-bearing *yogasana* is an appropriate way of building up bone density for practitioners of all ages, though for those with low bone density, the *yogasana* practice should be as low impact as possible (no jumping!).

Yin Yoga, where postures are held for longer periods while in sitting positions, counteracts ligament contracture by relaxing the yang muscles (superficial muscles, i.e. skin and muscles) so that the deeper, rarely touched yin areas open up, adjust and strengthen.

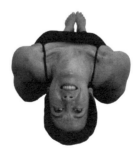

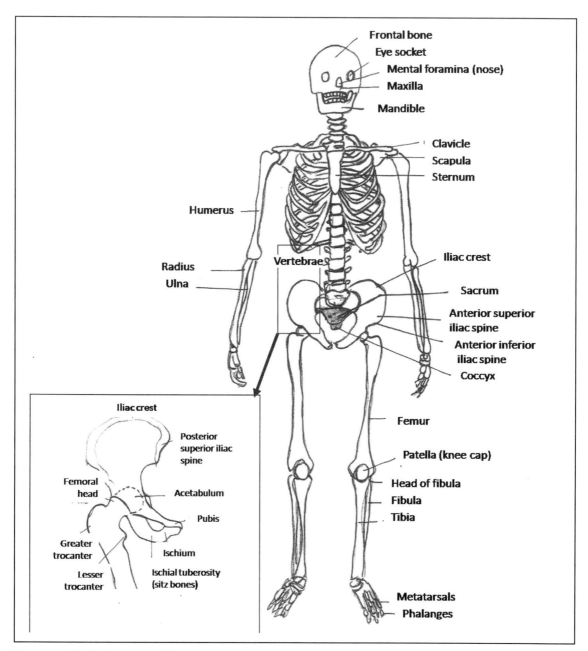

Diagram 3.2. **Main bones of the human body**

3.2.2. Joints

This is the juncture where the ends of two bones come together. Some joints are immoveable, others allow maximum angle of movement:

- Hinge joints allow for backward-forward motion, such as at the elbow and knee;
- Pivot joints allow rotary movements, such as turning the head from side to side;
- Ball-and-socket joints occur when the rounded end of one bone fits into the hollow of another, providing 3-dimensional rotation. These are found at the hip and shoulder.

The practice of *yogasana* may relieve stiff and painful joints: certain *yogasana* exert gentle pressure deep into the joints and bring vital circulation here (*pawanmuktasana*), the controlled *yogasana* stretches ease out joint tightness, and relaxation after an invigorating *yogasana* session brings relief to achy joints.

3.2.3. Ligaments

Ligaments connect bone to bone and are bands of tough, fibrous tissues. The main function of ligaments is to stabilize the joints. They are slightly stretchy (they look like criss-cross elastic bands) and are off-white in color because they have minimal blood circulation. Because of the limited blood supply to ligaments, torn and damaged ligaments do not heal themselves easily and almost certainly require surgery.

Ligaments which are damaged or weakened by the trauma of everyday living become too long, thus reducing the stability of the joints they bind around. Conversely, a lack of pulling action on the ligaments (i.e. stretching, or more accurately, stressing) reduces the ligaments' length in a process called contracture. Ligaments which are too short (as a result of lack of stress on the ligaments) will limit joint movements and often cause pain, such as in frozen shoulder syndrome (adhesive capsulate).

3.2.4.   Tendons

One of the most vulnerable areas when it comes to over-stretching tendons is the groin area. Thus, care should be taken when executing wide-legged *yogasana* such as *hanumansana* and the *utthita hasta padangustanasana*

Tendons connect bones to muscles. In general, tendons are less strong than ligaments. They are also less vascular than muscles and thus take longer to heal when irritated or injured. Overstretching tendons can result in painful inflammation known as tendonitis.

3.2.5.   **Muscle contraction**

Muscles are more elastic than connective tissue. The muscles work by lengthening or shortening to allow the bones to move. The movement direction is dependent on where the muscles attach and insert.

Concentric: Muscle fibers are shortening with contraction (in *urdhva dharunasana* = the hamstrings and gluteus muscles);

Eccentric: Muscles fibers are lengthening with contraction (in *urdhva dharunasana* = the quadriceps and hip flexors);

Isometric: Muscles contract and length is unchanged. (in *tadasana* = the quadriceps, hamstrings and core muscles).

3.2.6.   **Fascia**

Surya Namaskar at the beginning of any *yogasana* practice is a wonderful opportunity to stretch out the fascia.

Fascia is the bag that holds the body together. It is found in virtually every structure of the body, including wrapping muscles, organs, glands and blood vessels like cellophane. Gentle, slow and mindful practice of *yogasana* stretches the fascia, giving the muscles it wraps within its protective fold greater freedom to move and to grow in bulk. With age, fascia becomes tighter, and this can become limiting, especially in areas of past injuries.

3.3. Anatomical position and planes of movement

3.3.1. Anatomical position

The anatomical position is a reference point so that when describing a position everyone has the same point of reference, namely looking forward, the palms turned open to face the front, arms at the side and legs in a natural standing position.

3.3.2. Anatomical planes (*diagram 3.3*)
Movement of the body is based on whether the body is moving away or toward the anatomical position:
- Frontal Plane – divides the body front to back
- Transverse Plane – divides the body top and bottom
- Saggital Plane – divides the body left from right side.

3.3.3. Planes of movement (*diagram 3.3*)

The starting point is the anatomical position. The movement is based on the movement toward or away from the body in the different planes of movement:
- **Adduction**: movement toward body in frontal plane.
- **Abduction**: movement away from the body in frontal plane.
- **Flexion**: movement away from anatomical position anteriorly in saggital plane; alternately, bringing body parts closer together.
- **Extension**: movement away from the anatomical position posteriorly in the saggital plane; alternatively, bringing body parts farther apart.
- **Internal Rotation**: movement toward the body in the transverse plane.
- **External Rotation**: movement away from the body in the transverse plane.

3.3.4. Anatomical descriptions (*diagram 3.3*)

Anatomical positions are described based on different planes:
- Anterior – front of the body.
- Posterior – back of the body.
- Proximal – closer to the body center
- Distal – farther from the body center
- Medial – closer to the mid line of the body
- Lateral – farther from the mid line of the body.
- Superior – closer to the head.
- Inferior – toward the feet.

Diagram 3.3. **Planes of the body**

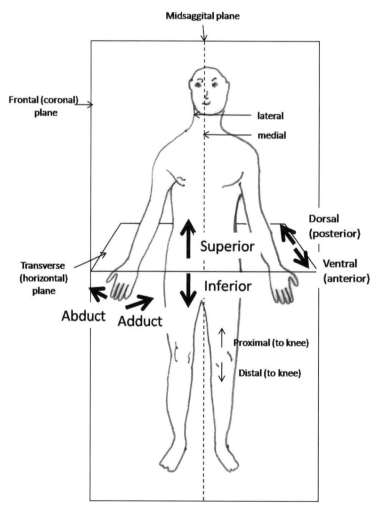

3.4. **The spine**

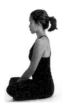

You are as old as your spine!

3.4.1. Function of the spine

The spine is the column that holds our body in its upright position. In addition, it is the brain's telegraph pole, transmitting messages to and from the muscles, glands, sensory and internal organs. It is also the anchor for many muscles of the body. The spine is vulnerable. It supports the weight of the upper body and houses the spinal nerves and the spinal cord.

3.4.2. Bones of the spine (*diagram 3.1*)

- 7 vertebrae in the cervical region
- 12 vertebrae in the thoracic region
- 5 vertebrae in the lumbar region
- 5 vertebrae in the sacral region fused into one.
- 4 vertebrae in the coccygeal region fused to form the coccyx.

3.4.3. Vertebrae (*diagram 3.1*)

A vertebra is an individual unit of the spinal column stacked on top each other. The vertebrae build up the spine. Although there are 5 different types of vertebrae (*section 3.4.2*), the architecture follows a similar blueprint:

- The body of the vertebra is the contact point for adjacent vertebrae, with the intervertebral discs (*section 3.4.4*) forming a layer of cushioning between the vertebrae;
- The processes radiating from the body are for muscle attachments;
- The intervertebral foramen is the canal where the delicate spinal cord is housed.

3.4.4. Intervertebral discs (*diagram 3.1*)

Of prime importance in spinal health are the intervertebral discs, which act to cushion adjacent vertebrae and preventing them from rubbing and shearing on each other's surface.

The intervertebral disc has two distinct components optimally designed for load bearing:
  i.   Nucleus pulposus (75% of load)
  ii.   Annulus fibrosis (25% of load)

Intervertebral discs are subject to a number of degenerative conditions, including aging, and forces which may cause them to bulge and rupture over time. High impact activities such as jumping back in *yogasana* before the arms and trunk have sufficient strength to carry the body weight accelerate damages to the intervertebral discs.

3.4.5. Curves of the spine

There are 4 natural curves of the spine. In the womb the spine is rounded into flexion known as the fetal position. From the instant of birth, when coming out of the birth canal, the forces of gravity act to begin the process of creating these 4 natural curves.

The 4 natural curves of the spine are:
  •   Cervical Concave Curve
  •   Thoracic Convex Curve
  •   Lumbar Concave Curve
  •   Sacrum Convex Curve

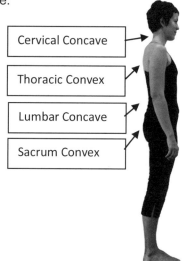

Cervical Concave

Thoracic Convex

Lumbar Concave

Sacrum Convex

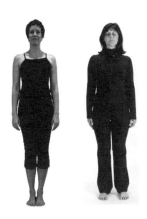

Tadasana is an excellent pose for learning to re-establish the natural curvatures of the spine:

- elongate the spine
- tuck in the chin
- lift the sternum
- bring navel in towards the back of the body
- lift the thighs and arches of the feet.

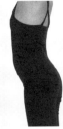

When excessive concave curves occur in the lumbar or cervical spine, it is known as a lordosis or sway back. This is seen in a forward head posture and protrusion of the abdomen (anterior tilt of the pelvis). *Yogasana* that realign the spine such as *tadasana* is ideal for teaching the body to find the correct neutral curves.

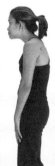

In a spine with excessive convexity of the thoracic spine, it is known as kyphosis. This is seen as a stooped posture and a rounded back. *Yogasana* that open up the heart center, such as *gomukhasana*, will counteract the kyphosis of the thoracic spine. These deviations may be caused by hereditary factors, spinal trauma or years of bad posture.

[REFER TO Book 2: Yoga Therapy]

3.4.6. Understanding the internal movement of the spine

The movement of the spine is identified in reference to the spinal curves. This should not to be confused with flexion and extension of the head or trunk.

- Spinal cervical extension is a reduction of the concave (lordosis) position of the spine. When the chin is tucked in the *yogasana*, the cervical spine lordosis will be flattened and the spine lengthened.

   - Thoracic extension is when we reduce the thoracic concavity or kyphosis. There are many *yogasana* that will reverse this curve and help lengthen the spine – *ardho mukha svanasana*, extended *balasana* and *ustrasana*.

76

> Forward bends are examples of trunk flexion; back bends are examples of trunk extension.
>
> Flexion and extension of the spine refer to the increasing or reduction of the spinal curve.

- Thoracic flexion is the rounding of the back and increase of the kyphosis. In Kundalini Yoga, spinal flex is a pose that focuses on flexion and extension of the thoracic spine.

- Lumbar extension is a flattening of the lumbar spine while lumbar flexion is an increasing of the lumbar curve. In forward bends, the lumbar spine extends as the convex curve is reduced. The opposite applies to back bends: the lumbar curve increases in back bends.

- In the full chakrasana, you see an extreme example of lumbar flexion, thoracic extension and cervical flexion.

- In the rag doll posture you see an example of lumbar extension, thoracic flexion and cervical extension (provided the person relaxes the head and tucks the chin).

3.4.7. Special considerations for the neck

The seriousness of the neck is because any injury to this region can be life-threatening.

Advanced yoga practice includes weight-bearing at the head. If there is insufficient strength in the trunk to maintain adequate alignment of the spine, then the area that will be most vulnerable is the neck.

In today's world where people experience a lot of tension, this tension often manifests itself in the muscles of the neck, in particular, the trapezius. Tightness in the trapezius is often seen as elevation across the shoulders. It is common to see a forward head posture (from too much computer usage or television-watching) which results in tightness of the levator scapulae muscles and hyper-lordosis of the cervical spine. Sometimes people may tip their head to one side instead of maintaining it at midline, and this is the result of the tightness in the sternocleidomastoid muscles.

In *yogasana*, effort should be made to lengthen the cervical spine along its natural curvature (*section 3.4.4*): shoulders relaxed, chin tucked and crown of the head lifted along the midline. If a practitioner cannot maintain good alignment, he should not attempt weight-

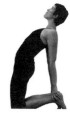

bearing exercises on the head, because his weight will be distributed in a detrimental way that will stress the neck.

Effort should be made to maintain good spinal alignment in all *yogasana* to safeguard the neck.

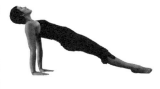

3.5. The Pelvis

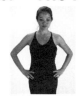

This is the bowl holding the sacred water of the Ganges!

3.5.1. Pelvic bones

Know the shape and construction of this "bowl" well, because it is the seat of our stability.

The pelvis (visualize this as a sacred bowl) is made up of three bones. The two coxal bones are mirror images and the third bone is the sacrum. The coxal bones join with the sacrum in the back. In the front the bones come together to form the pubic area. Together, the bones create the pelvic bowl. The function of the pelvis is to displace the upper body weight to the lower body. In standing, the weight is displaced to the legs and in sitting the weight is displaced to the ishial tuberosities.

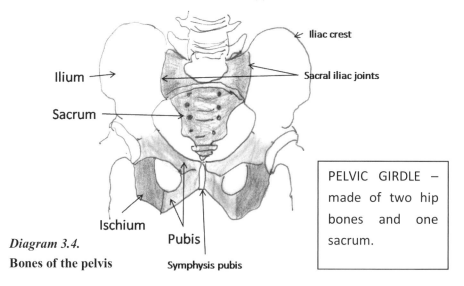

PELVIC GIRDLE – made of two hip bones and one sacrum.

Diagram 3.4.
Bones of the pelvis

78

1. Within the coxal bones, there are three parts that fuse together during adolescence: ischium, ilium and pubis.

2. The ilium attaches to the spine at the sacrum.

3. The sacrum is five-fused vertebrae and the coccyx is the tailbone that is attached at the end of the sacrum.

4. The sacral-iliac joints (SIJ) are the space between the sacrum and ilium bound together with the ligaments (*section* 3.5.2).

5. The space between the two coxal bones at the front is linked to each other by cartilage (*section 3.5.2*).

6. On the lateral surface of each coxal bone (where the ilium, ischium and pubis meet) is a deep socket called the acetabulum. This is where the head of the femur enters (ball and socket joint).

7. Stability of these bones is dependent on the integrity of the ligaments holding the bones together and the support of the muscles.

3.5.2.   Ligaments

The ligaments binding the three bones of the pelvis (*section 3.5.1*) together are as follows:

i.   The sacral-iliac joints (SIJ) are bound together by the anterior sacral iliac ligaments

ii.   The gap between the two coxal bones in the front is bound together by cartilaginous disc called the public symphysis.

The ligaments tie the two symmetrical pelvic bones together to create stability. In the back the pelvic bone connects to the sacrum of the spine and the lumbar vertebra of the spine with short and wide ligaments. This gives the pelvis its connection to the trunk.

The pelvis is connected to the lower extremities through the hip joint. Ligaments from the femur to the pelvis create the hip joint.

3.5.3. Muscles and movement

Movement of the trunk can come from either the movement occurring at the spine and pelvis or movement occurring at the hip and pelvis. In *yogasana,* the primary intention is to keep the spine straight and bend from the hip.

The ligaments tie the bones in place and the muscles allow the movement. When the muscles surrounding the pelvis are strong and balanced, the pelvis can move while maintaining optimal alignment.

In *yogasana* the focus is on movement occurring between the hip and pelvis. If there is tightness or weakness that leads someone to compensate the lack of movement in the lower pelvis with movement in the upper pelvis, the results may be an over-stressing of the ligaments between the pelvis and the lumbar/sacral region.

3.5.4. Alignment

Standing in *tadasana*, good alignment of the pelvis will be seen with the following:
- Iliac crests are even in height;
- One side of the pelvis is not rotated forward or backwards from the other side;
- The pubic bone and the anterior iliac spine are in the same plane.

For *yogasana*, the focus should be on the movement being on the hip joint while the spine remains straight. Therefore, for forward bending, the bend should initiate from the hips and the spine should be kept straight.

Childbirth stretches the ligaments binding the three pelvic bones. Once stretched, ligaments do not return to their original length. Stability is thus compromised. Care should be taken not to stretch ligaments beyond the point of stability. For example, in *janu sirsana,* if the practitioner has tight hamstrings or injuries, the weak link is the ligaments at the SIJ as the tight hamstrings prevent the pelvis from tipping forward as she is trying to bend her trunk into the extended leg. The key is to maintain a straight spine and allow the movement to be primarily from the hip joint. Overstretching from the lumbar sacral spine will lead to instability of the SIJ.

3.6. The Upper Extremities

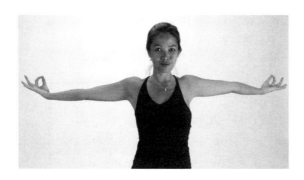

The alignment of the shoulder is based entirely on the alignment of the spine: elderly persons do not have full range of motion in the shoulders because their backs are rounded.

3.6.1. Bones of the upper extremities

The shoulder girdle is made up of the scapula (shoulder blade) and clavicle (collar bone). The upper arm is one large bone known as the humerus, and the forearm is made up of two bones (ulna and radius) which articulate allowing the rotation of the forearms.

The wrist is made up of eight small carpal bones arranged in two rows. The palm is made up of five metacarpal bones; each finger is made up of three phalangeal bones and the thumb has two.

3.6.2. Joints

The shoulder is the most mobile joint in the body. It is a ball-and-socket joint, which allows it to move in all directions. The elbow, however, only moves in one direction (flexion and extension) and is a hinge joint.

The wrist has two planes of movement: flexion-extension and ulna deviation-radial deviation.

When lifting the arm over the head, the ball part of the humerus must roll back and under the acromion (*diagram 3.5*).

Diagram 3.5. **The shoulder girdle**

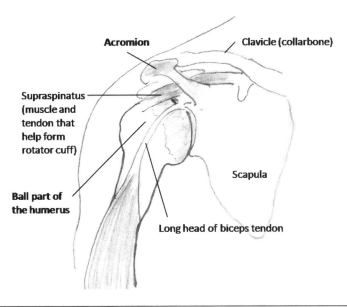

3.6.3. Muscles and movement

[REFER TO *section 3.12*]

Shoulder rotation is an important element of movement on the upper extremities. When the arm is lifted, it naturally rotates. This allows the humeral head to tuck under the acromion.

The standing *yogasana* are good opportunities for taking the arms through the upper range of motion. For example, in *trikonansana*, *parsvakonasana* and in *tadasana* with extended arms, the shoulders can be moved through the whole range using gravity as the only resistance.

On the other hand, in weight-bearing *yogasana*, the arms are strengthened using the body weight.

3.6.4. Alignment

The scapula, clavicle and humerus create the shoulder girdle. The strength of the shoulder girdle is important because it is the anchor and stability that allows the arm to freely rotate.

The elbow bends in one direction; in *yogasana*, a practitioner should be aware of hyperextension of the elbow (when the arms go beyond the straight position). For practitioners who have hyper-flexibility in their elbows, an effort should be made to keep a small inward bend at the elbows and not go beyond 0 degrees (*diagram*s *3.6* and *3.7*).

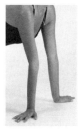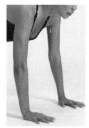

Diagram 3.6. Hyperextension of the elbows (left) and *diagram 3.7* keeping the eyes of the elbows facing forward with a slight bend to the arms (*right*)

3.7. The Lower Extremities

Your legs take you forward in life!

3.7.1. Bones of the lower extremities

The upper leg is made up of the femur, and the lower leg is made up tibia and fibula. The patella (kneecap) is a flat bone that sits in front of the knee joint. The quadriceps muscles come down and attach into the patella. The patella allows for the extension of the knee to be more efficient; in addition it offers additional protection for the knee.

There are seven tarsal bones that make up each foot. The largest of the tarsal bones is the calcaneus (heel). These bones articulate with the tibia and fibula to make the ankle joint. This part is called the hind foot. The forefoot is made up of the five metatarsals. Each toe is made up of three phalanges, and the big toe has two.

3.7.2. Joints

The hip joint is a ball-and-socket joint, and it is the most protected joint in that it is located deep into the body. The ball-and-socket allows for movement in all planes.

The primary movement of the knee is in one plane, namely extension-flexion (straightening and bending). When the knee is flexed, there is also some transverse rotation occurring at the joint.

The ankle joint is made up of the tibia, fibula and the talus, and is considered a hinge joint. The primary movements that are occurring are flexion-extension and inversion-eversion.

3.7.3. Muscles and movement

[REFER TO *section 3.1*]

Many *yogasana* require at least 90 degree flexion of the hip joint with the knee stretched straight out. In *dandasana*, the body needs to create a 90 degree angle: adequate flexibility of the hamstrings is required for this and many other *yogasana*.

To be successful in advanced *yogasana*, a person should be able to lie supine on the floor with one leg raised straight to 90 degree, the opposite hip fixed to the ground and pelvis in neutral position.

When there is hamstring tightness, there is probably associated tightness in the hip flexors and/or quadriceps. Both of these are two- joint muscles (they cross two joints), which is why they are prone to tightness. Hip extension is more difficult with the knee bent because the quadriceps are stretched across the two joints – this is seen in *urdhva dharunasana* and *natarajasana*. Hip flexion with the knee extended is more difficult because the hamstrings are stretched across the hip and knee joint, and this is seen in *hasta padangusthanasana A.*

3.7.4. Alignment

One of the most important things about the knee is making sure that it doesn't hyperextend. It is not uncommon to see the knee going into hyperextension in standing *yogasana* such as *trikonasana*. Effort must be made to keep the knee in the neutral position or move into slight flexion as a modification.

Hyperextension is more common in people with more flexibility or weakness. In these cases, the knees should never be locked in standing *yogasana*, especially on one-leg balancing. The tibia and fibula should be directly under the femur in a straight line so that the weight comes down directly to the ankle and is evenly distributed along the foot. Hyper-extending contributes to over-stretching the soft tissues in the back of the knee contributing to instability of the knee. Instructions for hyper-flexible practitioners should be to micro-bend or keep the knee soft.

The angle between the shaft of the femur and the femoral head as well as how the femoral head goes into the socket will determine the amount of rotation allowed at the hip. Generally, in adults, one should expect the amount of internal and external to be similar. Yoga can help to loosen tight muscles and soft tissues to make the rotation of the hip more even and symmetrical between left and right leg. However, one should also acknowledge that sometimes the bone structure is such that rotation might be limited. Limited rotation of the hips can be seen in practitioners whose knees come up to their ears in *baddha konasana*.

3.8. The muscular system and *yogasana*

3.8.1. Introduction

There are three different muscle types, each performing a different set of functions:
i.   cardiac muscles (which contract the heart);
ii.   smooth muscles (typically found in the viscera);
iii.   skeletal muscles (which we are most familiar with as they are principally the muscles that we use for movement).

Muscles that we will primarily be covering in this chapter are those that relate to movements for *yogasana*. For the beginner practitioner, these muscles function crudely as a group, not unlike a newly assembled orchestra, as they are not yet used to working together in harmony to deliver *yogasana*. This may be part of the reason why beginner practitioners (even those who are physically fit) suffer from muscle fatigue during and after a yoga class. It is only with dedicated practice that these skeletal muscles (and their supporting cardiac and smooth muscles) begin to move with minimal effort, like a finely tuned engine.

The main physical work of *yogasana* is about bringing consciousness to the muscles so that the body moves with grace and awareness. Many *yogasana* are done very slowly and the poses maintained for at least several breaths up to a few minutes. Weight-bearing exercises strengthen the muscles of the body. Thus, *yogasana* also build muscle strength and definition. *Vrksasana* and *adho mukha vrksasana* are two examples of *yogasana* that contribute to muscle strength and definition.

Yoga is closely associated with flexibility and stretching. Muscle fibers have great potential to increase their resting lengths, but there comes a point where they are overstretched and will eventually tear. However, the body has an inbuilt mechanism to prevent tearing: the tendon attaching the muscle to the bone resists stretching and is extremely strong. There are also mechanoreceptors in the muscles that trigger a contraction when they sense that a muscle is reaching its limit. But mindlessly competitive practices can cause muscle injury, obliterating the purpose of practicing yoga: *yogasana* is about cultivating awareness of the body, and every practitioner should learn to listen to his body first and foremost instead of being distracted by the superficial and the ego.

3.8.2. Workings of the muscles

Muscles move bones or joints by contraction, which is the process where the muscle length shortens. The terminology for the muscle which is contracting is agonist. This is the muscle 'doing the work'.

However, muscles almost always work in pairs, counterbalancing the action of its partner. So for every muscle that contracts, there is a corresponding muscle (or muscles) that relaxes or lengthens. For example, the quadriceps' opposite number is the hamstrings. Thus, in postures such as *urdhva dharunasana*, the quadriceps lengthen as the hamstrings shorten.

The counterbalancing muscle is known as the antagonist. Another set of oft-used terminology is abduction and adduction. Abduction is the process by which the limb is moved away from the central line of the body, whereas adduction is the process by which a limb is brought closer to the center of the body. For example, in *trikonasana*, you raise your arms into abduction to begin the *yogasana* and lower the arms in adduction as you finish the pose.

The amount of movement is dependent upon the location of the body part(s) and the joint(s) involved. The anatomical position is the reference point for defining the movement.

- Flexion - bending of the body toward itself. In a forward bend we bring our trunk closer to our legs, which is trunk flexion.

- Extension – moving to increase the angle between the body parts. When we straighten the elbow in triangle, we increase the angle between the forearm and upper arm. Extension for the shoulder and hip is defined as moving posteriorly (behind you) from the anatomical position. An example of the hip flexion and extension can be seen in *virabhadrasana I*, where the back hip goes into extension and the front hip into flexion.

- Rotation – when the movement is outward in the transverse plane, we have lateral/external rotation. A movement inward is medial/internal rotation (rotate towards the midline).

- Lateral Bending – is the side bending of the body in the frontal plane. This is seen in *trikonasana* where the body bends laterally.

3.8.3. Studying muscles

There is no substitute for dissection - it is difficult to get a good understanding of the human body from textbooks. It is only by peeling back layer upon layer of the body, or *annamaya kosha*, that the true miracle and complexity of the body is revealed to us.

Therefore, to facilitate that deep appreciation and understanding of human anatomy, the following sections have been organized as a dissection process. The information will be presented either according to geography and/or dissection order. A summary is given at the end of the chapter.

Study tip:

Do not worry about the names and functionality of the muscles in the first instance. Just imagine what they look like and where they are located within the body.

When you are comfortable with this, start working out how each muscle/muscle group work by getting on the mat and doing the *yogasana* yourself in order to feel those muscles working. It's the only way to learn!

3.8.4. Notes on the following sections

i. Only the main muscles for *yogasana* will be discussed. Small muscles, such as the fine muscles of the hands and feet, will be omitted;

ii. Though it can be argued that fasciae are as important for movement as muscles, they will be omitted in this chapter;

iii. The rich network of nerves, arteries and veins will also be omitted for the sake of simplicity and clarity;

iv. Plain English will be used to describe the location and positioning, such as 'neck region' instead of the more accurate 'medial third of the superior nuchal line';

v. If the geography is too complex to be described by words (for example, iv), diagrams will be used for illustrative purposes;

vi. The drawings are not to scale. They are ancient, from the author's Anatomy & Physiology classes at Manchester Medical School;

vii. The real purpose of the diagrams is to help you locate the muscles as well as to give you a rough idea of what they look like. You really need to do the suggested *yogasana* to understand the anatomy deeply!

Finally, this is Anatomy for yoga teachers, not medical students. Know how the muscles work in the context of *yogasana* instead of getting bogged down by facts and details which are not relevant for you to teach yoga safely and effectively.

3.9. Muscles of the Back

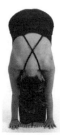

A strong and flexible back can do these two things: one, lift your heart to the sky and two, release the crown of your head to the earth.

Removing the skin and fascia of the back to just below the waist level, you will first come across the outermost muscles, namely the trapezius and the latissimus dorsi.

Diagram 3.8. **External muscles of the back**

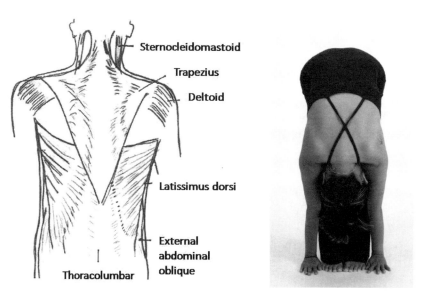

3.9.1. Trapezius (*diagram 3.8*)

The trapezius starts from the center of the back and is a triangular-shaped muscle.

The trapezius has three portions:
i.   upper – goes up towards the neck;
ii.   middle – goes to the upper thoracic;
iii.   lower – goes to the lower thoracic.

Each portion facilitates movements in specific parts of the upper trunk. The middle portion, when contracted, adducts the scapulae (drawing the arms back). The upper and lower portions work together to create a rotation of the scapulae upwards (contraction of the upper portion bringing the scapulae closer together while the lower portion shortens, pulling downwards). This rotation is critical when you move your arms upwards over your head.

Often, people overuse their trapezius muscles, and this is manifested in abnormally raised shoulders. Thus, it is important when doing arm raises in standing positions to:
1. raise the arms upwards and then
2. Pull the shoulders and shoulder blades down to engage the lower trapezius.

- Trapezius is used for arm balancing *yogasana*.

- In *urdva dharunasana*, they contract to pull back the arms and the scapulae, opening the chest.

- In *garudasana*, they stretch to draw the arms together at the front.

- To strengthen, lie on your stomach and lift your arms off the floor into the airplane pose.

- If you lift your arms straight out in front of you in *salambhasana*, you are engaging the upper trapezius; when arms are stretched straight behind in this yogasana, you are strengthening your lower trapezius.

3.9.2. Latissimus dorsi (*diagram 3.8*)

Latissimus dorsi (lats) looks shiny and its fascia is very different in that it is thick and dense. It starts in the lower spine: it is attached to the last six thoracic vertebrae through all the lumbar and sacral vertebrae (it goes down to the iliac crest). It inserts on top to underneath the armpits into the humerus.

There is some overlap between the top part of the lats and the trapezius at the back. *Parsvakonasana* gives you a nice stretch of the lats as well as strengthening it because you are holding your extended arm in position (working the muscle).

- In *urdva mukha svanasana*, the lats contract to draw the lower back up.

- In *adho mukha svanasana*, they stretch, elongating forward and lengthening.

- You can experience the lats in action when you put your arms together over your head with fingers clasped together and then bringing your fist down in front in wood-chopping motion.

- Lifting the legs and arms up into the air in *salambhasana* gives you an intense experience of the lats!

Peeling back the trapezius, you will see:

3.9.3. Rhomboids (*diagram 3.9*)

In *virabhadrasana II*, the rhombiods contract* to hold the scapulae in one plane, opening the chest laterally.
In *garudasana*, they stretch.

There are two rhomboid muscles, though they sometimes appear fused as one. Rhomboideus minor is above rhomboideus major. The rhomboids start from the middle and are attached to the scapulae at the other end. They hold the scapulae to the thoracic cage.

The rhomboids work very closely with the trapezius.

* The trapezius spans a larger part of the back than the rhomboids. Contracting the whole of the trapezius would arch the whole back, whereas the actions of the rhomboids are limited to the upper trunk.

Rhomboids

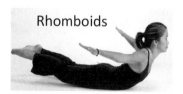

Trapezius

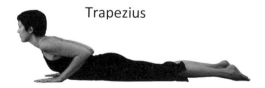

3.9.4. Levator scapulae (*diagram 3.10*)

In *jalandhara bandha*, the levator scapulae stretch to draw the chin downwards into a neck lock.

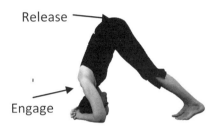

Release

Engage

Levator scapulae are on the same plane as the rhomboids. It is a long flat muscle starting from the upper cervical vertebrae. Its origin is covered by the overlapping of the sternocleidomastoid muscle. The levator scapulae end at the scapulae.

In most of *yogasana*, you want to engage this muscle bilaterally to keep the cervical spine lengthened.

Diagram 3.9. **Muscles of the upper back (after the trapezius and a segment of the rhomboideus minor had been removed).**

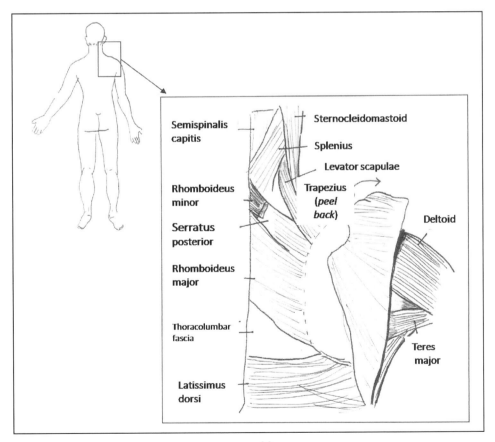

Diagram 3.10. **Levator scapulae**

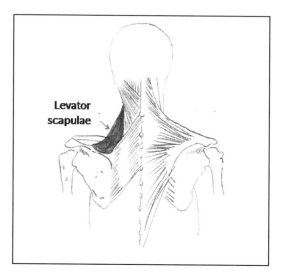

Levator
scapulae

Note on diagram *3.9* (*above*):

The rhomboideus muscles look like they are fused. The serratus posterior superior is deep to the rhomboids.

The serratus posterior inferior is covered externally by the latissumus dorsi.

Peeling back the latissimus dorsi, you will see:

3.9.5. Serratus posterior (*diagram 3.9*)

- The serratus are the muscles needed for *chaturanga dandasana* to hold the scapulae to the thoracic spine. If the scapulae are winged out, these muscles are not doing its work! Strengthen them by doing modified push-ups against a wall.

- In *garudasana*, they stretch to wrap the scapulae around the medial side of the body.

The serratus are fingerlike muscles that reach into the ribs and insert along the medial border of the scapulae.

Typically, they are antagonists to the rhomboids.

If you just raise your arms up with the scapulae snug against the thoracic spine, you've engaged your serratus. If you want to challenge these muscles further, go into the plank pose!

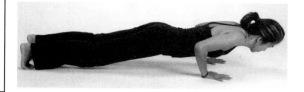

Moving down to the deep muscles of the back:

The deep muscles of the back extend from the skull to the pelvis and work together as extensors of the spine. The main group is the erector spinae.

3.9.6. Erector spinae

> * In backbends, such as *urdhva dharunasana*, they contract.
> * In forward bends, such as *uttanasana*, they stretch.
> * In dynamic cat-cow, we are working on the gentle lengthening and contracting of the erector spinae along the entire spine.

This is a big group of muscles, and it starts from the spinous processes of all the lumbar vertebrae, the sacrum, posterior sacroiliac ligament and the posterior part of the iliac crest. These muscles run parallel to the spine.

Beneath the erector spinae are:

3.9.7. Transversospinalis muscles

> Sufi grind (kundalini yoga) is good for maintaining the flexibility of the spine by consciously working on the individual vertebra by moving the fine transversospinalis muscles.

These are the small muscles that criss-cross the spine and connect one vertebra to the other. They look like elastic bands that tie the vertebrae together. Their main function is to give stability to the trunk.

There are two groups of transversospinalis muscles:

1. Rotators (long and short)
2. Multifidus

3.10. **Abdominal muscles**

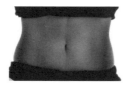

Fire in the belly gives you the drive to succeed in life!

3.10.1. **Rectus abdominis**

The rectus abdominis is the outermost muscle of the abdomen and is responsible for flexion movement of the trunk. The muscle runs straight from the lower ribs to the pubic bone. The rectus from the left and right side of the body comes together in the midline creating the linea alba. The rectus has three fibrous bands traversing the muscle to create the "6 pack abs" look.

If the pelvic girdle is fixed, contraction leads to forward bends such as *uttanasana*. A stronger effect of the contraction of rectus abdominis is seen in *tolasana*. It is stretched in backbends such as *urdhva dharunasana*.

The abdominals are stretched in *yogasana* such as camel or other backbends that lengthen the distance between the anterior ribs and pelvis.

The muscle is strengthen in yogasana such as boat pose where the abdominal muscle generates tension co-contracting with the spinal extensors to keep the trunk long and straight.

3.10.2. **Internal and External Obliques**

The obliques run in a diagonal pattern, and when they contract they pull the trunk into a rotational pattern to the left or right. The fibers of the two oblique muscles – the external and internal oblique muscle, run in a diagonal pattern opposite of each other. The external oblique runs from the lower ribs down and inward to the iliac crest and pubic area. The internal oblique runs from the iliac crest up and inward to the lower ribs and linea alba.

The obliques work together on opposite sides of the body to create the line of pull for rotation. For rotation of the trunk to the right, the internal oblique on the right works with the left external oblique to create the motion. For rotation of the trunk to the left, the internal oblique on the left work with the external oblique on the right.

The oblique muscles will be lengthened in *yogasana* such as a twist. The external oblique will lengthen when the trunk rotates one direction and the pelvis rotates the opposite direction. In this same posture the internal oblique on the opposite side will be lengthened.

The obliques will be strengthened in *yogasana* such as revolved triangle. In this posture, the obliques will be lengthened and must also work hard to maintain balance.

The origin of the external oblique muscle is higher on the ribs than the internal oblique muscle insertion on the ribs. Contraction of the external oblique draws the chest toward the hip.

Contraction on the one side of the internal oblique muscles and extension of the other side facilitate deep twisting *asana* such as *pavritta trikonasana.*

3.10.3. Transverse abdominals

The transverse abdominals are the deepest group of the abdominals and run from the sides to the center like a belt. When you draw your belly to the navel, you are engaging you transverse abdominals which then act to stabilize your pelvis.

Maintaining "naval to the spine" during yogasana will work your transverse abdominal muscle.

3.10.4. Breathing and the abdominals

The abdominals provide support to keep the internal organs within the chest cavity. They are also responsible for maintaining the internal pressure needed for respiration (the respiratory system is based on the change in pressure between the inhale and the exhale). Upon inhaling, the diaphragm contracts and presses downward on the abdominals. Lower pressure in the lungs is created and the air flows into the lungs. With exhalation, the diaphragm relaxes, creating increased pressure in the lungs and air flows out of the lungs. The abdominals act as the walls of a container in which this pressure system is able to function.

Pranayama such as breath of fire or *kapalabhati* breathing will work to strengthen the abdominals.

Diagram 3.11. **External musculature of the abdominal wall**

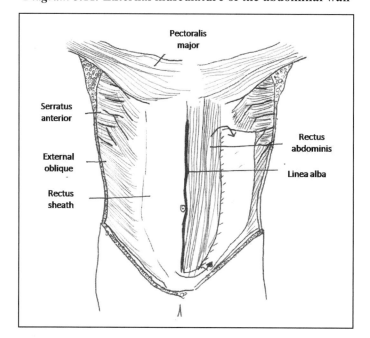

3.10.5. Diaphragm

The diaphragm is the major organ of inspiration. The contraction and relaxation of this muscle varies the pressure in the thoracic cavity facilitate respiration (*section 3.10.4).*

The diaphragm looks like a dome when it is pulled up, and a flying saucer when relaxed. The tendon is in the middle, with muscles surrounding it. This sheet of muscle is stuck to the walls of the abdominal cavity. The diaphragm is controlled by the phrenic nerve.

3.11.   Muscles of the lower extremities

[REFER TO *section 3.7*]

Below the diaphragm, towards the back of the body are these two major muscles, namely quadratus lumborum and the psoas:

3.11.1.   Quadratus lumborum

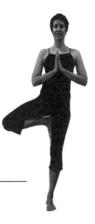

It is part of the posterior abdominal wall and starts from the middle of the iliac crest and inserts into the vertebrae. This is a really deep muscle, and is very close to the erector spinae (therefore, they often work in tandem).

In *parsvakonasana*, the quadratus lumborum is deeply stretched.

If this muscle is weak, you would not be able to keep the pelvis level in *Vrksasana.*

3.11.2. Psoas muscles (psoas major and iliacus)

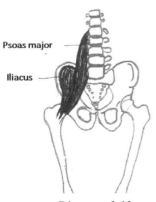

Psoas major
Iliacus

Diagram 3.12.
Psoas major and iliacus

Psoas major starts from the vertebrae of the lower back, and the iliacus starts from the inside of the iliac crest. Both merge to form one tendon that is attached to the proximal femur. Psoas is like a suspension bridge between the trunk and the leg. Releasing psoas is the key to many *yogasana* and plays a key role in maintaining the body's stability (especially in inversions).

Contraction on the one side facilitates *utthita trikonasana*.   In   backbends   such   as *urdhvadharunasana*, the psoas is stretched to open up the pelvic area.

3.11.3. Tensor fascia latae (TFL)

(Discussed first, because the gluteus maximus inserts into it)

Running along the outside of the leg from the pelvis to the knee is the illiotibial band (ITB). The ITB provide knee stability during movement. Inserting into the band one third way down the thigh is the TFL. The actions of the TFL are hip abduction, flexion and medial rotation.

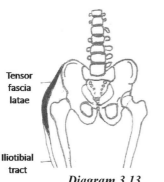

Tensor
fascia
latae

Iliotibial
tract

Diagram 3.13.
**Tensor fascia latae and
iliotibial tract**

- In *supta kurmasana,* the tensor fascia latae is stretched.

- In *ardha chandrasana,* the tensor fascia latae is contracted to bring the leg off the ground.

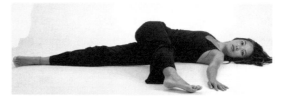

3.11.4. HIP ABDUCTORS

Hip abductors abduct the lower limbs, and some may internally rotate the hips. They are very important stabilizing muscles. We engage these stabilizers when walking and running.

The legs start from the gluteal region (or the buttocks). The gluteal region is made up of gluteus maximus, g. medius and g. minimus. The top part of the thigh is held in place at the side by the iliotibial band.

Gluteus maximus

Gluteus maximus is a very large muscle, which plays an important role in keeping the trunk erect. It is very thick and fleshy. Its origin is the sacroiliac region, and then the fibers fan out diagonally to insert into the iliotibial band of the fascia latae as well as the femur bone.

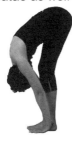

Stretching the gluteus maximus in *uttanasana*

- In *ustranasana*, the gluteus maximus contracts to stabilize the sacroiliac region, to support the backward bend of the trunk.
- In *purvottanasana*, it contracts to push the trunk upwards.
- In *uttanasana*, it stretches.

Gluteus medius

Gluteus maximus overlaps gluteus medius, which is a smaller muscle. It starts from the ilium and inserts into the femur.

Its basic action is hip abduction and stabilizing. For example, contracting the maximus outwardly rotates the hips, and the counter-action of the medius balances this out. It steadies pelvis so the body maintains balance in one-legged yogasana.

- Working with the tensor fascia latae (synergist), the gluteus medius contracts and brings the leg off the ground in *ardha chandrasana.*
- In *padmasana,* the gluteus medius is stretched.

Gluteus minimus

This is the deepest of the gluteal muscles. It starts from the ilium and inserts into the femur. Its function, principally, is to assist the medius. On a finer scale, it tilts the pelvis in walking.

3.11.5. THE EXTERNAL HIP ROTATORS

Simply put, their function is to turn the feet outward. In standing *yogasana*, they help to stabilize the pelvis and knees. They originate from the back of the pelvic bone and cross the back of the hip to insert on the upper femur. The external rotators are as follows:

1. Quadratus femoris
2. Piriformis
3. Obturator internus/externus
4. Gemellus inferior/superior

Diagram 3.14. **External hip rotators (*left*) and with quadratus femoris (*right*)**

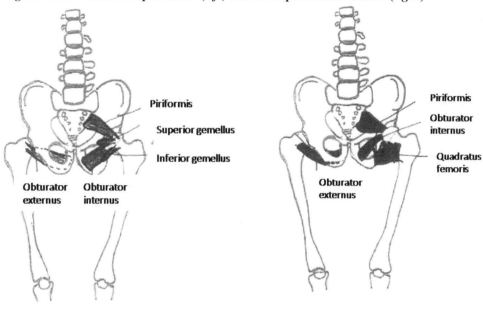

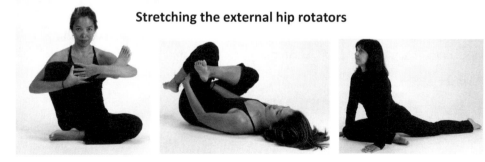

Stretching the external hip rotators

3.11.6. THE ADDUCTORS

The adductors are a group of muscles that connect the inner thigh bone to the pelvis via the pubic bone or the ischium. They adduct the leg (moves towards midline of the body) as well as stabilize the hip and legs (especially in inversions).

The adductors are:

1. Adductor Magnus
2. Adductor Longus
3. Adductor Brevis
4. Pectineus
5. Gracilis

Pectineus and gracilis are smaller in size than the adductors and are located deeper into the leg. The gracilis is the longest of the adductors.

Diagram 3.15. **The adductor muscles**

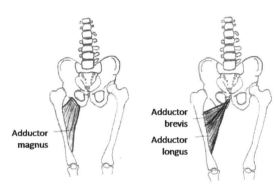
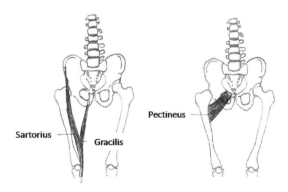

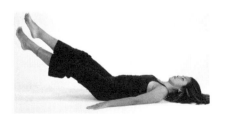

Strengthening and stretching the adductor muscles.

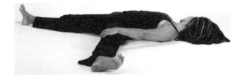

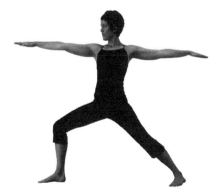

In *virabhadrasana II*, the adductors are simultaneously strengthened and stretched.

- In *prasaritta padottanasana*, the adductors are stretched, and they are engaged to stabilize the body in the forward bend.

- In *utkatanasana*, they contract.

- The pectineus are stretched in *baddha konasana*.

- The gracilis flexes the knee, and medially rotates the tibia relative to the femur. Rotating the feet in *upavisatha konasana* flexes the gracilis.

- In *parsvakonasana*, the adductors in the back leg are all stretched. The deepest stretch for all the adductors occurs in *upavistha konasana*, whilst in *tittibhasana*, they are all contracted to press the legs against the elbows.

3.11.7. Quadriceps

The quadriceps is the front muscle of the thigh, so called because this muscle has four heads:

1. rectus femoris
2. vastus lateralis
3. vastus medialis
4. vastus intermedius

> *one of the most important functions of the quadriceps is to keep the kneecap in alignment.

They all combine to form a tendon that inserts into the patella (kneecap). Unlike the vastus muscles, the rectus femoris starts from the iliac crest at the front of the pelvis. The others start at the femur.

Diagram 3.16. **The quadriceps muscles**

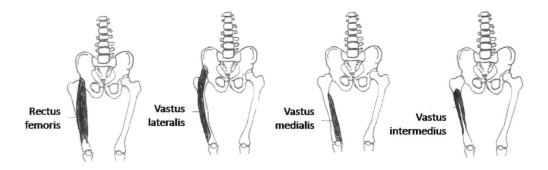

Rectus femoris   Vastus lateralis   Vastus medialis   Vastus intermedius

In general, this group of muscles is an antagonist to the hamstring. Therefore, in *uttanasana* and most standing forward bends, the quadriceps should contract. *Virabhadrasana I* and *II* strengthen the quadriceps. In backbends such as *Urdhva dharunasana*, they are lengthened and stretched. Quadriceps also functions to extend the knee and flex the hip.

3.11.8. Hamstrings

Hamstring is the name given to the back muscles of the thigh. Their function is to extend the hip and flex the knee joints. There are three groups of muscles which make up the hamstring:

1.   Semitendinosus
2.   Semimembranosus
3.   Biceps femoris

The semitendinosus and semimembranosus are in the inner section of the thigh. The biceps femoris is in the outer section. Starting from the sitting bone, they all insert into the tibia and fibula. Biceps femoris has two heads (one attaches at the sitting bone, the other one on the femur).

In *uttanasana* and most standing forward bends, all three groups of muscles that make up the hamstrings are stretched, especially the biceps femoris. Semitendinosus and semimembranosus are stretched more intensely in lateral leg stretches such as *Upavistha konasana*.
In *urdhva dharunasana*, they contract.

Diagram 3.17. **The hamstrings (back view of the lower leg)**

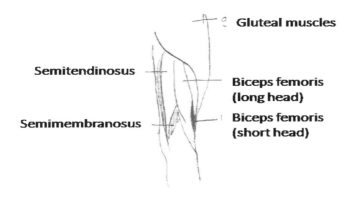

Gluteal muscles

Semitendinosus

Biceps femoris (long head)

Semimembranosus

Biceps femoris (short head)

3.11.9. Gastrocnemius, soleus and tibialis posterior

They are the muscles of the calves. This is a very powerful muscle group that are used in walking, and therefore gets a lot of work-out, which makes them short and tight. Gastrocnemius is just under the skin, the soleus lies beneath it. With the plantaris, they join together to form the Achilles tendon, which is the thickest and strongest tendon in the body.

Together with the tibialis posterior, the gastrocnemius and soleus plantarflex the foot. The soleus flexes the foot when the knee is bent.

Diagram 3.18. **Muscles of the calf**

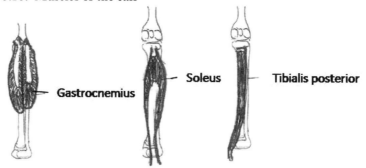

Ardho mukha svanasana is the ubiquitous calf stretch. However, for students with tight calf muscles, try *virabhadrasana I, II* and *Pavritta trikonasana*, focusing on grounding the back ankle.

In *pascimottanasana*, these muscles are stretched to point the toes to the sky, and in *purvottanansana*, they contract to keep the foot on the ground.

3.11.10. Sartorius

Sartorius is the longest muscle in the body, and the name means 'tailor'. It looks like a ribbon, and flexes the thigh and leg and rotates the leg medially and the thigh laterally.

- In *baddha konasana*, it is stretched.
- In *padmasana*, it is contracted.

3.11.11. MUSCLES OF THE FOOT

Proper alignment of the feet is one of the most important aspects of *yogasana*. The foot has several types of movement:

• Dorsiflexion (drawing the toes up towards the knee)
• Plantar Flexion, point the toes
• Inversion adduction of the foot (turning the foot in)
• Eversion abduction of the foot (turning the foot out)

Flexors
These are the deep muscles of the back leg that flex the toes.
- Flexor hallucis longus (FHL)
- Flexor hallucis brevis (FHB)
- Flexor digitorum longus

> Spreading toes consciously in *tadasana* and grounding the foot in standing poses activate the flexors.

Extensors
These are muscles in the front part of the leg. They extend the foot and toes.
- Extensor digitorum longus
- Extensor hallucis longus
- Tibialis anterior

> In *utkatanasana*, these muscles are strengthened.

Evertors
These are located on the outside of the leg.
- Peroneus longus (fibularis longus)
- Peroneus brevis

> In *Virabhadrasana III* and *Ardha Chandrasana* press out with all four corners of the foot.

Invertors
- Anterior Tibialis
- Posterior Tibialis

3.12.   Muscles of the upper extremities

[**REFER TO** *section 3.6*]

3.12.1. Deltoids

Deltoids are the muscles of the shoulder, and are what that give shoulders the rounded look.

- Anterior* (front head) – raises the arm forward
- Lateral (side head) – abducts arm
- Posterior* (back head) – draws the arm back

*Anterior and posterior deltoids are antagonists.

- Anterior section is used in *chaturanga dandasana* (contraction, to bear weight).
- In *virabhadrasana II*, lateral section contracts to abduct arms in position.
- Posterior section is used in *purvottanasana* to pull back the scapula.

3.12.2. Scapula region

Geographically, this is generally defined as teres major, teres minor, infraspinatus and the upper part of the upper head of the triceps branchii. They stabilize the shoulder. All of these are partially covered by the posterior part of the deltoid.

However, a more functional classification is rotator cuff. This is the name given to this group of muscles:

i. subscapularis
ii. infraspinatus
iii. supraspinatus
iv. teres minor

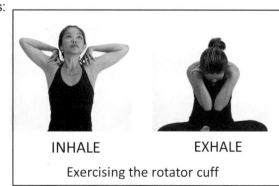

INHALE   EXHALE

Exercising the rotator cuff

Note: Rotator cuff injury is the common cause of shoulder pains. Damage to rotator cuff is seen in competitive swimmers, cricket players and any sort of intense wrenching of the arms, and also due to degeneration of the tendons (an effect of aging).

[REFER TO *Book 3*: YogaSense™ Shoulder Opening Routine]

- In *gomukhasana*, the subscapularis and infraspinatus work antagonistically. In the upper arm, the infraspinatus contracts and the subscapularis relaxes. In the lower arm, the subscapularis contracts and the infraspinatus relaxes.

- In *virabhadrasana II*, the supraspinatus contracts. Teres minor rotates the arm outward, whilst teres major extends the arm backward and pull the arm down.

3.12.3. ARMS

Technically, the arms are part of the superior extremity, which refers to the shoulder (deltoid and scapula regions – *section 3.12.1*), arms (brachium), forearms (antebrachium), wrists (carpus) and hands (manus).

The brachium region divides the arm into the flexor region (characterized by biceps) and the extensor region (characterized by triceps).

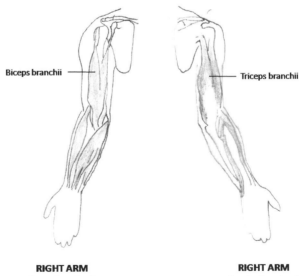

Biceps branchii

Triceps branchii

*Diagram 3.19.*Biceps and triceps of the right arm

**RIGHT ARM
(anterior view)**

**RIGHT ARM
(posterior view)**

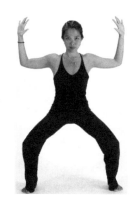

Biceps

The flexor region's main muscles are the biceps, brachialis and coracobrachialis. The coracobrachialis starts from the coracoid process of the scapula and inserts in the middle of the humerus.

The biceps is so called as it has two heads (the muscle divides into two), which are the short head and the long head. Both the long and the short heads start at the scapula, and then contracting to form one tendon which inserts into the radius. The brachialis lies deep underneath the biceps (but does not insert on the radius). It is an elbow flexor.

Contraction of the biceps

In the goddess pose (*pictured*), the biceps contract to maintain arms at right angles.
In *purvottanansana*, the biceps are stretched by the lift of the torso.

In *adho mukha svanasana*, the triceps are stretched (antagonistic to the action of the biceps). The triceps contract in *urdhva mukha svanasana*.

Triceps

The triceps are located at the back of the arms. Triceps mean 'three heads'. The long head starts at the scapula, the medial and short heads at the humerus. They all combine to insert into the ulna.

The main muscles lower down the arm are the radialis and ulnaris, which act to flex and extend the wrist as well as supporting the action of the muscles of the forearms. Because of their details and complexity, as well as the fact that they are not the prime movers in *yogasana*, we will not be covering them in this book.

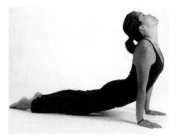

Contraction of the triceps

Moving to the triangles of the neck:

3.12.4. Sternocleidomastoid

This muscle is the main muscle of the neck, located on both sides of the front of the neck. It originates from the sternum (sterno) and clavicle (cleido), and ending in the skull just behind the ear (mastoid).

Straining this muscle may result in seemingly unrelated symptoms such as dizziness and nausea. The sternocleidomastoid muscle can be strained in accidents (whiplash injury), turning one's head to one side a for prolonged period or a fall/trauma.

- In *purvottanasana*, the
- sternocleidomastoid muscle extends and supports the head.
- In *jalandhara bandha*, the sternoclaidomastoid contracts to hold the head forward in a neck lock.

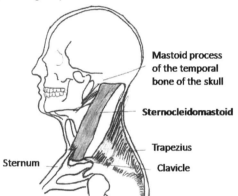

Mastoid process of the temporal bone of the skull

Sternocleidomastoid

Trapezius

Sternum

Clavicle

Diagram 3.20. **Sternocleidomastoid muscle**

Moving to the front of the body:

3.12.5. PECTORAL REGION (front of body)

Removing the superficial fascia and breast tissue, we expose:

Pectoralis major
This is a large flat, triangular muscle covering the chest. It consists of a small clavicular portion (originating from the medial clavicle) and a large sternocostal portion (originating from the sternum). The origins of this muscle are clavical, sternum and costal cartilages. It inserts into the humerus.

Beneath the pectoralis major is the **Pectoralis minor** which originates from the third, fourth and fifth rib and inserting into the scapula.

These are the muscles needed for *chaturanga dandasana*. It is exercised in push-up type repetitive activity. Pectoralis are stretched across the chest in purvottanasana.

Contraction causes protraction, horizontal flexion and arm flexor.

3.12.6. THORAX

The thoracic region consists of 12 thoracic vertebrae, the sternum, 12 pairs of ribs and their costal cartilages. The spaces between the ribs are filled with intercostal muscles. These muscles hold up the ribcage and move it in respiration.

The external intercostal muscles: 11 pairs of thin muscular sheets that run down and forward around the thoracic wall.
The internal intercostal muscles: also 11 pairs but in the inside of the ribcage.

External intercostal muscles are used in the inhalation part of deep abdominal breathing.

Internal intercostal muscles are used in the forced exhalation of *kapalabathi*.

3.13. Summary notes: muscles covered in this chapter

Muscle/muscle group	Function(s)	Notes
Abdominal: external oblique	Flexes and laterally bends the trunk	
Abdominal: internal oblique	Flexes and laterally bends the trunk	Anterior fibers run up and medially, perpendicular to the fibers of external abdominal oblique
Adductor brevis	Adducts, flexes and medially rotates the femur	
Adductor longus	Adducts, flexes and medially rotates the femur	
Adductor magnus	Adducts, flexes and medially rotates the femur; extends the femur	
Biceps branchii	Flexes the forearm and arm (long head); supinates	
Biceps femoris	Extends the thigh; flexes the leg	One of the hamstring muscles
Deltoid	Abducts arm; anterior fibers flex and medially rotate the arm	Main abductor of the arm, assisted by the supraspinatus
Diaphragm	pushes the abdominals inferiorly, increasing the volume of the thoracic cavity (inspiration)	Muscle of respiration

Muscle/muscle group	Function(s)	Notes
Erector spinae	Extends and laterally bends the trunk, neck and head (except the spinalis, which only extends the trunk and neck)	Separated into three columns of muscle: • iliocostalis • longissimus • spinalis
Gastrocnemius	Flexes leg and plantar-flexes foot	the calcaneal tendon of the gastrocnemius and soleus is the thickest and strongest tendon in the body
Gemellus, inferior	Laterally rotates the femur	
Gemellus, superior	Laterally rotates the femur	
Gluteus maximus	Extends the thigh; laterally rotates the femur	
Gluteus medius	Abducts the femur; medially rotates the thigh	
Gracilis	Adducts the thigh; flexes and medially rotates the thigh; flexes the leg	
Iliacus	Flexes the thigh; if the thigh is fixed, it flexes the pelvis at the thigh	
Iliopsoas (psoas)	Flexes the thigh; flexes and laterally bends the lumbar vertebral column	

Muscle/muscle group	Function(s)	Notes
Infraspinatus	Laterally rotates the arm	infraspinatus, supraspinatus, teres minor and subscapularis are the rotator cuff muscles
Intercostal	Keeps the intercostals space from blowing out or sucking in during respiration	
Latissimus dorsi	Extends the arm and rotates the arm medially	
Levator scapulae	Elevates the scapula	
Obturator externus	Laterally rotates the thigh	
Obturator internus	Laterally rotates and abducts the thigh	
Pectineus	Adducts, flexes and medially rotates the thigh	
Pectoralis major	Flexes and adducts the arm; medially rotates the arm	
Pectoralis minor	Draws the scapula forward, medially and downward	
Piriformis	Laterally rotates and abducts thigh	
Psoas major	Flexes the thigh; flexes and laterally bends the lumbar vertebral column	

Muscle/muscle group	Function(s)	Notes
Quadratus lumborum	1. Laterally bends the trunk; fixes the 12th rib. 2. Elevates the pelvis.	1. When the pelvis is fixed. 2. When the trunk is fixed.
Quadratus femoris	Laterally rotates the thigh	
Quadriceps femoris	Extends the knee; rectus femoris flexes the thigh	composed of 4 muscles: rectus femoris vastus lateralis vastus intermedius vastus medialis
Rectus abdominis	Flexes the trunk	
Rectus femoris	Extends the leg; flexes the thigh	Part of the quadriceps femoris muscle
Rhomboideus major	Retracts, elevates and rotates the scapula inferiorly	
Rhomboideus minor	Retracts, elevates and rotates the scapula inferiorly	
Sartorius	Flexes, abducts and laterally rotates the thigh; flexes leg	
Semimembranosus	Extends the thigh; flexes the leg	One of the hamstring muscles
Semitendinosus	Extends the thigh; flexes the leg	One of the hamstring muscles
Serratus anterior	Draws the scapula forward; the inferior fibers rotate the scapula superiorly	

Muscle/muscle group	Function(s)	Notes
Serratus posterior inferior	Pulls down lower ribs	Muscle of respiration
Serratus posterior superior	Elevates the upper ribs	Muscle of respiration
Soleus	Plantar flexes the foot	
Sternocleidomastoid	Initiates abduction of the arm, then the deltoid muscle completes the action	
Tensor fascia latae	Flexes, abducts and medially rotates the thigh	
Teres major	Adducts the arm, medially rotates the arm; assists in arm extension	Teres major inserts beside the tendon of latissimus dorsi, and assists latissimus in its actions
Teres minor	Laterally rotates the arm	Part of the rotator cuff muscles
Tibialis anterior	dorsiflexes and inverts the foot	Acts as both an antagonist (dorsiflexion/plantar flexion) and a synergist (inversion) of the tibialis posterior
Tibialis posterior	plantar flexes the foot; inverts the foot	Acts as both an antagonist (dorsiflexion/plantar flexion) and a synergist (inversion) of the tibialis anterior

Muscle/muscle group	Function(s)	Notes
Tibialis posterior	plantar flexes the foot; inverts the foot	Acts as both an antagonist (dorsiflexion/plantar flexion) and a synergist (inversion) of the tibialis anterior
Transversus abdominis	Compresses the abdomen	
Trapezius	Elevates and depresses the scapula (depending on which part of the muscle contracts); rotates the scapula superiorly; retracts scapula	
Triceps branchii	Extends the forearm; the long head extends and adducts arm	
Vastus intermedius	Extends leg	Part of the quadriceps femoris muscle
Vastus lateralis	Extends leg	Part of the quadriceps femoris muscle
Vastus medialis	Extends leg	Part of the quadriceps femoris muscle

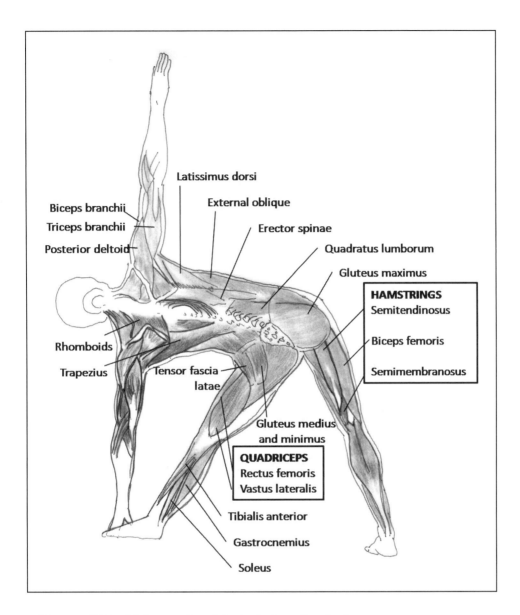

Latissimus dorsi

Biceps branchii

Triceps branchii

Posterior deltoid

External oblique

Erector spinae

Quadratus lumborum

Gluteus maximus

HAMSTRINGS
Semitendinosus

Biceps femoris

Semimembranosus

Rhomboids

Trapezius

Tensor fascia latae

Gluteus medius and minimus

QUADRICEPS
Rectus femoris
Vastus lateralis

Tibialis anterior

Gastrocnemius

Soleus

Diagram 3.21. **Main muscles of the body in action during *yogasana***

3.14. Treatment for overstretched/torn muscles

- The R.I.C.E. (Rest, Ice, Compress, Elevate) technique is one of the most common ways to treat muscle injury:

- Rest the muscle until the pain decreases. For sore muscles, gentle stretching helps.

- Apply ice even if you are going to see a doctor: place crushed ice in a plastic bag and wrap with a moist towel.

- Wrap the injured area with an elastic bandage to help control swelling and provide support. Begin wrapping at the farthest point away from the body and wrap toward the heart. Don't wrap too tightly, and remove bandage if there is numbness or tingling.

- Raising the injured area above your heart will allow gravity to help reduce swelling by draining excess fluid.

Early mobilization of the injured lower limb is vital for the correct rehabilitation of the muscle. This includes stretching and strengthening exercises throughout the pain free range. These can aid with decreasing the swelling in the area. In addition, exercise will ensure that any new material will be laid down in correct orientation thus reducing the risk of subsequent injuries.

See a sports injury specialist.

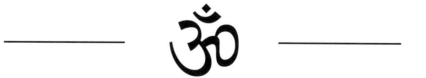

CHAPTER FOUR

Physiology

OVERVIEW OF THE CHAPTER

4.1   The basic concepts
4.2   Main systems of the body
4.3   Common ailments and symptoms
4.4   High risk categories
4.5   Important points for the yoga teacher

4.1.   The basic concepts

4.1.1. Physiology

Physiology is the understanding of: i. the way the systems integrate together; ii. how the systems communicate with each other; iii. how the internal environment is maintained stable (homeostasis).

Physiology is the science of the body in good health, and encompasses the body's mechanical, physical and biochemical functions. The study of physiology involves the body, the organs of the body and the cells in which the organs are made up of. Anatomy and physiology are closely related fields of study: anatomy is the study of structures of the body and physiology is the study of their functions.

The approach to physiology in this book is through the understanding of the main systems of the body affected by *yogasana*, and expanding on this to understand the symptoms of commonly encountered ailments, illnesses and diseases. Although this approach is less stringent compared to rote textbook learning of medical students and science undergraduates, it nevertheless provides a practical way for yoga teachers to grasp the basics of this complex and vast subject.

4.1.2.   Organization of the human body

The body is extremely complex. But the bottom line is, it is made up of cells. These are the building blocks of the human body, and a human body is built from an estimated 100 trillion cells.

The body works like a well-oiled engine because of the superb communication and coordination among its systems.

4.1.3.   Main cellular structures

Cells, though different in forms and functions, generally have the same basic architecture:

Nucleus

The nucleus contains the chromosomes (genetic material) of the cell. Each chromosome consists of a single molecule of deoxyribonucleic acid (DNA). DNA is the 'instruction manual for the human body', as it contains the genetic instructions required for the development and functioning of all known living organisms. It is also used for the long-term storage of genetic information.

Nucleolus

This is contained within the nucleus and important for the translation of genetic information into proteins.

Mitochondrion (*plural* mitochondria)

This is the cell's powerhouse, where cellular energy is generated from biochemical processes.   In addition, mitochondria also perform other important cellular functions such as cellular signaling, cellular differentiation, cell death, the control of the cell cycle and cell growth.

Ribosomes, endoplasmic reticulum (ER) and Golgi apparatus

These are the sites of protein manufacture, packaging and transportation. They are synonymous to an efficient factory!

Diagram 4.1. **A typical cell**

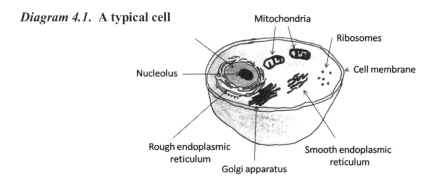

The key thing to note is that these cells are bathed in fluid, called the extracellular fluid (ECF).   From this fluid, the cells absorb nutrients and oxygen, and excrete waste products through the venous or lymphatic system. In the human body, the ECF is of two types:

i. blood plasma that circulates in the circulatory system with other components that make up blood;

ii. interstitial fluid that bathes the cells.

In an average young adult male, 18% of the body weight is protein and related substances, 7% mineral, 15% fat and 60% water.

4.2. **Main systems of the body**

4.2.1. Introduction

In unicellular organisms (such as amoebas), each cell is capable of independent existence. As unicellular organisms evolved into complex multicellular organisms (such as human beings), various cell groups took on specific functions. For example, the function of the gastrointestinal system is to digest and absorb food for the body's usage.

In the Western view, the human body is organized into inter-related systems, the main systems being:

i. Nervous
ii. Immune
iii. Lymphatic
iv. Endocrine
v. Digestive
vi. Circulatory
vii. Respiratory
viii. Urinary
ix. Genital
x. Integumentary
xi. Musculo-skeletal

Table 4.1. gives a summary of the main functions of these systems.

Table 4.1: **Summary of the main functions of the body's systems**

Classification	Main function(s)
Nervous	Command center of the body, responding and reacting to internal and external stimulation. The brain and the spinal cord are the anchors of the nervous system, from which nerves, ganglia and parts of the receptor and effector organs branch out. Sympathetic and parasympathetic divisions, which act to accelerate and to slow down the body respectively.
Immune	Defense system of the body, which is influenced by the Nervous System. Factors such as stress compromise the efficiency of the Immune System.
Lymphatic	Its main role is combating infection through its infection-fighting cells (known as white blood cells). The lymphatic system also carries lymph, which is a clear fluid that comes from the blood, containing the white blood cells, protein, water and minerals.
Endocrine	Regulator of the body's activities by secretion of hormones into the bloodstream. These hormones travel to the tissues and organs of the body and affect important functions such as growth, sleep, hunger. The pituitary gland is the gland that secretes hormones that regulate the activities of other hormone-secreting glands.
Digestive	Its function is the mechanical and chemical breaking down of food into its basic building block (called amino acids) which can be assimilated by the body for fuel.
Circulatory	Transporter of nutrients (including oxygen) to the cells of the body and waste products from the cells to the appropriate organs of excretion. The blood is the main mode of transportation, pumped round the body by the heart.
Respiratory	Breathing is the vital life process. Respiration is the process of bringing oxygen into the body and excreting carbon dioxide to the external environment.

Classification	Main function(s)
Urinary	Its role is the production, storage and excretion of urine; also a pH-regulator.
Genital	The sexual and reproductive organs of the body
Integumentary	This is the protective outermost layer of the body, which is both our barrier and link to the external world.
Musculo-skeletal	Also known as the locomotor system, it confers movement via muscular and skeletal actions.

4.2.2. The nervous system

A healthy nervous system keeps all the muscles, organs and tissues of the body working efficiently, giving you a sharper sensory perception, fostering calmness in your approach to life and filling your body with energy and vitality. *Yogasana* stretch and purify the bundles of fibers that make up the large nerves, and this has the effect of clearing toxins from the system, keeping the nervous system healthy, responsive and efficient.

Neurons

This is the typical unit cell of the nervous system. A neuron processes and transmits information to enable the integration and communication between different parts of the body and the maintenance of a stable internal environment. A neuron works by virtue of its responsiveness to stimuli (for example, light, pain, pressure, etc). Upon sensing a stimulus, it communicates to the central NS via chemical and electrical means. The central NS then processes the information it receives from the neuron and duly sends instructions for action to the relevant parts of the body (*diagram 4.2*).

Afferent neurons are responsible for sending information to the central nervous system and efferent neurons are responsible for information leaving the central nervous system.

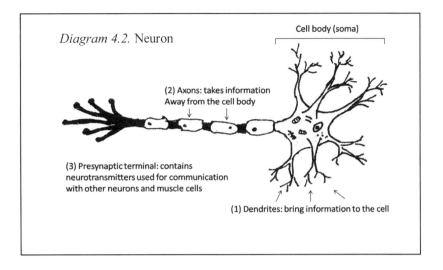

Diagram 4.2. Neuron

Cell body (soma)

(2) Axons: takes information
Away from the cell body

(3) Presynaptic terminal: contains
neurotransmitters used for communication
with other neurons and muscle cells

(1) Dendrites: bring information to the cell

Organization of the nervous system

The nervous system (NS) is the command centre of the body, as it is composed of the brain and spinal cord (known as the central NS), with nerves, ganglia, receptor and effector organs branching out from the core (known collectively as the peripheral NS).

The peripheral NS is subdivided into the autonomic NS and the somatic NS. The autonomic NS is further subdivided into the sympathetic NS and the parasympathetic NS.

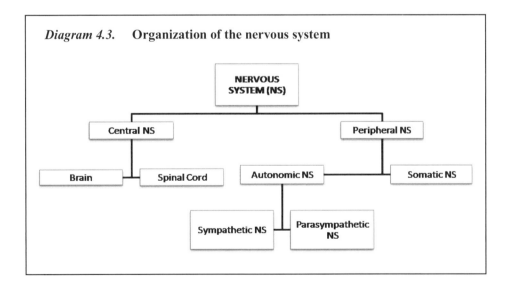

Diagram 4.3. Organization of the nervous system

THE CENTRAL NERVOUS SYSTEM

The brain gives us the ability to experience, rationalize and feel.

It's also our thread to Universal Consciousness, our immortality.

One of the most powerful mantras in Kundalini Yoga is "Wahe Guru", or consciousness is ecstasy.

The brain

In Western anatomy, the central NS is the seat of consciousness, because it is here that the brain sits. The brain is a complex organ, and because if its complexity, it is extremely fragile. Deprivation of oxygen kills the brain quicker than other major organs in the body. There is a close physiological relationship between the mind (the thinking part of the brain) and the body. A good illustration of this is our posture. Our posture is our emotional signature. For example, a stressed person's body is tight, bunched up, compressed. A person who is depressed often has a concaved trunk, with the chest collapsing and the eyes to the ground.

There is also a close psychological relationship between the mind and the body, which is evidenced by medical research on the effects of placebo. "If you think you are well, then you are" is a simple statement that is truer than it appears.

Because of the close relationship between the mind and body, the practice of *yogasana* can create a circle of well-being that encircles the body. Take the example of *tadasana*, often considered the first pose in *yogasana*: Our feet connect us to the ground, and this grounding motion gives us a feeling of connection, of security, stability. For a student prone to anxiety attacks, the best *yogasana* would be standing still in *tadasana*, feeling his feet on the ground, and concentrating on taking in deep breaths, channelling that breath from the earth to the heart. As he exhales, he focuses on letting go of the stressor while maintaining strong contact to the ground through his feet.

The lowering of the blood pressure while in *tadasana* also aids the relaxing effect of this *yogasana*.

Remove your shoes and stand with your bare feet grounded to the earth. Draw a deep breath to the heart center and feel the earth's calming energy. Hold that breath. Exhale and release all your tension to the earth. Relax. *Just be.*

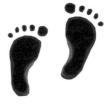

Spinal cord

The second component of the central NS is the spinal cord. In yogic anatomy, the spinal cord is known as the *merudanda*, the column that extends from the base of the skull to the coccyx. In Western anatomy, the spinal cord is comprised of nerve tissues to support its prime function as a communication channel. It is often likened to telegraph poles. The key feature of the nerves in the spinal cord is that unlike other tissues such as bone, they do not heal or regenerate (though research is ongoing for spinal cord regeneration).

THE PERIPHERAL NERVOUS SYSTEM

The peripheral NS is subdivided into the autonomic NS and somatic NS. The autonomic nervous system is further divided into the sympathetic and parasympathetic system. The autonomic system is primarily involved in maintenance of body functions and organs. The somatic NS receives external stimuli from skin, striated muscles, and connective tissues and also through the eyes and ears via two cranial nerves. The somatic system controls the response of the voluntary movements of the body by utilizing the skeletal muscles.

Autonomic NS

The terminology autonomic NS was first coined because it was thought that this system functions automatically, independent of outside control. This, of course, is not a view held in yogic anatomy. Much of *yogasana* is about working on the autonomic NS through alignment and the corresponding effects on the body's energetics to maintain good health.

> The Autonomic NS helps you to adapt to changes in your environment. It adjusts or modifies some bodily functions in response to stress.
>
> Cultivate calm. Meditate.

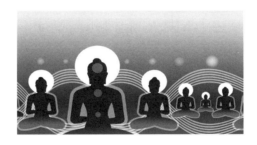

The autonomic NS is about helping the body to adapt to changes in the internal environment (often as a result of changes in the external environment such as temperature). This process is known as homeostasis. Impaired ability to adapt to those changes not only impacts the body physically, but mentally, too. The autonomic NS is the means by which smooth muscles, cardiac muscles, glands and viscera are controlled. The viscera have various receptors in them, such as osmoreceptors, baroreceptors, chemoreceptors, etc., that respond to changes in the internal environment. The afferent neurons send information from the visceral to the central nervous system through the sympathetic and parasympathetic pathways. The components of the NS communicate with each other by means of chemical messengers called neurotransmitters. The main neurotransmitters in the NS are acetylcholine, noradrenaline, dopamine, serotonin and various peptides. In the brain, imbalances in the level of different neurotransmitters result in mood disorders.

Sympathetic NS

The sympathetic nervous system is perhaps most commonly associated with engaging the body in a fright-fight-flight response. The sympathetic system is always active even when the body is at rest, working on processes such as digestion. When doing challenging *yogasana,* the body moves into short-term sympathetic dominance. With regular practice the body adapts to these challenging *yogasana,* the sympathetic dominance becomes less intense. This is why *sarvangasana,* which is a restorative *asana,* is initially stressful for the new student, and its therapeutic values can only be realized after a period of practice.

Because of its do-or-die *modus operandi,* the components of the sympathetic NS are fully integrated and work as a team, that is to say, an accelerated heart rate (due to anxiety, stress or fear, among others) is accompanied by the tensing of muscles, a heightened state of awareness and shallow, rapid breathing. These are the responses that send the body into a ready-to-fight mode, which would cause long-term health problems if the occurrence is regular and prolonged.

Long term physical manifestations of stress include hypertension (a big killer), heart problems, compromised auto-immune system, headaches, backaches, disturbed sleep patterns, anxiety, depression and a whole host of other problems.

If we use the analogy of the body as a car, the sympathetic NS acts as an accelerator in the body, while the parasympathetic NS is the brake.

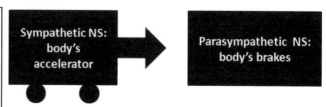

Diagram 4.4. **Depiction of the body's sympathetic NS and parasympathetic NS.**

Parasympathetic NS

Conversely, the parasympathetic NS is involved in activities that calm or goes to the throat area, lungs, heart and digestive organs. The motions of the chest in respiration stimulates the vagus nerve (and thence, heart rate), with inhalation inciting sympathetic activity of the heart (heart rate increases). This micro fluctuation of the heart rate between sympathetic and parasympathetic dominance is known as respiratory sinus arrhythmia. On a more macro scale, in relaxation after a challenging series of *yogasana,* the body moves into parasympathetic dominance to regain status quo. However, in cases where there is extreme parasympathetic dominance, which may result in depression, *pranayama* can be used as the key for unlocking sympathetic activities.

Changing the body from sympathetic dominance to parasympathetic dominance is one of the aims of *yogasana. Pranayama* is key to this transformation. Consciously slowing down the breath will increase the parasympathetic NS influence in the body and will reduce the sympathetic NS influence on the body. Danucalov, Simões, Kozasa and Leite (2008) showed that certain yogic practices (namely meditation) have the effect of reducing the body's metabolic rate while others (namely energizing *pranayama*) speeds the metabolic rate up compared to the rest state.

One of the aims of *yogasana* when it comes to the autonomous NS is bringing the two spheres of sympathetic NS and parasympathetic NS closer together to enable an easy transition between the two. As the sympathetic NS and parasympathetic NS affect every single tissue of the body, we can through *yogasana*, affect literally every cell of our body.

Diagram 4.5. **The transformation effects of *pranayama* on the autonomic NS**

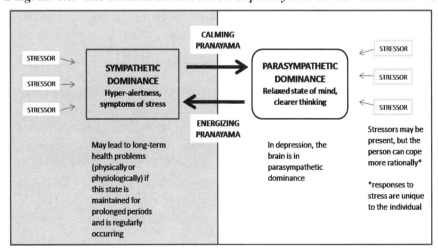

The model proposed in *diagram 4.5.* has been corroborated by research (Brown and Gerbarg, 2005) which shows that certain yogic breathing techniques (Ujjayi and Bhastrika *pranayama*, *Chapter 7: Techniques*) can alleviate anxiety, depression, everyday stress, post-traumatic stress and stress-related medical illnesses. Mechanisms contributing to a state of calm alertness include increased parasympathetic drive, calming of stress response systems, neuroendocrine release of hormones, and thalamic generators.

4.2.3. The immune system

The immune system is the body's defense system, and it works by recognizing and killing foreign invaders and neutralizing toxins. Recognition of foreign invaders is by the immune system's marauding cells (which act like a police patrol). These "police" cells are the neutrophils, monocytes and the lymphocytes. These cells are able to identify foreign invaders by their protein coat. The cells that do the killing are the white blood cells known as phagocytes (composed of cells such as neutrophils, macrophages and eosinophils) which are made in the bone marrow and found in lymph, blood and tissue.

The workings of the immune system are influenced to a large extent by the nervous system. Anatomically, the components of the immune system (thymus, lymph nodes and spleen) are threaded with the branches of the autonomic NS. Biochemically, stress leads to the production of chemicals that affect organs such as the adrenal glands, with the final outcome being the inhibition of the immune system's functions. An example of this is a stressed-out or fatigued person who is more prone to coughs, colds, sore throats and other ailments symptomatic of a compromised immune system.

Extrapolating this effect, it is obvious to see how mental attitude can affect the overall health of a person. If a person feels that the whole world is against them, that life is about fighting and there is no support available, his body then resides in the fight-or-flight realms, namely in the sympathetic mode, which could result in life-threatening illnesses such as hypertension and heart diseases, as well as being perpetually vulnerable to common symptoms. A study of yoga philosophy and other similar texts will help to shift the mindset and perception, which is the first step on the road of wellbeing.

Conversely, an overactive immune system results in asthma, allergy attacks and auto-immune conditions. Rheumatoid arthritis is caused when the cells of the body's immune system attack the cartilage in the joints. In Acquired Immune Deficiency Syndrome (AIDS), the whole immune system is under attack by the human immunodeficiency virus (HIV) virus.

A balanced *yogasana* class can contribute significantly to wellbeing, because it stimulates the parasympathetic NS, which releases the neurotransmitter acetylcholine. Acetylcholine is known to strengthen the immune system. Therefore, ensure that your students have sufficient time for relaxation at the end of a class!

Savasana after a *yogasana* class is good for your parasympathetic NS!

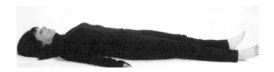

4.2.4. The lymphatic system

The lymphatic system is comprised of lymph (clear fluid bathing the cells), the lymph vessels (for transporting lymph) and the lymph nodes (for storing lymph). Lymph is formed from arteriole pressure squeezing fluid from the blood as the blood flows into fine capillaries in the vicinity of the cells. Lymph has about the same composition as blood plasma, and contains the all-important, infection fighting white blood cells. In addition, lymph carries debris and bacteria, and moves around the body in lymph vessels.

As the lymph vessels are a mode of moving fluids through the body back to the venous circulation, care must be exercised when doing inversions for a person suffering from cancer to prevent the spread of cancerous cells around the body. Cancer sufferers should seek guidance from an experienced teacher who understands the pathology of cancer, and should never practice *yogasana* without consulting the oncologist first.

4.2.5. The endocrine system

The endocrine system is the name given collectively to the organs which secrete hormones that regulate the body's function. It produces effects as wide-ranging as growth, tissue function, and sexual appetites.

Almost all glands are controlled by the brain, and as the human body evolved in size and complexity, the Endocrine System became a means of communication between the command center and the organs.

The Western map of the endocrine system corresponds closely to the chakra system described by yogic anatomy, though these two views evolved independent of each other. This is discussed in further detail in the section on Yogic Anatomya & (Ayurv *Chapter* 6).

4.2.6. The digestive system

Digestion is the process of breaking food down into smaller components that can be taken up by the individual cells of the body which will use these food components for the basic processes of life.

The human digestive system looks like a bag of approximately 10 meters in length, starting from the mouth and terminating at the anus. When food is added into the bag, digestion occurs, aided by the digestive chemicals inside the bag and the muscular action of the muscles surrounding the bag.

Digestion actually begins in the mouth, with the mechanical process of chewing and the chemical reaction between the enzymes in the saliva and the food. The process of digestion intensifies in the stomach, where the action of very strong chemicals, including hydrochloric acid, breaks down food. Meat requires greater acidity and muscular activity to digest, which explains why one feels tired after a heavy meal.

Digestion continues in the small intestines, where food is broken down into its molecular components. It is here in the small intestines that the molecular components of food are absorbed and transported to the cells that need them. The indigestible remainder of the food travels down to the colon or large intestines. The main activity taking place here is the absorption of water. A diet rich in fruits and vegetables will result in stools that are easily expelled as the fiber content in fruits and vegetables provides the 'exercise' needed by the colon to expel waste.

Other organs and glands that lie outside the bag also support the digestion by producing enzymes for the process, such as the pancreas and liver. Bodily secretions are enhanced by the parasympathetic NS. The sympathetic NS, on the other hand, facilitates muscular contraction and spasm. Therefore, a practitioner should not eat a heavy meal at least three hours before a class.

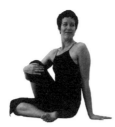

The impact of *yogasana* such as twists aids the muscular action of digestion.

4.2.7. The circulatory system

The Circulatory System is about the circulation of blood (and in it, the nutrients, waste products, energy, debris and heat) around the body in a network of arteries, capillaries and veins, which are also known as the vascular system.

The center of the circulatory system is the heart as described in *Chapter 6: Yogic Anatomy & Ayurvĕda*. The heart, or the *anahata* chakra, is the home of the soul and the seat of our consciousness, compassion and love. In the body, the role of the heart is to ensure that blood (and its precious cargo) gets to distant cells and tissues to sustain life. The pumping of the heart creates the necessary blood pressure to facilitate the flow. This action is facilitated by the muscles of the heart, known as the myocardium. The myocardium beats at its own pace, without the need for external stimuli.

Because of the heart's continuous activity, the supply of blood to the heart is very important. An efficient heart is one that pumps slow and steady, allowing the chambers (i.e. atria and ventricles) to fill up fully before pumping, therefore exerting less effort to pump the same volume of blood. Research has shown that yoga relaxation is associated with a significant improvement in cardiac health of healthy yoga practitioners (Khattab, Khattab, Ortak, Richardt and Bonnemeier, 2007). Regular aerobic exercises (like *Surya Namaskar*) strengthen the myocardium and thereby decreasing heart rate. Emotions, too, play a significant role in affecting heart rates

4.2.8. The respiratory system

Research has shown that yogis and athletes have better pulmonary function than people who lead sedentary lifestyles (Prakash, Meshram and Ramtekkar, 2007).

"If you breathe better, you live better" was a comment made by one of my trainee teachers, Myriam Aguilar, years ago. Indeed, this echoes the views of ancient sages and mystics, who believed that breath has profound impact on life. Our breath is our link to the Universal Consciousness. From the vastness of the unmanifested Universe to the smallest cell in our body, our breath touches the infinite and the infinitesimally small. Raghuraj and Telles (2008) showed that unilateral nostril yoga breathing practices (*nadi sodhana*) have an immediate effect on the body's blood pressure. Therefore, *pranayama*, or breathing consciously, forms one of the eight limbs of yoga.

Breath is primal, instinctive and natural, yet one has to marvel at its complexity. It involves:

1. Movement of the Abdomen
2. Movement of the Pelvic Floor
3. Movement of the Sacrum, Coccyx and Lumbar Spine
4. Movement of the Spinal Column
5. Movement of the Hips
6. Movement of the Shoulder Girdle and Arms

The primary muscles involved in breathing are the intercostals, diaphragm and abdominal muscles. The lungs are the main respiratory organ. The heart lies in between the lungs, more to the left. Thus, it is advisable for students to lie on the right side to decrease pressure on the heart.

4.2.9. The urinary system

The urinary system - comprised of the two kidneys, two ureters, the bladder and the urethra – is an excretory system that produces, stores and eliminates urine from the body. The kidneys filter out water-soluble waste products from the blood. It also regulates electrolytes (ions such as Na+, K+ and Ca+) to maintain the acidity and alkalinity of the blood. This is an important homeostasis function, as enzymes have a very narrow pH-tolerance. The activities of kidneys are controlled by hormones, namely the renin-angiotensin-aldosterone system.

4.2.10. The genital system

The genital system refers to the reproductive organs of the body. In yogic anatomy, the male reproductive/sexual system lies in the *mooladhara* (or base) chakra, as this corresponds to the location of the testes. In women, it is the *svadisthana* (or second) chakra that corresponds to the reproductive/sexual system, because this is where the ovaries and womb are found (*Chapter 6: Yogic Anatomy & Ayurvĕda*).

The reproductive/sexual organs are influenced by hormones, such as the gender-based steroids, androgen and oestrogen. The gonads are the male glands responsible for the growth and development of the sexual organs as well as sexual behavior.

4.2.11. The integumentary system

The integumentary system refers to the system that creates a protective layer around us, namely the skin. The skin, our interface to the world outside, protects the more delicate and vulnerable structures of our body. It is the largest organ of the body and also contains sweat glands, hair and nails. Exposure to sunlight provides most humans with their vitamin D requirement (UV rays trigger vitamin D synthesis in the skin).

The skin is well supplied with blood vessels and sweat glands to facilitate its function as the body's chief heat regulator. It is also rich in sensors. In stretching *yogasana*, these sensors are activated, giving the practitioner clues as to what is happening deeper down, namely at the muscular level.

In *yogasana*, manual adjustments from the teacher often help the practitioner enormously in refining his alignment. The teacher's touch on a specific point brings the practitioner's awareness into the posture (*Chapter 8: Teaching Methodology*).

4.3.   Common ailments and symptoms

Note that this is discussed more comprehensively in *Book 2: Yoga Therapy.*

4.3.1.   The parameters of *yogasana*

There is a lot going on inside the body which is invisible to the naked eye, and indeed, to sophisticated medical imaging machines. Activities

When the body shows signs of fighting an infection, do not do any inversions.

Do not do any challenging *yogasana*. Opt for total rest to give your body the chance to recover.

at cellular level remain largely undetected until they have gathered sufficient momentum to manifest as symptoms, which is what we experience as discomfort, illness and disease. In fact, some diseases such as Alzheimer's begin as far back as twenty years before the first symptoms are observed.

Depending on the severity, *yogasana* can, to a certain extent, alleviate discomfort, but specific illnesses and diseases are best treated by targeted means, such as with the appropriate medicine. The section on Yoga Therapy (*Book 2*) deals with using *yogasana* to support the body's intrinsic healing mechanisms.

4.3.2. Fever

The main thing to remember about fever is to keep the body cool (through frequent sponging) and drinking lots of water.

The body's normal temperature when measured orally is generally 98.6 degrees Fahrenheit. This may fluctuate by about 1°F throughout the day. A person is considered to be feverish when her body temperature rises to 100°F or more. Fever is one of the body's most generic responses to any activity that moves it out of its narrow, optimal functioning band (for example, infection).

The underlying cause of fever is the body fighting an infection. If the infection is local (for example, toothache), there will be localized swelling and a rise in temperature. If the infection is more global (for example, when the body is under attack by foreign invaders), the body's overall temperature rises.

A student with fever should not attempt *yogasana*, other than relaxation in *savasana*.

4.3.3. Stress

Early on in our evolutionary path, the stresses encountered by our ancestors were real threats, such as lions jumping at them or poisonous snakes falling from branches of trees. Stress, as you can see, is not

137

necessarily a bad thing, as it is a survival mechanism (a little stress now and then is actually good!). However, in the modern world, most threats are imagined rather than actual, given that lions no longer roam the streets. Stress also has a strong emotional link.

In response to modern versions of these threats, our bodies go into the fight-or-flight mode, with the sympathetic NS dominating the parasympathetic NS. With the sympathetic NS having the upper hand, our body moves into the state of heightened awareness – breathing becoming shallow and fast, muscles bunching up, pupils of the eye dilating. In a prolonged state of stress there is the potential to damage the body physiologically (such as weakening the immune system, opening the body up to a whole host of attack)Yoga is effective as a stress moderator by the following mechanism:

i. study and understanding of yoga philosophy
ii. *pranayama* that slows the body down
iii. restorative *yogasana* such as *pascimottanasana*

4.3.4. Hypertension

Blood pressure in the body is controlled to a large extent by the heart. Locally, blood pressure is caused by the constriction and dilation of the muscles of the blood vessels and through the effect of hormones. When a body meets with stress, the sympathetic NS kicks in to vasodilate the muscles of the heart and striated muscles, while closing down the blood flow to other 'non-essential' parts of the body. Because there is relatively more closing down of blood vessels than vasodilation, the overall impact is an increase of the blood pressure. The heart has to work harder to pump blood under high pressure. If this state of high blood pressure and high heart rate is maintained, hypertension is the outcome. Hypertension can kill through strokes, heart attacks, heart failures and arterial aneurysm. It may also cause the kidneys to fail.

As most cases of hypertension is idiopathic (arising from unknown causes), *yogasana* is beneficial for those suffering from hypertension.

Apart from stress, other causes of hypertension have been linked to too much salt in the diet, alcohol and obesity.

Savasana is the generic effective *yogasana* for hypertension, though if the hypertension is caused by atherosclerosis, *yogasana* has minimal effect.

138

Inversions should not be taught to students with hypertension.

4.3.5. Persistent headaches

Headaches are experienced by most people at some stage or other in their lives, often as a reaction to tiredness, over-stressing the eye-muscles and lack of sleep, to name but a few common causes. Such casual headaches may be dealt with simply by getting adequate rest and relaxation, taking a break from intense activities and readdressing recent changes.

A common cause of persistent and frequently occurring headaches is bad posture. A person who has weak core muscles, exacerbated by depression or an introspective personality, will demonstrate a posture where the chest collapses into itself, and the back looks like a hump. In this posture, tightness in the neck, shoulder and head area will bring about muscle tension headaches.

Yogasana that will alleviate this condition include:
• strengthening of the core muscles
• chest-openers such as *setu bandhasana*, *garudasana* and *gomukhasana*.

Bhatia, Dureja, Tripathi, Bhattacharjee, Bijlani and Mathur (2007) showed that yoga as a part of a program (namely non-steroidal anti inflammatory drugs, botulinum toxin injections and a yogic lifestyle course) help patients with chronic tension type headaches.

> Persistent headache should be investigated by a physician as it could be a symptom of something more severe.

However, persistent headaches may have deeper underlying causes. The seemingly generic "headache" could be the symptom for many different underlying illnesses, and therefore should be investigated with the guidance of a qualified physician. The most common causes of persistent headaches are mood-related disorders, namely depression and anxiety attacks.

4.3.6. Depression

Depression is on the rise, and is often referred to as the malaise of the modern world. In its most extreme form, it leads to suicide. However, mild depression has the power, too, to destroy by robbing its sufferers of rationale, family and quality of life.

There are strong indications that depression is genetically linked. Depression can be broadly divided into one of the two categories:

Exogenous depression
Exogenous depression is caused by something happening on the outside, such as a traumatic event or prolonged period of stress. This external aggravation puts the body's mechanism into the fight-or-flight mode, which releases chemicals into the bloodstream, and this upsets the normal neurotransmitter levels in the brain. When the aggravation is removed, the sufferer often returns to status quo. However, in some cases, the depression remains and becomes pathological.

Meditation and a study of yoga philosophy (or similar literature) could often aid the recovery from exogenous depression.

Endogenous depression
In endogenous depression, the imbalances in the neurotransmitter level occur without an external trigger. In both cases of depression, the parasympathetic nervous system dominates over the sympathetic. Medical intervention is often the only way to redress the imbalances in the neurotransmitter level.

Medical intervention involves addressing the imbalances of the neurotransmitter levels. Supporting this would be *yogasana* that helps the body regain more sympathetic dominance:
i. back-bending *asana*
ii. chest-openers
iii. strong *pranayama*
iv. relaxation with the eyes wide open.

Note: Other major areas of mood disorder are compulsive disorder and bipolar (though these do not demonstrate the symptom of persistent headaches).

There is still some stigma attached to mood disorders. In many cultures, depression is suffered in silence without the benefit of physician, psychologist or psychiatrist care. The personal nature of mood disorders makes the sufferer feel isolated, alone and guilty, which exacerbate the illness. Mood disorders can be cured or controlled through proper care protocol. Encourage your practitioners to seek help if needed.

Though yoga should not be seen as the magic pill for mood disorders, the benefits of yoga practice are undoubtedly manifold for the sufferer and could support medical intervention enormously. A study evaluating the influence of yoga in relieving symptoms of depression and anxiety in women suggests that yoga can be considered as a complementary therapy or an alternative method for medical therapy in the treatment of anxiety disorders (Javnbakht, Hejazi Kenari and Ghasemi, 2009).

4.3.7. Migraine

Unlike the previous two categories where the headache is the symptom of muscular contraction, migraine is caused by over-pressurisation of the blood vessels of the brain. Migraines are characterized by light and noise sensitivities, and by nausea.

Apart from medical intervention, ways of alleviating migraines are:
i. relaxation with eyes covered, in a darkened, silent room
ii. minimal or zero motion.

Localized pain
Localized pain, in particular, behind the eye, is another classical symptom of vascular headache. *Yogasana* that reduce blood pressure may bring relief to this type of headache:
 i. mild inversions with head on the floor, such as the dolphin pose
ii. *adho mukha svanasana* with head supported on a block.

The causes of migraines are multi-faceted, and could be as wide-ranging as hormonal ("time of the month") to dietary (chocolate is a common culprit). A qualified and appropriately trained yoga therapist will be able to guide her client towards a better understanding of his body to elicit the appropriate course of action.

4.3.8. Frequent sore throats, fevers, coughs and colds

The underlying cause of frequent illnesses is a weak immune system. A weak immune system is likely to be caused by fatigue, stress, an over-dominance of the sympathetic NS, change of environment (often resulting in stress) and poor diet. Changing the destructive patterns or removing the stressor, addressing the lifestyle issue and making positive changes in one's life is by far the most effective means of strengthening the immune system.

Yogasana to support this include:
i.   Rigorous *yogasana* to wake the body up
ii. Followed by long restorative *yogasana* and plenty of rest
iii. *Pranayama* to shift to parasympathetic dominance.

4.3.9. Influenza ("flu")

Influenza is often confused with the common cold. Both are the result of viral attack on the body, which results in runny nose, sore throat, mild fever, tiredness and a cough. The difference between influenza and the common cold is the severity of the former relative to the latter. Influenza can also lead to complications such as pneumonia. When the body is under viral attack, the best cure is plenty of rest and plenty of fluids.

4.3.10. When it is not appropriate to attend yoga

Yoga is a system of wellness, and a general yoga class caters to those who are in a good state of health. If in doubt, a teacher should refuse to take a practitioner on until a physician's note is presented.

Practitioners should NOT attend yoga class if they are:
- Suffering from acute pain and discomfort (for example, torn muscles)
- Infectious (for example, conjunctivitis, spluttering cough)
- Recovering from surgery (including caesarean births)
- Having a fever
- Using recreational drugs
- Under medical care.
    Open sores should be covered up with bandages or plasters

4.4. High risk categories

4.4.1. Diabetes

Diabetes is a metabolic disorder where the sugar content in the body is either too high or too low. It is often treated with insulin.

In the diabetic, the blood sugar level may fluctuate between very high levels (hyperglycaemia) and to dangerously low levels (hypoglycaemia), with death as an outcome. Moderate *yogasana* can help a diabetic student, but care must be ensured that he is not hyper or hypo at any time (ensure that he does not come to class with an empty stomach and has taken his insulin).

4.4.2. Cancer

Cancer is the name given to the condition where cells in the body have gone mad, dividing disorderly and behaving malignantly. This happens when the immune system is under-active, and fails to check the abnormal proliferation of cells.

Moderate *yogasana* is beneficial for strengthening the immune system, though it is counter-beneficial to work the body too hard (eliciting a sympathetic response). Accumulating evidence supports the beneficial impact of complementary therapies (such as acupuncture, yoga, meditation and physical activity) on physical and emotional symptoms associated with cancer treatment (Cassileth, Gubili, and Simon Yeung, 2009), though Smith and Pukal (2008) suggested that further research in this area is warranted.

For students with active cancer, inversions should not be done as it may encourage the cancerous cells to migrate to other parts of the body (though there is no conclusive evidence).

4.4.3. Recovery from surgery (including caesarean births)

Surgery involves cutting through layers of skin, fat, muscles and ligaments. Because of the many layers of tissues involved, students should not attempt *yogasana* until at least the third month after surgery. Gentle walking is a good form of exercise in the meantime.

4.4.4. **Slipped disc and other trauma of the spine**

Slipped disc is one of the most common forms of back injury and refers to prolapsed or herniated disc. Intense forward bends such as *uttanasana* or *pascimottanasana* are not advisable. Positions involving pelvic flexion such as *supta padangusthanasana* are also contraindicated.

Because of the complexity, it is best that students with slipped disc avoid *yogasana* altogether and opt for alternative forms of gentle exercise such as swimming.

Practitioners with severe scoliosis, lordosis and other spinal abnormalities seeking yoga as a cure should study *yogasana* under the supervision of a teacher of yoga therapy.

4.4.5. **Senior citizens**

Human bodies change dramatically with age. *Yogasana* should support the stage of life a person is in and not cause the body undue stress or possible damage by inappropriate *yogasana*.

Because of the wide-ranging outcomes and the highly individualized nature of these outcomes, it is difficult to generalise the effects of growing old. In general, senior citizens should remain mobile, fit and alert as possible to maintain their quality of life. There are not many forms of exercise as suitable for senior citizens as *yogasana*. Research has shown that a specialized yoga program (shorter duration and modified to accommodate reduced flexibility) improves the physical fitness in senior citizens after a 24-week period (Chen, Chen, Hong, Chao, Lin and Li, 2008).

Points to remember when teaching yoga to senior citizens include:
- Bone weakness – fractures occur easily
- Decreasing heart and lung fitness - do not do *yogasana* that are too challenging or that require intensive cardio activity
- Decreasing range of motion – stretching is important!
- Decreasing efficiency in digestive function
- Increase in chronic diseases such as heart disease, diabetes and hypertension.

Care should be taken to ensure the comfort and safety of your practitioners in this category, as they are more prone to dizziness, falling and exhaustion.

4.4.6. Pregnancy

A pregnant practitioner should attend a specialized prenatal yoga class. The primary reason is that the aims of a prenatal yoga class is different from a standard yoga class – the aims of a prenatal class are typically bonding with the baby, pain management, vocal intonation, empowerment and exploring optimal birth positions.

Gentle yoga or restorative classes are not a proxy for prenatal yoga. This is because certain seemingly calming postures such as twists should not be done in pregnancy, and beyond the second trimester, pregnant women should not lie flat on their back. All in all, prenatal yoga is a complex field, one which is too complicated to be covered within the scope of this book. Thus, all pregnant practitioners should be referred to an appropriately qualified prenatal yoga teacher.

4.5. Important points for the yoga teacher

4.5.1. Managing your practitioners' expectations

Yoga is a system of wellness, and a general yoga class is for maintaining that wellness. Practitioners seeking to heal specific ailments through yoga should seek the advice from a teacher trained in yoga therapy.

Yoga is not a quick-fix solution. Practice of yoga should be consistent and devoted, and over a long period of time to deliver results. In addition, diet, positive thinking, practicing karma yoga and following the yoga code of ethics are all vital parts of the equation leading to mental, emotional, spiritual and physical wellbeing. A practitioner attending *yogasana* class for an hour once a week while neglecting all other factors will not get the benefits of yoga.

4.5.2. Yoga is not the cure for everything

There is a role for medical science, even for hard-core yogis. For example, if you have a broken bone or a fracture, there is no other way but to get the bone set properly in a hospital, after the appropriate X-rays have been taken. Even though bones are natural healers (newly generated bone cells will cover both ends of the broken bone until it is as good as new), you will still need a cast or pins to ensure that the break heals properly. Similarly, other localized injuries or specific major illnesses (such as meningitis, leukaemia and cancer, to name a few) are best dealt with using the capabilities of modern science. In these cases, yoga and other holistic approaches have an important role to play, namely, in maintaining the wellness of the rest of the body, mind and soul and thus aiding recovery.

4.5.3. Yoga is not suitable for everybody

Unless you are teaching a VERY gentle class or a specialized class, yoga could be contraindicated for these categories of students:
1. Recovering from surgery (minimum: 3 months before resuming yoga, or till cleared by the surgeon)
2. Slipped disc or other spinal trauma and abnormalities (for example, scoliosis)
3. Under medical care and / or medication for high blood pressure and other serious illnesses
4. Using recreational drugs.

For some individuals, even with the safeguards in place, yoga is not a suitable form of exercise. For example, according to Bertschinger, Mendrinos and Dosso (2007), yoga can be dangerous for individuals with glaucoma (disease of the optic nerve).

4.5.4. You are a yoga teacher, not a doctor

In the United States, the law forbids the yoga teacher to function as a doctor as well, imposing a clear cut demarcation of responsibilities. Whatever jurisdiction you practice in, it is prudent and moral to limit your advice only to yoga and matters directly related to yoga, because that is the scope of a yoga teacher.

References

Bertschinger, D.R., Mendrinos, E., & Dosso, A. (2007). Yoga can be dangerous--glaucomatous visual field defect worsening due to postural yoga. *Br J Ophthalmol.* 2007 Oct;91(10):1413-4.

Bhatia, R., Dureja, G.P., Tripathi, M., Bhattacharjee, M., Bijlani, R.L., & Mathur, R. (2007). Role of temporalis muscle over activity in chronic tension type headache: effect of yoga based management. *Indian J Physiol Pharmacol.* 2007 Oct-Dec;51(4):333-44.

Brown, R.P., & Gerbarg, P.L. (2005). Sudarshan Kriya yogic breathing in the treatment of stress, anxiety, and depression: part I-neurophysiologic model. *J Altern Complement Med.* 2005 Feb;11(1):189-201

Cassileth, B.R., Gubili, J., & Simon Yeung, K. (2009). Integrative medicine: complementary therapies and supplements. *Nat Rev Urol.* 2009 Apr;6(4):228-33.

Chen, K.M., Chen, M.H., Hong, S.M., Chao, H.C., Lin, H.S., & Li, C.H. (2008). Physical fitness of older adults in senior activity centers after 24-week silver yoga exercises. *J Clin Nurs.* 2008 Oct;17(19):2634-46.

Danucalov, M.A., Simões, R.S., Kozasa, E.H., & Leite, J.R. (2008). Cardiorespiratory and metabolic changes during yoga sessions: the effects of respiratory exercises and meditation practices. *Appl Psychophysiol Biofeedback.* 2008 Jun;33(2):77-81. Epub 2008 Mar 4.

Javnbakht, M., Hejazi Kenari, R., & Ghasemi, M. (2009). Effects of yoga on depression and anxiety of women. *Complement Ther Clin Pract.* 2009 May;15(2):102-4. Epub 2009 Mar 20.

Khattab, K., Khattab, A.A., Ortak, J., Richardt, G., & Bonnemeier, H. (2007). Iyengar yoga increases cardiac parasympathetic nervous modulation among healthy yoga practitioners. *Evid Based Complement Alternat Med.* 2007 Dec;4(4):511-7.

Prakash, S., Meshram, S., & Ramtekkar, U. (2007). Athletes, yogis and individuals with sedentary lifestyles; do their lung functions differ? *Indian J Physiol Pharmacol.* 2007 Jan-Mar;51(1):76-80.

Raghuraj, P., & Telles, S. (2008). Immediate effect of specific nostril manipulating yoga breathing practices on autonomic and respiratory variables. *Appl Psychophysiol Biofeedback.* 2008 Jun;33(2):65-75. Epub 2008 Mar 18

Smith, K.B., & Pukall, C.F. (2008). An evidence-based review of yoga as a complementary intervention for patients with cancer. *Psychooncology.* 2008 Sep 26. [Epub ahead of print].

CHAPTER FIVE

The Brain and the Mind

OVERVIEW OF THE CHAPTER

5.1   The philosophical-physiological perspective
5.2   The brain: the Western perspective
5.3   Anatomy and physiology of the brain
5.4   Effects of yoga on the brain
5.5   The mind and science
5.6   The yogic mind
5.7   Yogic practices for a healthy brain and mind

5.1. **The philosophical-physiological perspective**

5.1.1. **Dualism**

What is the distinction between the rich, verdant inner world of thoughts, feelings, fantasies and emotions and the scientific, highly sophisticated workings of the neurons of the brain (*section 4.2.2*)? These two very different events take place in the same location, namely, within the gray matter enclosed inside our skulls.

Take colors, for example. Are they "out there", in the petals of a flower, the glow of someone's cheeks, and the drabness of a concrete block? Or are they merely our visceral, emotional perception, born within us, without any connection to the outside world?

It is said that no two people ever see the same rainbow. And, yes, this fact is true scientifically. A rainbow is made up of the diffraction of light through millions of raindrops. And since raindrops are constantly in motion, and the eyes of two people cannot occupy the same place in space at the same time, each observer sees a different rainbow.

5.1.2. **The yogic perspective**

People often use the words "brain" and "mind" interchangeably. However, from the yogic perspective, the brain is an organ of the body where important biochemical reactions take place; the mind, on the other hand, is characterized by *vritti* (Koay, 2008). For the yoga practitioner, the question of how the mind can affect the workings of the brain and the rest of the body underpins the practice of *yogasana* and the yogic lifestyle.

5.2. **The brain: the Western perspective**

5.2.1. **The scope**

The brain is a remarkably intricate organ. Even though it only weighs approximately 3 pounds in an adult, it is responsible for all of our thoughts, memories, dreams, fantasies, as well as keeping us alive. It is the seat of our consciousness. The brain receives stimuli from the internal organs, receptors on the surface of the body and the sensory organs. It then reviews the stimuli, before reacting to correct the position of the body, the movements of the limbs and the functioning of the internal organs. All in all, it functions as mission control for the whole body.

The brain is one of the most complicated parts of the body to study. In this book, it is covered at a basic level, namely, to the level sufficient to facilitate the understanding of the relationship between the brain, the mind and yoga.

5.2.2. Brain biology

The brain is extremely vulnerable. It is encased within the skull and suspended in the cerebrospinal fluid. Despite its protective casings, the brain is susceptible to mechanical damage such as from a blow to the head.

If blood flow to the brain is interrupted for more than about 10 seconds, loss of consciousness may result. Lack of oxygen, abnormally low glucose levels in the blood and presence of toxic substances can cause brain damage within minutes.

The brain is susceptible to diseases as wide-ranging as Parkinson's and Alzheimer's to depression and schizophrenia. It is also susceptible to poisoning by viral agents and neurotoxins.

5.3. Anatomy and physiology of the brain

5.3.1. Major internal parts of the brain

To study the brain, we divide and classify it into several strata, bearing in mind that there is a high degree of overlap in its overall functionality.

The main regions of the brain are the cerebrum, cerebellum and brainstem.

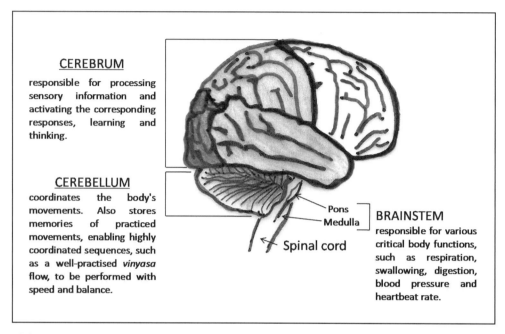

CEREBRUM

responsible for processing sensory information and activating the corresponding responses, learning and thinking.

CEREBELLUM

coordinates the body's movements. Also stores memories of practiced movements, enabling highly coordinated sequences, such as a well-practised *vinyasa* flow, to be performed with speed and balance.

Pons
Medulla
Spinal cord

BRAINSTEM

responsible for various critical body functions, such as respiration, swallowing, digestion, blood pressure and heartbeat rate.

Diagram 5.1. **Main regions of the brain and their functions (midsaggital plane)**

Brainstem

The brainstem is the lowest in brain development hierarchy, and is the primitive/vegetative part of the brain. It is responsible for various critical body functions, such as respiration, swallowing, digestion, blood pressure and heartbeat rate. As such, if there is severe damage to the entire brainstem, these automatic bodily functions stop and death is the result. The brainstem also helps adjust posture.

Cerebellum

The cerebellum lays just above the brainstem and coordinates the body's movements. With the information it receives from the cerebrum and the basal ganglia about the position of the limbs, the cerebellum helps the limbs move smoothly and accurately. It does so by constantly adjusting muscle tone and posture.

The cerebellum interacts with areas in the brainstem called vestibular nuclei, which are connected with the organs of balance (semicircular canals) in the inner ear. Together, these structures provide a sense of balance. The cerebellum also stores memories of practiced movements, enabling highly coordinated sequences, such as a well-practiced *vinyasa* flow, to be performed with speed and balance.

<u>Cerebrum</u>

At the top of the hierarchy is the cerebrum, which is generally accepted to be the seat of our consciousness. It is responsible for processing sensory information and activating the corresponding responses, learning and thinking. The cerebrum is the largest part of the brain.

5.3.2. The surface of the cerebrum (cerebral cortex)

The outer portion of the cerebrum (often referred to as the "gray matter") is called the cerebral cortex. To fit the relatively large surface area of the cerebral cortex into the skull, it is densely folded. This is known as cortical folding or gyrencephalization.

The cerebral cortex is divided into right and left hemispheres. The right hemisphere controls the left side of the body and vice versa.

The two hemispheres of the brain are connected by a band of tissue called the corpus callosum. It is believed that the right hemisphere is associated with creativity, spatial ability, face recognition and music, while the left is associated with calculations and logical abilities.

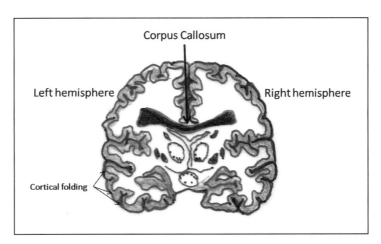

Diagram 5.2. **Transverse slice of the brain**

To visualize the cerebral cortex, imagine a thick wrapping that wraps itself over and around most of the structures of the brain, to the depth of between 1.5mm to 5mm. This area is gray, enclosing the "white matter" beneath (*section 5.2.6*).

The cerebral cortex is the most highly developed part of the human brain and is responsible for thinking, perceiving, producing and understanding language. According to the Western perspective, this is the seat of our consciousness.

5.3.3. Cerebral cortex lobes

The cerebral cortex is the information-processing part of the brain. It is divided into lobes, with each lobe having a specific set of functions (*diagram 5.3*):

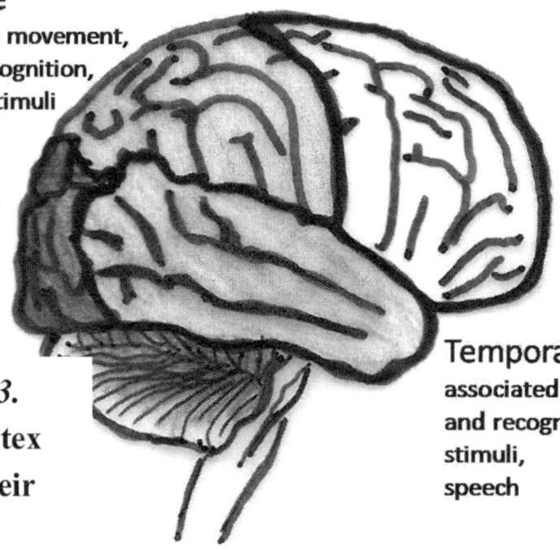

Parietal lobe
associated with movement, orientation, recognition, perception of stimuli

Frontal lobe
associated with reasoning, planning, parts of speech, movement, emotions, and problem solving

Occipital lobe
associated with visual processing

Temporal lobe
associated with perception and recognition of auditory stimuli, memory, and speech

Diagram 5.3.
Cerebral cortex lobes and their functions

5.3.4. Beneath the cerebral cortex

Underneath the gray matter is the white matter, which consists mainly of nerve fibers that connect the nerve cells in the cortex with other parts of the nervous system. Together, this makes up the cerebrum.

Diagram5.4.
Transverse slice showing gray and white matters of the brain

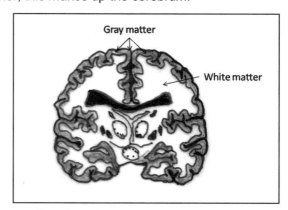

Gray matter

White matter

Collections of nerve cells—the basal ganglia, thalamus, and hypothalamus—are located at the base of the cerebrum. The basal ganglia coordinate movements. The thalamus generally organises sensory messages to and from the highest levels of the brain, providing a general awareness of such sensations as pain, touch and temperature.

The hypothalamus, through the secretion of hormones, coordinates many bodily functions, such as control of sleep and wakefulness, maintenance of body temperature, and regulation of appetite and the balance of water within the body.

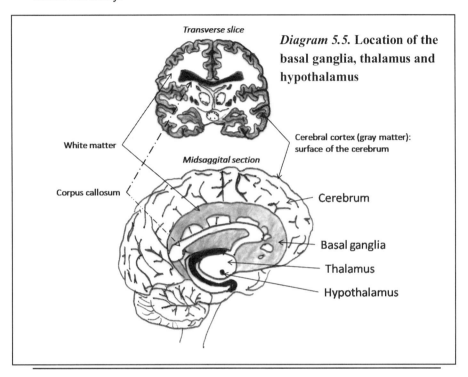

Diagram 5.5. Location of the basal ganglia, thalamus and hypothalamus

5.3.5. The limbic system

The limbic system is buried under the cerebrum. It is often referred to as the intermediate (or paleopallium) brain. Evolution-wise, this structure is relatively old compared to other parts of the brain. It is also our emotional seat. It influences the endocrine system and the autonomic nervous system (*Chapter 4: Physiology*).

The main components of the limbic system are:

Hypothalamus

This is the body's thermostat (*section 5.2.6*). The hypothalamus is also responsible for regulating hunger, thirst, responses to pain, levels of pleasure, sexual satisfaction, anger and aggressive behavior.

Thalamus

The thalamus is the relay station to the cerebral cortex (*section 5.2.4*), where most of the brain's information processing takes place.

Hippocampus

This is where new experiences are converted into long-term memories. If this area is damaged, a person lives in an altered reality, where everything she experiences at present fades into nothingness, while old memories before the hippocampus was damaged remain clear.

Amygdala

The amygdala is responsible for generating negative emotions such as anger, fear, aggression and those associated with the fight-or-flight response.

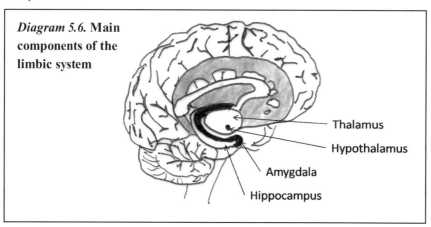

Diagram 5.6. Main components of the limbic system

- Thalamus
- Hypothalamus
- Amygdala
- Hippocampus

5.4. **Effects of yoga on the brain**

5.4.1. **Accepted benefits of yoga**

There has been a renaissance in the last decade or two in the practice of yoga as an alternative to modern, Western medical science. Kjellgren,

Bood, Axelsson, Norlander, Saatcioglu (2007) showed in a pilot study that participants may improve their wellness by learning and applying a program based on yoga and yogic breathing exercises.

New research is constantly emerging on the benefits of yoga to physical, mental and emotional health. With science, each piece of new research is reviewed, scrutinized, tested and challenged by the proponent's peers over a period of time before it becomes valid and widely accepted by the community.

5.4.2. Emotional management

Our emotional state has a real, tangible effect on the physical body. A common example is comfort eating, where a person eats to compensate for his lack of direction in life, low self-esteem or unhappiness. This could lead to excessive weight gain, which has a detrimental effect on health.

In addition constant stress can overload the immune system and cause long term damage to one's health.

The amygdala is the part of the brain responsible for generating these negative feelings. Therefore, for peace, calmness and serenity to return to a troubled mind, keeping busy on a non-emotional task is an effective antidote. On a higher level, mastery of the Yoga Sutra (*Chapter 2: Philosophy, Ethics & Lifestyle*) would enable one to dissociate oneself from the machinations of the turbulent mind, accepting that none of the material world is real. Happiness can be cultivated when the amygdala is quietened, pure love cultivated and a sense of direction in life established. That is one of the aims of yoga.

5.4.3. Improving basic vital life functions

The brainstem is involved in the basic vital life functions such as cardiovascular system control, respiratory control, pain sensitivity control, alertness and consciousness. Regular practice of physical *yogasana* and *pranayama* over a period of time improves cardiovascular and respiratory functions. Yoga is also known to keep the brain alert; an experienced practitioner generally tends to breathe deeper, hence taking more oxygen into the body.

The pilot study of Michalsen, Grossman, Acil, Langhorst, Lüdtke, Esch, Stefano and Dobos (2005) showed that an intensive 3-month Hatha Yoga program is effective in reducing stress and associated psychological outcomes in mentally distressed women.

Note (1): it is not clear how yogasana *practice impacts the brainstem, but there is much evidence to support the fact that physical exercise improves both cardiovascular and respiratory functions.*

Note (2): Classical neuroscience states that the brainstem is basically a fixed and unchanging structure, but new research shows that it can be rewired by music training (Northwestern University, 2007).

5.4.4. Changing perspectives on life

The frontal part of the cerebral cortex is believed to play a key role in the integration of both behavioral acts and autonomic reactions. In fact, because of the extensive neurological functions associated with it, the cerebral cortex is thought to play an important role in integrating the activities of the entire body systems (Udupa, 1996).

Consciousness, self-awareness and self control (housed in the frontal lobes) are all awakened by the study of yoga philosophy or other spiritual texts. As one journeys deeper into one's Self, the external world ceases to exert its hold and one is thus freed to a large extent of the trivialities of daily life. A yogi adept in the yogic philosophy will be able to stop her train of thoughts before it catalyzes a chain of negative reactions which cascade down her body, setting off an avalanche of detrimental physiological effects (increased stress level, depression, hunger pangs) or destructive actions (hurtful words, rash actions, irreversible damage to relationships).

5.4.5. Physical coordination

Physical coordination enables one to move effortlessly and with grace. The motor cortex, at the back of the frontal lobes also allows you to consciously move your muscles. The cerebellum (*section 5.2.3)* co-ordinates muscles to allow precise movements and to control balance and postures.

A constant and dedicated practice of *yogasana* creates 'body intelligence', where the body responds effectively and efficiently to external situations.

The ability to move with grace infuses us with self-confidence and joyful movement.

5.4.6. Right-left hemisphere balancing

The communication between the two hemispheres of the brain, each with its own distinct functions, is facilitated by the corpus callosum. Despite their distinct functions, almost all tasks require both hemispheres and their interactions (Robin, 2002).

Research has supported the theories that breathing practices affect hemisphere laterality (Robin):

- Breathing through the right nostril (left hemisphere of the brain) increases the heart rate, systolic blood pressure and consumption of oxygen, as appropriate for the stimulation of the sympathetic nervous system (*diagram 4.5)*. Verbal performance is also enhanced during right nostril breathing;

- Spatial task performance (associated with the right hemisphere) is enhanced during left nostril breathing, and the body shows reduced perspiration, too, with left nostril breathing (characteristic of parasympathetic dominance);

- Alternate nostril breathing or *nadi sodhana* (*Chapter 7: Techniques*) has been practiced for thousands of years by ancient yogis for improving their general state of health.

Pranayama and *yogasana*, especially in cross-patterning postures, open up and strengthen the bridge between both hemispheres of the brain to create a more balanced individual (as opposed to being strongly left or right brain dominant).

Indeed, as mentioned earlier in this section, the fluidity of the left hemisphere–right hemisphere interaction elevates our experience of an activity from pleasurable to profound. For example, a new practitioner to yoga engages his left brain when he first starts attending yoga classes. He busies himself with the technicalities of each posture and concentrates on processing the multitude of instructions he receives from his yoga teacher. He uses his logic to analyze and to record each new experience. These are all left brain activities.

After a long period of practice, when the practitioner is familiar with the postures, he begins to feel his *yogasana*. He moves intuitively and his breath flows. He feels his yoga singing within him. The artistry of his movements – movement in meditation – involves right brain dominance, and serves to elevate his practice from the physical to a spiritual level where his mind, body and soul become one. This is the moment of serendipity when yoga becomes a part of the practitioner's life. The musical analogy is when (and if) a competent and experienced musician moves up from being very good to the maestro level.

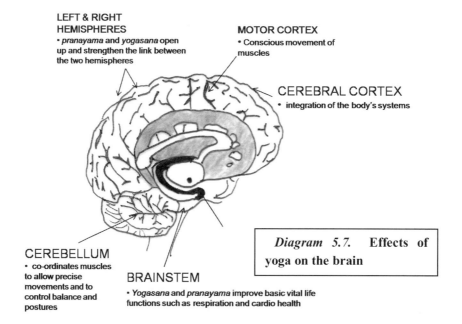

LEFT & RIGHT HEMISPHERES
• *pranayama* and *yogasana* open up and strengthen the link between the two hemispheres

MOTOR CORTEX
• Conscious movement of muscles

CEREBRAL CORTEX
• integration of the body's systems

CEREBELLUM
• co-ordinates muscles to allow precise movements and to control balance and postures

BRAINSTEM
• *Yogasana* and *pranayama* improve basic vital life functions such as respiration and cardio health

Diagram 5.7. **Effects of yoga on the brain**

5.5.   The mind and science

5.5.1.   Introduction

What is the mind? Is it the seat of the human soul, the creator of our reality, or is it something more mechanical, more rational? Plato and Descartes proposed that the mind is a separate entity from the brain (the brain is considered part of the body). This argument is known as dualism. Subsequent philosophers and scientists have argued that the mind is a result of the brain's functioning, and is nothing more than the workings of the anatomical brain. According to this second thread of argument, the mind ceases to exist when the brain stops functioning (Hebb, 1974).

Farthing (1992) defines mind as "the functioning of the brain to process information and control action in a flexible and adaptive manner". From the Western perspective, perhaps the simplest distinction between the brain and the mind is that the brain is studied by dissection while the mind is studied through observation.

The science of the mind falls mainly within the jurisdiction of psychology and psychiatry, with many branches emanating from these two established ones. Common ailments of the mind include schizophrenia, depression, anxiety, psychotic and personality disorders. An average of 1 million people commit suicide every year, (accounting for 1.5% of all deaths worldwide). Most people who die by suicide have psychiatric disorders, notably, mood, substance-related, anxiety, psychotic, and personality disorders, with comorbidity being common (Hawton and van Heeringen, 2009). Understanding the workings of the human mind is indeed an important science.

5.5.2. Psychology

According to the *Concise Oxford Dictionary*, psychology is the scientific study of the human mind and its functions. Obviously, the human mind cannot be studied by dissection of the brain. The method employed is studying human behavior to elicit the workings of the mind.

Broadly, the study of psychology can be divided into these three main branches (Huit, 1996):

- Cognition and reasoning– "knowing" from perception and ideas;
- Emotion and affect – emotional interpretation of cognition and reasoning;
- Conation or volition – connection of knowledge and effect on behavior; associated with the issue of "why."

A psychologist would investigate the nature, functioning and potential of an individual's mind. This would involve understanding the subject's awareness, attention, intention, imagination and concentration. The psychologist would then develop techniques for the individual to become aware of these functions, and to also strengthen and expand their use and control.

On the remedial side (namely, clinical psychology), the psychologist would diagnose and treat disorders of the brain, emotional disturbances, and behavior problems. On the commercial side, a social psychologist would look at how the actions of others influence the behavior of an individual, and use it to design products and marketing strategies. Today, the services of psychologists are widely used ranging from sports and education to artificial intelligence research and criminology.

5.5.3. Psychiatry

Psychiatry is the study of mental disorders and their diagnosis, management and prevention. The main difference between a psychiatrist and a psychologist is the educational route that each takes. A psychiatrist is trained as a medical doctor, and is therefore a holder of a Doctor of Medicine (M.D.) degree, before receiving additional, specialized training in psychiatry. He is therefore qualified to prescribe medications to treat disorders of the mind.

A psychologist holds a doctorial degree obtained by research and dissertation. Because a psychologist has strong grounding in research instead of medicine, she is well-trained to analyze information and draw conclusions from her sessions with her clients. Her educational route would also have given her a background in analyzing the effectiveness of the various forms of treatment in use and making a judgement as to which works for a particular client.

5.5.4. Application of psychology and psychiatry

Unlike broken bones, disorders of the mind cannot be so easily fixed. Accurate diagnosis is the first major hurdle. For example, an individual who demonstrates certain abnormal behavior traits could be suffering from any number of closely related disorders: anxiety attacks, strong dislike of new places and new people, unexpected bursts of violence, "down" mood, all of which could either be symptoms of bipolar disorder, depression, autism or even neurological causes, such as having micro-seizures in the brain. It is not uncommon that two highly qualified professionals in these fields would arrive at different conclusions.

Once the disorder had been narrowed down or isolated to the most probable cause, the mode of treatment (whether counseling or by medication or both) is prescribed.

5.6. The yogic mind

5.6.1. The mind according to the Yoga Sutra of Sri Patanjali

The mind is where Western science meets centuries-old yogic anatomy. One of the definitive pronouncements of Sri Patanjali's Yoga Sutra is:

yogaschittavritti nirodhah [Yoga Sutra 2,I]

The practice of yoga is to still the fluctuations of the mind, known as *vritti*. These fluctuations have been identified by Sri Patanjali as understanding, misunderstanding, imagination, sleep and memory:

pramanaviparyayavikalpanidrasmrtayah [Yoga Sutra 6, I]

According to Sri Patanjali, we are defined - and distracted - by the construct of the mind, which is widely known as the ego. The ego drives us to act in uncharacteristic ways, and sometimes to take actions lacking in integrity. The need to acquire material things is a good example. Human beings are driven to reach out and grab for more, as instructed by the hungry mind. To have more and to surround ourselves with the external symbols of our success have become symptomatic of modern life. Even on the roof of poor homes, big satellite dishes are mounted on the roofs, the "wealth" of the householder is thus proudly displayed to his neighbors.

But material things do not buy ever-lasting happiness – they are only temporary distractions to satiate an insatiable mind. Eternal bliss can only be found when the incessant chattering of the mind is quietened and the true self within is known:

tada drashtuh svarupe avasthanam [Yoga Sutra 3,I]

5.6.2. Anatomy of the mind

The actual brain structure holds little importance in yogic anatomy, except as housing or scaffolding for three important glands, namely the pineal, hypothalamus and pituitary glands (*Chapter 6: Yogic Anatomy & Ayurvĕda*).

Like modern Western anatomy, the mind has its own architecture which is known as subtle anatomy, or anatomy of light. The mind cannot be seen directly but its presence can be constructed from its machinations (known as *vritti*). A large part of the yogic journey is self-study and the study of relevant texts (or *svadhyaya*) to understand one's mind, then applying the principles of practice to move towards a state of equilibrium and stillness. Thus, yogic anatomy of the mind shares many common foundations with the science of psychology.

In yogic anatomy, the individual mind is called *citta*. It is part of the Universal Mind, known as *cit*. The relationship between *citta* and *cit* is analogous to the relationship between a drop of water and the vast ocean from which the drop of water comes from. The boundary that stops our individual mind from merging with its limitless potential is the ego. The ego has the same effect on the mind as a water container does on a handful of water: water encased in the container is trapped by the solid boundary of the container and is not free to assume its own shape and form. The water becomes defined by its container – the water becomes the shape, colors and textures of its container and loses its natural fluidity and beauty. The practice of yoga frees the mind from its container, so that it can merge with the Universal Mind and achieve its potential. When a person reaches this stage of freedom, his mind is said to be in the superconscious state.

5.6.3. States of consciousness

There are four levels of consciousness in the human mind:
1. The unconscious
2. The subconscious
3. The conscious
4. The superconscious

The conscious mind: Feel it with *yogasana*

The conscious mind
The conscious mind is the part of you that is awakened, that drives your thoughts and actions, and that makes you the unique person that you are. No two persons are identical, because the conscious mind creates an individual who is as unique as fingerprints, shaped by his history, acquired knowledge, learned responses and life's experiences. *Yogasana* works by heightening the awareness of bodily sensations in the conscious mind.

The subconscious mind: Experience it with meditation

The subconscious mind

The subconscious mind sits below the conscious. Thoughts from this level are intangible, vague impressions that sometimes penetrate the barrier. It is in meditation that thoughts and images from the subconscious surface.

The unconscious mind

The unconscious mind is where our primal and basic instincts arise from. In psychoanalysis, the unconscious is a technical term meaning 'that part of the psyche that cannot be directly observed'.

We would say that an inanimate object is unconscious, but according to several ancient philosophies, everything has consciousness. In a rock, that consciousness is buried deep in the unconscious, so inanimate objects such as rock appears unconscious.

The superconscious mind

As with the unconscious mind, not much is known about the superconscious mind. And because it is such an unknown entity, myths and theories about the superconscious mental state are plentiful. It is commonly believed that once the superconscious state is achieved, the person experiences abundance, bliss and amazing abilities.

It is also believed that Leonardo da Vinci was one of the most prolific geniuses ever lived because he managed to tap into his superconscious mind.

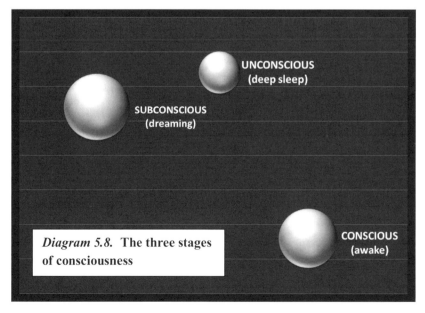

Diagram 5.8. **The three stages of consciousness**

5.6.4. Moving through the states of consciousness

Each day, we move through the three stages of consciousness smoothly and organically, as we move from deep sleep (unconscious) to the dreaming state (subconscious) to being awake (conscious).

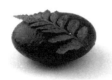

 state

When we are awake, the gross state is experienced – we do things, we say things, we interact. This is characterized by the five elements of Earth, Water, Fire, Air, and Space in their <u>gross</u> form (*bhuta*). It is from these elements that all physical things are built. This gross realm is born from the subtle realm of the subconscious state.

Subconscious state

In the subconscious state, the gross state retreats and the subtle state rolls forward in a dreamlike flow. This is the domain of the five elements of Earth, Water, Fire, Air and Space in their <u>etheric or subtle</u> aspect (*tattva*). These five subtle elements map onto the five similar ones in the gross form (*bhuta*) of the conscious state.

In meditation, one sometimes encounters the same experience as the dreaming state. Though it is an achievement for the practitioner to experience the nuances of this subtle state, she has to let go of those sensations to reach deeper into her Inner Self.

Unconscious state

In deep sleep, we let go of all sensations as the mind moves towards the unconscious state. This is the causal realm, where nothing is manifested yet.

The practice of Yoga Nidra delivers its practitioners an experience of this state: there is nothing there but emptiness, like a blank canvas waiting to be painted.

<u>The superconscious mind</u>

Not much is known of this realm.

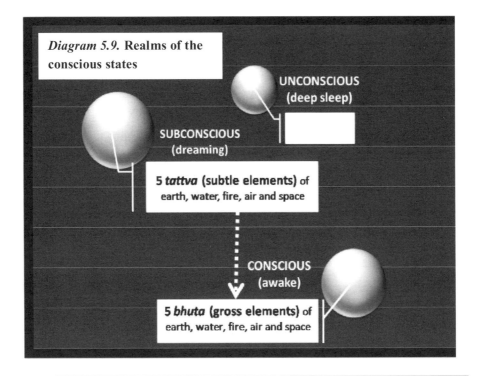

Diagram 5.9. **Realms of the conscious states**

UNCONSCIOUS
(deep sleep)

SUBCONSCIOUS
(dreaming)

5 *tattva* (subtle elements) of earth, water, fire, air and space

CONSCIOUS
(awake)

5 *bhuta* (gross elements) of earth, water, fire, air and space

5.6.5. Birth of the mind

[REFER TO *section 2.2.2*]

From the yogic perspective, the transformation of subtle elements into the gross is as seamless as moving from a dreamlike state into the wakeful state. According to Samkhya philosophy, the individualized mind is born of the unmanifested state, or *Brahma*:

From *Brahma* to *purusha* and *prakriti*
From the unmanifested state known *Brahma* (*Chapter 2: Philosophy, Ethics & Lifestyle*), *purusha* and *prakriti* come into being.

From *purusha* and *prakriti* to *Mahad*
The potential energy of *purusha* and the creative will of *prakriti* coming together set forth a chain of events which begins with the creation of *Mahad*, the first expression of creation. *Mahad* is the supreme intelligence that manifests itself in every being, infusing it with its intrinsic intelligence. You only have to look at the complexity of cellular functions (*Chapter 4: Physiology*) to marvel at how something as tiny as a single cell could operate with the efficiency and complexity of a major factory. *Mahad* is *cit*.

<u>From *Mahad* to *ahamkara* and *buddhi*</u>

From the pure, undifferentiated intelligence known as *Mahad* comes another level of existence, namely the sense of "I am", or *ahamkara*. *Ahamkara* is the ego. You experience the ego each time you look at an external object or another person and register that separateness in your mind. With the creation of the boundary, *Mahad* becomes *buddhi*, which is individualized reasoning powers and intellect, or the individual mind.

5.6.6. From mind to matter

According to Samkhya philosophy (*Chapter 2: Philosophy, Ethics & Lifestyle*), from the vibrations of cosmic *prana*, the sleeping matter is agitated to split into three parts. These three parts become the universal qualities, known as *guna*. The *guna* are of three different flavors (Koay, 2006):

Table 5.1. **The three universal qualities**

Guna	Analogy	Taste description	Quality
Sattva	Perfectly ripe apple	Purity and freshness	Spiritual, light
Rajas	Unripe apple	Sour and tart	Fire, movement, change
Tamas	Over-ripe apple	Heavy and rotting	Darkness, inertia

Extrapolating from *Table 5.1*, the qualities of *tamas* are those that are associated with inertia and heaviness. The heaviness of *tamas* brings inactivity, sleep and unconsciousness. It is darkness, confusion.

But there is no such thing as a bad thing in Yoga Philosophy. Everything has to exist in balance with each other, and the Universe is in equilibrium. Without *tamas*, nothing is tangible; all our experiences are ethereal and fleeting.

Tamas gives us our sensory experiences of the material world (the inorganic universe) through our perception of sound, touch, form, taste and odor (*diagram 5.11*). It is the mass that creates the objects of our sensory experiences.

Diagram 5.10. Tamas and sensory perceptions

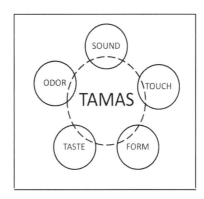

While *tamas* is inertia and unconsciousness, *sattva* is the light of consciousness; it is potential energy. Rajas is characterized by movement and change, like the intense activity going on inside an unripe apple; it is kinetic energy, or energy of movement and change (*diagram 5.12*):

Diagram 5.11. The energetic properties of the three gunas

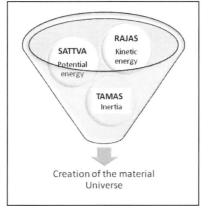

From Albert Einstein's $E = mc^2$, arguably the most famous equation of all time, energy and mass are interchangeable, that is to say, mass and energy are the same thing:

$E = m\,c^2$, where

• E = energy
• m = mass
• c = the speed of light in a vacuum (celeritas), (about 3×108 m/s)

The kinetic energy of *rajas* is the catalyst for the creation of our Universe, in the same manner that the cosmic vibrations of *prana* gave rise to the three *guna*. From *sattva*, the organic universe is born. The organic universe is the being that is us: the mind, the five sensory faculties (*jñānendriya*) and the five motor faculties (*karmendriya*). (*diagram 5.13*) From *tamas*, the inorganic universe of the five objects of sensory perception (*tanmātrā*) is born. These five *tanmātrā* are the qualities of the five gross elements (*bhuta*) (*diagram 5.14*)

Diagram 5.12. **The creation of the organic universe**

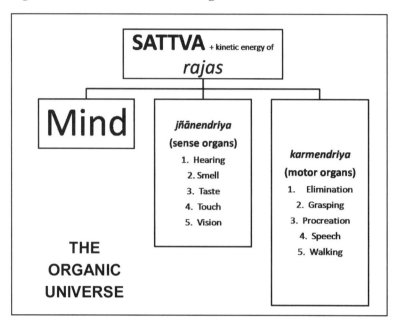

Diagram 5.13. **The creation of the inorganic universe**

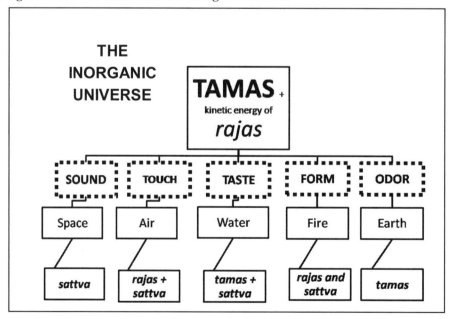

5.6.7. Manifestations of the mind

As discussed in *section 5.6.5*, with the creation of the sense of 'I-ness' or *ahamkara*, the supreme intelligence (*Mahad*) is differentiated into individual intelligence (*buddhi*).

From the interaction of *sattva* and *rajas, manas* is born. *Manas* receives impressions from the recording facilities (*jñānendriya*) (*diagram 5.13*). Together, the *ahamkara, buddhi* and *manas* form a system which is equivalent to the Western physiological models (*Chapter 4: Physiology*).

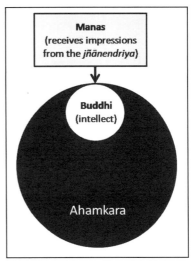

Diagram 5.14. Ahamkara, buddhi and *manas*

How this system operates in real life

Your *jñānendriya* are assailed by the sensory inputs of your workplace: your colleagues and the external badges that they wear: new car, foreign holidays, designer clothes, expensive perfume. Your *manas* processes this information and passes it to your *buddhi*. Your *buddhi* reasons that your colleagues are more successful than you.   Your *ahamkara* screams, "Damn! I will have to take out a bank loan to buy an expensive new car and better designer clothes to show my colleagues I am as good, if not better, than they."

Because of faulty perception and spiritual laziness, human beings become obsessed with unimportant things (for example social status, material possessions and external signs of success) to the extent that they live each day of their lives unconsciously (existing each day instead of living life to the full).

The unimportant things are all mere dressings for the ego: the more you have, the larger your ego. When your ego becomes so large that it shadows the real you, this situation is known as *asmita*. You lose sight of the true meaning of life when your ego is so huge and demanding that it prevents light from shining on you.

Diagram 5.15. Asmita.

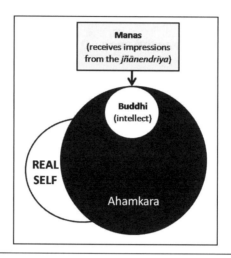

5.6.8. Pathology of the ego

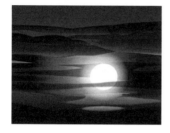

The machinations of the mind (*vritti*) cloud the True Self that lies within.

Vritti sarypyam

itaratra

[Yoga Sutra 4, I]

The ego is largely a construct of the mind. On the positive side, ego gives us a sense of self-pride, drive and ambition. It is our identity. But fuelled by a society that celebrates excess, the negative side of the ego becomes more prevalent. In a world that has lost its values, the ego drives us to mindlessly grab for more in our misguided quest to be "successful" (Koay, 2008).

Feeding the rampant ego could suck all the energy and resource out of a person. The typical man living in the pressurized modern world has his conscious mind exhausted by the demands of the modern lifestyle – salary, mortgage, pension, school tuition, job promotion, pay rise, new car, vacations, an "improved" lifestyle and so forth. These become his world view, as his mind is in the lowest level of consciousness (*mudha*).

In this state of mind, he limits the breadth of his reality to these benchmarks. He fixes his perspectives on these false values. His vision narrows. He goes through life like a zombie. Fixated on grabbing more, he neglects the other areas of his life. The areas that he neglects in his pursuit of a false god may well be his health, the relationship with his family, his spiritual wellbeing and personal growth.

Living in the modern world, chances are his familial ties are not strong, and he has not invested enough in his faith or his community to be able to draw the support he needs from them when things go wrong in his life, or when the benchmark he sacrifices his life for is not realized. He is cut loose with no life jacket.

What we then see is the scourge of modern life that medical science is not always successful in treating. According to Hindu scriptures, this is the age of Kali, or the age of darkness. We see diseases such as degenerative diseases, cardiovascular conditions, drug abuse, stress, anxiety attack, depression, insomnia, obesity and other dietary ailments on the rise. Pills, injections and other quick fixes typified by Western medicine do not address the underlying problem within, and solution – if any – is often temporary and superficial in nature.

LIVE PATANJALI!
Yoga Wisdom for Everyday Living

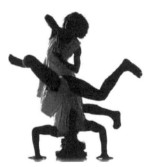

Yoga silences the chattering of the mind.

yogaschittavritti nirodhah

[Yoga Sutra 2, I]

Following the yoga path does not mean renouncing modern life. In fact, in the renaissance of yoga, yogis were urged to be householders instead of pious hermits living in remote caves. These ancient yogis were exhorted to live their yoga in the "real" world. This is because the world exists to set us free.

It is in the world that we see the workings of yoga. Although yoga is not the cure for all modern diseases, practicing Yoga Philosophy is effective in helping one manage one's life better. With a yogic frame of mine, one is better equipped to cope with the challenges of modern, pressurized living. Yoga Philosophy also provides an internal infrastructure and value system that are thousands of years old. Self-study and study of spiritual texts (*svadhyaya*) ensures that one has a self-checking mechanism and a moral compass in a world that has lost its values.

The physical practice of *yogasana* has been shown to improve health (Kjellgren, *et al*), and health is an important component in a yogic life, because the body is our soul's earthly vehicle.Being a yogi means never surrendering your consciousness, because consciousness is ecstasy. It means being awake, aware and conscious every waking moment of your life. consciousness (*anu*) to universal consciousness (*vibhu*), from merging your *citta* with its source, *cit*.

5.7. Yogic practices for a healthy brain and mind

5.7.1. How yoga works

Yoga equips practitioners with effective tools to deal with the challenges of modern society. A *yogasana* class creates a certain amount of challenge, pressure and stress for the yogi, and it is through applying the principles of yoga, as outlined in Patanjali's Yoga Sutra, that the yogi learns how to meet these challenges, pressures and stress with grace and equanimity. Lessons learned on the mat are transportable to real life, and this is one of the most important contributions of yoga to the modern world.

The mind and the brain thrive on information. *Svadhyaya* provides *sattvic* (pure) food for the conscious mind and meditation gives expression to the deep subconscious mind. Yoga is about eradicating the barriers between the conscious and subconscious levels. On the one hand, reflex actions are brought to the conscious realm so that the yogi has a better mastery of his body. On the other hand, by continuous and long practice, *yogasana* brings deliberate, conscious actions to the subconscious level. This allows the yogi to flow through his *vinyasa* with minimal conscious effort, leaving the conscious mind free to enjoy the sensations of the *yogasana*.

5.7.2. The practices

Within the eight limbs of *ashtanga yoga*, one will find all the necessary components for living a happy, healthy and spiritual life:

1. *Yama* (the basis of *karma* yoga – yoga of action)
2. *Niyama* (the basis of *karma* yoga – yoga of action)
3. *Asana* (the basis of *karma* yoga – yoga of action)
4. *Pranayama* (the basis of *jnâna* yoga – yoga of knowledge)
5. *Pratyhara* (the basis of *jnâna* yoga – yoga of knowledge)
6. *Dharana* (the basis of *jnâna* yoga – yoga of knowledge)
7. *Dhyana* (the basis of *bhakti* yoga – yoga of love and devotion)
8. *Samadhi* (the basis of *bhakti* yoga – yoga of love and devotion)

The path of *ashtanga yoga* has been covered in detail in Chapter 2 (*Chapter 2: Philosophy, Ethics & Lifestyle*).

Regular physical exercise (*yogasana*)

Make exercise a part of your daily lifestyle!

There is evidence indicating that regular practice *yogasana* or other similar form of physical exercise has profound benefits on the brain function (van Praagh, 2009).

With old age, the brain goes into decline and is often beset by diseases such as Alzheimer's and Parkinson's. However, it is never too early to start making regular exercise a part of your life to safeguard your brain's health. Research has shown that early life physical activity may delay late-life cognitive deficits (Dik, Deeg, Visser, and Jonker, 2003).

Mental exercise (*svadhyaya*)

Learn something new everyday

Keeping the mind challenged with activities such as learning a new language or doing crossword puzzles keeps the brain active.

Healthy diet (*sattvic*)

Eat well

Pinilla (2006) showed that dietary factors are a powerful means to influence brain function on a daily basis. Diets rich in omega-3 fatty acids, vitamin E or the curry spice curcumin benefit cognitive function. Conversely, saturated fat increases metabolic distress and reduces learning and memory.

Meditate (*dhyana*)

Meditation: start with 3 minutes a day

For centuries, meditation has been practiced for cultivation of well-being and emotional balance.

Recent studies show that meditation may affect multiple pathways that could play a role in brain aging and mental fitness (Doraiswamy and Xiong, 2003). Although its mechanisms are at an investigational stage, it is proposed that meditation may reduce the risk of cerebrovascular disease and age-related neurodegeneration (Doraiswamy, *et al*, 2003).

A happy frame of mind (*sukha*)

Be happy!

The concept of happiness as a factor is often overlooked in therapeutic terms. However, some evidence has emerged recently suggesting that improvements in patient status can result from interventions to improve the patient's level of happiness in diseases, including epilepsy, Huntington's disease, multiple sclerosis, Parkinson's disease and stroke (Barak and Achiron, 2009).

Diagram 5.16. **Yogic practices for a healthy brain and mind.**

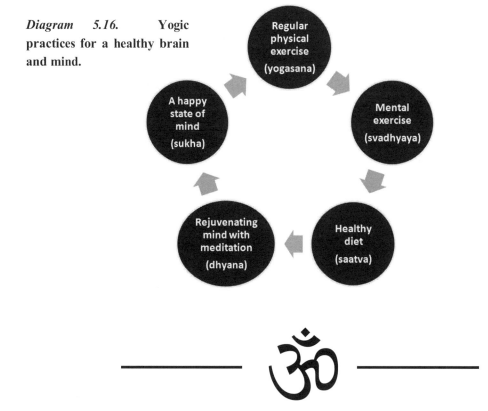

References

Barak, Y., & Achiron, A. (2009). Happiness and neurological diseases. *Expert Rev Neurother.* 2009 Apr;9(4):445-59.

Dik, M., Deeg, D.J., Visser, M., & Jonker C.(2003**).** Early life physical activity and cognition at old age. *J Clin Exp Neuropsychol.* 2003 Aug;25(5):643-53.

Doraiswamy, P.M., & Xiong, G.L. (2003). Does Meditation Enhance Cognition and Brain Longevity? *Ann N Y Acad Sci.* 2007 Sep 28. [Epub ahead of print]

Farthing, G. W. (1992). *The psychology of consciousness.* NJ, USA: Prentice Hall

Hawton, K.., & van Heeringen, K. (2009). Suicide. *The Lancet,* Volume 373, Issue 9672, 1372 – 1381.

Hebb, D. O. (1974). What psychology is about. *American Psychologist, 29,* 71-79.

Huitt, W. (1996). The mind. *Educational Psychology Interactive.* Valdosta, GA: Valdosta State University. Retrieved April 24, 2009, from http://chiron.valdosta.edu/whuitt/col/summary/mind.html

Kjellgren, A., Bood, S.A., Axelsson, K., Norlander, T., & Saatcioglu F. (2007). Wellness through a comprehensive yogic breathing program - a controlled pilot trial. *BMC Complement Altern Med.* 2007 Dec 19;7:43.

Koay, J. (2006). *The Kundalini Yoga Cookbook.* London, UK: Gaia Octopus.

Koay, J. (2008). *Live Patanjali! Yoga Wisdom for Everyday Living.* London, UK: Sun Yoga.

Michalsen, A., Grossman, P., Acil, A., Langhorst, J., Lüdtke, R., Esch, T., Stefano, G.B., & Dobos, G.J. (2005). Rapid stress reduction and anxiolysis among distressed women as a consequence of a three-month intensive yoga program. *Med Sci Monit.* 2005 Dec;11(12):CR555-561. Epub 2005 Nov 24

Northwestern University (2007, March 13). Music Training 'Tunes' Human Auditory System. *ScienceDaily.* Retrieved April 24, 2009, from http://www.sciencedaily.com /releases/2007/03/070312152003.htm

Pinilla, F.G. (2006). The impact of diet and exercise on brain plasticity and disease. *Nutr Health.* 2006;18(3):277-84.

Robin, M. (2002). *A Physiological Handbook for Teachers of Yogasana.* USA: Fenestra Books.

Solomon, R. (1980). The opponent-process theory of acquired motivation: The costs of pleasure and the benefits of pain. *American Psychologist, 8,* 691-712

Udupa, K.N. (1996). *Stress and Its Management by Yoga.* India: Motilal Banarsidass.

Van Praagh, H. (2009). Exercise and the brain: something to chew on. *Trends Neurosci.* 2009 Apr 4. [Epub ahead of print]

CHAPTER SIX

Yogic Anatomy & Ayurvĕda

OVERVIEW OF THE CHAPTER

6.1   Anatomy of light
6.2   Ayurvĕda
6.3   The three *dosha*
6.4   *Dhatu, ojas* and *tejas*
6.5   *Prana* and *agni*
6.6   Energy conduits of the body
6.7   The *chakra* system
6.8   The subtle bodies
6.9   The yogic way to good health

6.1. Anatomy of light

6.1.1. Introduction

Yogic anatomy is the anatomy of light. While much of early Western anatomy's body of knowledge was gleaned from dissection of cadavers, yogic knowledge in this field has been based on the study of living bodies.

Over the centuries, the observations made by early healers were verified by generations of practitioners, and this long process of testing, observing and verifying gives yogic anatomy as much legitimacy as Western anatomy. Yogic anatomy has stood the test of time, though its exact workings have never been elucidated.

Indeed, with the advent of dissection, several key features of yogic anatomy were found to correlate with the Western view. Yogic anatomy also shares many similar concepts with ancient Eastern healing sciences, such as chi, meridians, yin and yang, among others.

6.1.2. Advent of modern Western medicine

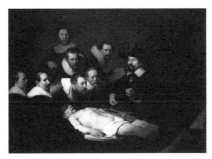

Diagram 6.1 "Anatomy Lesson of Dr. Nicolaes Tulp" by Rembrandt van Rijn, 1632.

Early European medicine was largely folk medicine-based. Its practices were largely built on superstitions and beliefs that were handed down, often with little proof of the efficacy of a particular treatment other than hearsay and blind faith. Cures and remedies were based on plants, charms, and rituals unique to a specific folk culture. Medicine in the Dark and Middle Ages were often associated with witchcraft and shamanism.

In early times, physicians rarely came in physical contact with the patients and made their diagnoses from looking at flasks of urine from the patients (Fischer, 2005), from which a skilled physician could allegedly divine over 1,000 diagnoses. There was, of course, no systemized training for medical professionals at that time.

Early anatomy classes were public events no different to a pantomime, where the paying public came in their hordes to watch a charismatic surgeon chopping up a dead body or sawing away some body part of a live patient. (Prior to the discovery of anesthesia, limbs were sawed off with the patient conscious and forcibly held down by assistants, while the surgeon sawed away and the public gaped).

These early surgeons shared the same professional strata with barbers and other craftsmen, rather than with "gentlemen" physicians. The surgeons belonged to the professional guild of the Barber-Surgeons' Company rather than a medical association. Indeed, there had always been differences between surgery and medicine from the Middle Ages and the Renaissance (Fischer).

Early scientists, with their clear and thorough methodology (experimental design, research protocol, data-gathering and analysis) began changing the face of the medical establishment by establishing common principles of good practice for both physicians and surgeons.

One of the biggest killers in early times was infections. Doctors did not know about germs, the invisible killer and patients often died of sepsis. Some of the early fathers of change in this field were:

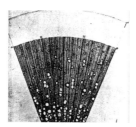

- Antonie van Leeuwenhoek (1632-1723) who first observed cork cells under a microscope and then widened his field of study to the understanding of micro-organisms.

Diagram 6.2. Microscopic section through one year old ash (*Fraxinus*) wood. Drawing of Antonie van Leeuwenhoek.

- Ignaz Semmelweis (1818-1865) who expanded the scope of Leeuwenhoek's work and introduced hygiene standards for physicians attending birthing women;

- Joseph Lister (1827-1912) proved the principles of antisepsis. He introduced carbolic acid to sterilize wounds and surgical instruments, thus cutting down death by sepsis dramatically.

Modern Western medicine has advanced to great heights today, to the extent that it appears more like science fiction! We can put tiny cameras and robots into human bodies, surgeons are able to perform operations remotely and spare body parts can be grown in laboratories are amongst the feats of modern Western medicine. The great drawback is, of course, that in becoming so specialized, modern Western medical science has become compartmentalized, sacrificing the benefits of a more holistic approach and a more integrated treatment protocol. Going to your local general practitioner with symptoms that fall outside the common and you will be referred to a stranger, a specialist, who has never seen you before; if the aforesaid specialist could not figure out what is wrong with you, you are passed on to the next. Thus, it is not uncommon for a person suffering from a less-than-straightforward ailment to see several specialists who work independent of each other, with no one professional pulling together a whole care package.

Current thinking is leaning towards a more interdisciplinary approach towards healthcare, with traditional ('alternative') medicine such as homeopathy being offered alongside conventional healthcare. In the United Kingdom, the London Homeopathic Hospital became a part of the University College London Hospitals in 2002, and its services are available under the National Health Service, as part of the government's commitment to integrate complementary and conventional care.

6.1.3. Foundations of holistic medical sciences

Medical sciences from its earliest inception were simply practices to maintain the continuity of life. From the earliest communities of cave dwellers, rituals surrounding the management of births, diseases and deaths had formed the cornerstone of this art.

One of the oldest cave arts ever discovered (Lascaux, France, portrayed the use of plants as medicine, which shows that medicine had been practiced as far back as 13,000 and 25,000 BC (from radiocarbon dating the Lascaux cave drawings to ascertain the age). From the common roots that the holistic sciences share with the Western branch, the Eastern medical sciences remain largely unchanged (except to refine its age-old practices).

6.1.4. Branches of the holistic medical sciences

The holistic medical sciences are frequently referred to as complementary medicine or alternative therapies. Increasingly, they are being practiced alongside conventional medicine to deliver an integrated healthcare system, though some physicians still maintain a closed mind about non-Western practices.

6.2. Ayurvĕda

6.2.1. An introduction

If yogic anatomy is mapped onto modern Western anatomy, then the equivalent to physiology as discussed in this chapter is Ayurvĕda. Ayurvĕda is the oldest healing system in the universe. It is the medical science that predates all medical knowledge.

Ayurvĕda is a large and complex field that rarely a book can do justice to, let alone a chapter within a book. The purpose of this discourse is therefore no more than the briefest introduction to this science.

Ayuh is life, and *véda* is knowledge. As such, Ayurvĕda is about understanding life, its nature, scope and purpose. It goes beyond what is here and now to seeking out the Creator, knowing the Creator and expressing that Divinity in our everyday life. It is therefore about the body, mind and soul. Ayurvĕda is living science, because new knowledge and methods are added to its corpus of ancient wisdom. Its main objective is to achieve optimal health and well-being through a comprehensive approach that addresses mind, body, behavior, and environment. The main difference between Ayurvĕda and Western medicine is that in Ayurvĕda, there is no specialization of fields as there are in Western medicine, for example, cardiology, oncology, urology, etc. In Ayurvĕda, the belief is treating the whole person, and treating each person as an individual, and perhaps most importantly, imparting personal responsibility for one's health.

An Ayurvĕda physician gets to know the patient and works in partnership with the patient to deliver an integrated healthcare system based on the patient's individual constitution, stage of life, lifestyle and state of health, with attention paid to the health of mind, body and soul. Yoga as a practice is often integrated into Ayurvĕda.

This chapter will only cover Ayurvĕda to the level and depth required to give readers an appreciation of this integral part of yogi science, and how it relates to the path and in the life of a serious yoga practitioner. A complete treatise on Ayurvĕda is outside the scope of this book.

6.2.2. Origins of Ayurvĕda

Ayurvĕda did not originate from the minds of men, of mere mortals. Deep in Indian history, the *rishi* (or seers) and sages who lived ascetic lives in remote caves and mountains meditated for long periods, and pure wisdom and knowledge came to them when they were deep in meditation. This knowledge was passed on to their disciples. At its dawn, Ayurvedic knowledge was passed down in oral tradition, from one heart to another, throughout the ages. The knowledge was held in nuggets called Sutra, which are not unlike Sri Patanjali's Yoga Sutra (*Chapter 2: Philosophy, Ethics & Lifestyle*). These nuggets were assimilated by the students, became a part of them, and in time, they were handed over to the next generation, often by oral transmission.

The knowledge was written down into scriptures called Vedas, or bodies of knowledge. Ayurvĕda is contained in the Vedas. The three classic books of Ayurvĕda are *Charaka*, *Sushruta* and *Vagbhata*.

6.2.3. Ayurvĕda in the Western world

Ayurvĕda is widely practiced in India, and is slowly gaining recognition by the Western medical professionals (*Note 2 at the end of this section*). Modern scientific research methods have been applied to Ayurvĕda to study is effectiveness in managing and treating various diseases such as cancer (Balachandran and Govindarajan, 2005).

Whereas Western allopathic medicine is excellent in handling acute medical crises, Ayurvĕda demonstrates an ability to manage chronic disorders that Western medicine has been unable to (Sharma, Chandola, Singh and Basisht, 2007).

Sharma *et al* (2007) proposed that Ayurvĕda may be an effective treatment for cardiovascular diseases (17 million deaths annually worldwide), cancer (22 million diagnosed in 2000) and diabetes (171 million diagnosed in 2000), because modern Western medicine in some instances has even contributed to the ill health of the patients who utilize it though toxic side effects and other iatrogenic disorders (Sharma *et al*, 2007).

Turmeric, the common spice used in cooking (also known as curcumin, Latin name *Curcuma longa*), has been shown in various scientific research to have medicinal qualities. Most notable are its anti-inflammatory properties and its role as a therapeutic agent in wound healing, diabetes, Alzheimer's, Parkinson's, cardiovascular and pulmonary diseases, and arthritis.

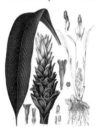

Diagram 6.3.
Image from Koehler's Medicinal-Plants 1887

Ayurvĕdic pharmaceutical science was collated from the various scriptures by Săranghadhara. There has been an upsurge in demand for Ayurvĕda-based remedies because synthetic drugs are considered to be unsafe (Subhose, Srinivas and Narayana, 2005). However, the wide-scale manufacture of these traditional herbal medicines needs to be developed further with the participation of practitioners from both the allopathic and non-allopathic systems to optimize the risk-benefit profiles of Ayurvĕdic medicines (Gogtay, Bhatt, Dalvi and Kshirsagar, 2002).

Note 1: Ayurvĕdic medicine does not lend itself to the over-the-counter approach, as Ayurvĕda only works when it is specially prescribed for the individual by a trained physician after a thorough consultation. The prescription handed out alongside dietary advice and lifestyle changes, amongst others.

Note 2: Though widely practiced by Asian Indians living in the United States, Ayurv ĕda has not crossed into the mainstream yet. Satow, Kumar, Burke and Inciardi (2008) conducted a survey of 64 Asian Indians living in North Carolina and though 95% of the participants were aware of Ayurĕda, 78% had knowledge of Ayurvedic products or treatments, and about 59% had used or were currently using Ayurĕda, only 18% of those using Ayurvĕda had informed their Western medical doctors.

6.3. **The three** *dosha*

6.3.1. **The foundations**

Ayurvĕdic medicine is based on an individual's characteristics and body frame rather than oriented toward treating disease or sickness. According to Sharma *et al* (2007), treatment of disease with the *Ayurvĕda* method is highly individualized and depends on the psychophysiologic constitution of the patient. There are different dietary and lifestyle recommendations for each season of the year. In addition, an individual's program is tailored according to the psychophysiologic constitution of the patient.

From the interplay of energies between the five gross causative elements known as *bhuta* (*section 5.6.6*), the organic and inorganic universes are born. From the Unmanifested Universe, the vibrations of *prana* created Space (also known as Ether). From the flow of Space, Air came into being. In turn, the flow of Air caused friction, and the resultant heat and light brought Fire into being. Fire burned, and liquefied certain ethereal elements, which became Water. Water solidified to become Earth. Earth is the mother of all beings, alive and inanimate (*Diagram 6.4*):

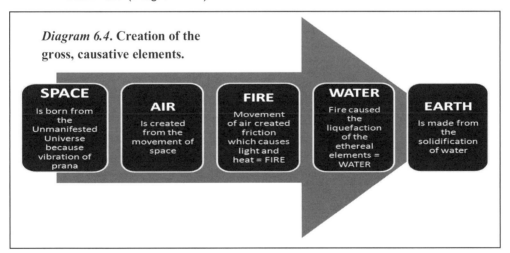

Diagram 6.4. **Creation of the gross, causative elements.**

SPACE — Is born from the Unmanifested Universe because vibration of prana

AIR — Is created from the movement of space

FIRE — Movement of air created friction which causes light and heat = FIRE

WATER — Fire caused the liquefaction of the ethereal elements = WATER

EARTH — Is made from the solidification of water

The five gross causative elements of Earth, Water, Fire, Air and Space are organized into three basic types of energy or functional principles. The name given to this organizational principle is *dosha*. There are three *dosha*, namely *vata, pitta* and *kapha* from the five *bhuta* (*Diagram 6.5*):

Diagram 6.5. **The three *dosha* from the five *bhuta*.**

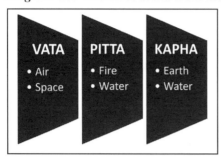

The *dosha* support life; they are forces that can sometimes go out of balance. For example, if they are not expelled efficiently from the body, their over accumulation causes a disequilibrium and disease and sickness may result.

From these five *bhuta*, too, human beings are created and organized into the three *dosha* types.

6.3.2. *Dosha* and their attributes

The most revered Ayurvĕdic text, the *Charaka Samhita*, which was written by the ancient physician Charaka, stated that all elements (both organic and inorganic), and actions as well as thoughts, have their own definite attributes. According to *Ayurvĕda*, there are twenty basic attributes, arranged in ten opposite pairs. These pairs function together, like night and day, and must be in balance with each other. These twenty attributes underpin the practice of Ayurvĕda, from pharmacology to food preparation, from the inorganic to the organic, and from thoughts to actions.

Diagram 6.6. **Dosha and their attributes**

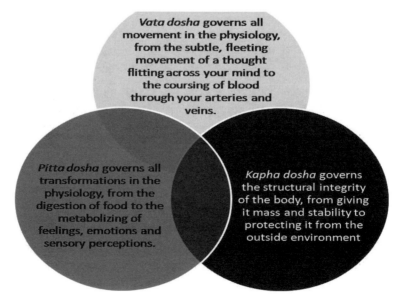

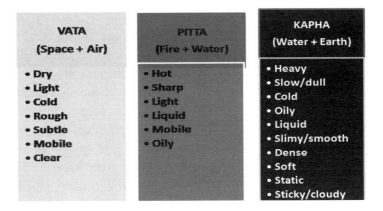

VATA (Space + Air)	PITTA (Fire + Water)	KAPHA (Water + Earth)
• Dry • Light • Cold • Rough • Subtle • Mobile • Clear	• Hot • Sharp • Light • Liquid • Mobile • Oily	• Heavy • Slow/dull • Cold • Oily • Liquid • Slimy/smooth • Dense • Soft • Static • Sticky/cloudy

6.3.3. *Doshic* signature

Each of us is a microcosm of the Universe: the elements of Space, Air, Fire, Water and Earth are expressed in us and play a role in our anatomy and physiology. These elements pair up to form our *dosha* signature. A person's combination and proportions of *vata, pitta* and *kapha* are determined at conception (genetics, emotional state of parents and other factors at the moment of conception) but are also affected by external factors such as diet, state of mind and lifestyle. A person's combination and proportions of the three *dosha* at birth is his *prakriti.*

For example, a person could be mainly *kapha* with small proportions of *vata* and *pitta* in her *doshic* makeup, or a person could have all three *dosha* in equal proportions. The degree of variation in the *dosha* proportions affects that person's predisposition to health, behavioral traits and outlook in life.

But two persons with the same *dosha* composition will not necessarily have the same characteristics, because within the *dosha*, there are sub-*dosha* which account for the micro-differences. Also, within *dosha*, there are different characteristics. For example, a *vata*-dominant person may be cold, whereas another person of similar *doshic* make-up may be dry. Overall well-being depends on keeping the *dosha* in balance. Any imbalance among the *tridosha* causes a state of unhealthiness or disease. Though diet can rarely affect the genetics, proper management of lifestyle, appropriate food intake and attitude can improve a person's wellbeing tremendously.

For example, a person whose dosha is in equal proportion under normal circumstances may become too *vata* if she has recently undergone an emotional trauma. Alternatively, she may become too *kaphic* if she had been eating too much unhealthy food and neglects exercising her body. *Dosha* imbalance is manifested in the physical body as sickness and disease. A person seeking medical advice from an Ayurvĕdic physician would have to fill in detailed questionnaires to ascertain the *doshic* signatures of his physical and mental states before a course of treatment can be prescribed. This may include yoga, meditation, traditional massage, dietary changes and herbs.

6.3.4. Characteristics of *vata*

Vata is air and movement. Therefore, its attributes are mobile, clear, light, subtle, cold, dry and rough. *Vata* individuals are good motivators, good at starting projects but often move on instead of seeing something to completion. To be close to a *vata* individual, you have to be prepared for change!

An individual who is *vata*-dominant physically typically has:

- slender frame
- lightweight bone structure
- dry, rough or dark skin
- brown / black hair coloring
- large, crooked or protruding teeth, thin gums
- small thin lips and mouth
- dull, dark eyes

Vata is found throughout the body, especially in the head region, respiratory sites and in the small intestines and colon, where it plays an important role in digestion. Thus, the main functionalities of *vata* are respiration, digestion, movement and thoughts.

A person with *vata* as her main mental constitution is like the breeze. There is often a lightness and swiftness in their step and laughter. They are light sleepers, too. *Vata* individuals are quick and lively in thought, speech and action, and they make friends easily. They thrive on change, and are creative and enthusiastic.

When the *vata* is out of balance, emotionally the individual may experience:

Vata-balancing foods:
- Pureed soup
- Basmati rice
- Mung beans
- Comfort foods like stews
- Blanched nuts

Eat less dried food like crackers and less raw. Eat more sweet, sour and salty.

- anxiety and a feeling of being overwhelmed
- rushing around like a headless chicken but unable to slow down
- sleeplessness
- tendency to forget things, though short term mental activities are fine

Physically, she may experience one or more of the following:
- dry, chapped lips
- dry skin
- brittle hair (with split ends if long)
- abdominal gas
- poor digestion and decreased bowel movement.

Factors that exacerbate *vata* imbalance include eating too much dry or raw food and ice cold drinks. A hectic daily schedule, too much travel and too much mental activity also make this imbalance worse.

6.3.5. Characteristics of *pitta*

Pitta is predominantly fire with some water in it. It is the energy that creates heat in the body and fires the body up for digestion (it is the source of the flame, but not the flame itself). Its attributes are heat, lightness, sharpness, acidity, oiliness and liquidity. *Pitta*-dominant individuals often have low tolerance for heat and tend to gravitate towards cooler climes. A *pitta* individual makes an inspired leader.

An individual who is *pitta*-dominant physically typically has:
- medium height and build
- fair to reddish complexion and hair coloring
- small yellowish teeth, soft gums
- green or grayish eyes
- average sized mouth

Pitta is mainly located in the lower stomach and small intestine. It is also found in blood, gallbladder, spleen, liver, eyes, sweat, sebaceous secretions and gray matter of the brain. Its main functions are digestion, maintenance of body temperature and regulating eyesight.

188

When the *pitta* is out of balance, emotionally the individual may experience:

- jealousy
- rampant ambition
- obsession with sex
- temper outburst over minor incidences
- Irritability and frustration

Physically, he may experience one or more of the following:

- excess stomach acid and heartburn
- hair loss
- disturbed sleep pattern
- constant thirst
- increased sensitivity to heat
- skin breaking out in spots or patches

Factors that exacerbate *pitta* imbalance include emotional trauma, over-exposure to heat, poor dietary behavior (skipping meals or irregular mealtimes) and eating too much hot, spicy food.

**Pitta*-balancing food:*

- Use ghee as cooking medium
- Pears
- Mangoes
- Milk and milkshakes
- Carrots
- Leafy greens
- Asparagus
- Basmati rice
- Almonds

Eat more sweet, bitter and astringent

6.3.6. Characteristics of *kapha*

Kapha is Water and Earth. Like water and earth, *kapha* is characterized by heaviness, stability, coldness and softness. It is unbounded, flows freely and offers lubrication and protection. A *kapha* individual makes a good friend. They are loyal, sweet and easy-going. In a relationship, stability is their hallmark and their love of the home.

An individual who is *kapha*-dominant physically typically has:

- large frame with well-padded joints
- tends to be overweight
- thick and pale-colored oily skin
- strong white teeth
- rich, wavy hair
- blue eyes
- full lips / large mouth

Kapha-balancing foods:
- Clear soups
- Bean casseroles
- Steamed broccoli or cauliflower
- Green apples
- Dry cereal
- Salt free crackers

Cut down on sweet, salty and sour!

Physically, she may experience one or more of the following:
- excessive sweating
- oily skin and hair
- feels uncomfortable in hot and clammy environments
- mental fatigue even well-rested
- difficult to be roused (lack of motivation)
- heaviness around head, throat and chest
- clinginess and finds it hard to deal with change
- prefers to be spectator instead of participant

Factors that irritate the *kapha dosha* include a diet of too much deep-fried, sweet and heavy food (especially late at night), ice-cold foods and beverages, having too much daytime sleep and lack of exercise.

6.4. *Dhatu, ojas* and *tejas*

6.4.1. *Dhatu*

When *Vata*, *Pitta* and *Kapha* are in balance in the body, these three *dosha* are referred to as *dhatu* (from the Sanskrit word *dha* which means to "hold in place, keep in place"). This is yogic anatomy's equivalent to Western anatomy's model of the tissue, namely the grouping of cells that perform the same function. From the five *bhuta*, eight *dhatu* are made (*Table 6.2*), with each *dhatu* playing a vital role in growth, reproduction and survival.

Dhatu	Western anatomy equivalent
Rasa "juice of life"	Plasma (liquid part of the blood, excluding red blood cells)
Rakta	Red blood cells
Mamsa	Muscle
Meda	Fatty tissue
Ashi	Bone and cartilage
Majja	Marrow, nerve tissue and connective tissue
Shukra	Male reproductive tissue
Artava	Female reproductive tissue

Each *dhatu* has its own fire, or *agni*, and the *agni* must be strong to maintain the health of the *dhatu*. If one *dhatu* is not functioning well, it will slowly affect others, because the body functions as one completely integrated unit.

As in the Western model of physiology, the capillaries carry nutrients (product of digestion) from the gastrointestinal tract to the tissue. From the end product of digestion, we get the first *dhatu*, when heated with *agni*. This is the *ahara rasa,* the first *dhatu*.

Ahara rasa then matures and becomes nutrients for the second *dhatu,* Some of the *rasa* is also transformed into red blood cell (*rakta*, the second *dhatu*).

Each *dhatu* is created successively (each step takes five days of cooking by *agni*), and undergoes the same process of receiving nutrition, transformation from immature (*asthayi*) *dhatu* to mature (*sthayi*) *dhatu*, and producing end-products. Because each *dhatu* is dependent on its predecessor for its creation, the appropriate quantity and quality of each *dhatu* and its functioning must be balanced for perfect health to be achieved.

All these activities need *agni* to take place. Thus, this internal fire is of central importance in the maintenance of good health according to the principles of Ayurvĕdic Medicine (section *6.5*).

6.4.2. Ojas

Ojas is the essence of life. It is the pure essence of the *dhatu*. When *ahara rasa* (*6.4.1*) is transformed into *rasa dhatu* and other by-products, *ojas* is also created. Every single *dhatu* has the ability to make its own *ojas*. This is localized *ojas*. The *dhatu* in the body is also bathed in collective *ojas*.

Ojas helps to maintain healthy *agni*, and conversely, the quality of *ojas* is influenced by the quality of *agni*. External factors which influence the quality of *ojas* are stress (working too hard on physical activity), lifestyle (too much sex), state of mind, relationships, over-exposure to unhealthy environment and chronic wasting diseases. In the Western view, *ojas* is the immune system.

6.4.3. Tejas

Tejas is the rays of the sun and the solar energy in food (the life energy is *prana*; the protective energy is *ojas*). *Tejas* is what that gives color to our eyes, hair, skin, and aura. This is the first quality of *tejas*. A person with strong *tejas* has bright eyes, clear skin, shiny hair and a bright aura surrounding him.

Ojas, tejas and *prana* combine to form the aura that shields us from harm coming from the outside world. *Ojas* is the substance of the aura, *tejas* is its color and *prana* is its vitality. As thought is the movement of *prana* through time, *tejas* is the form of the thought. It is the intelligence that makes us conscious individuals – it is up to us to find our path to enlightenment.

6.5. *Prana* and *agni*

6.5.1. *Prana* and *agni*

Prana with capitalized 'p' is Life Force. The pulsations of *Prana* in the unmanifested Universe led to creation (*section 5.6.5*). Without *Prana*, there would have been no life.

Prana is not air: the air that we breathe in is *prana* without the capitalization (*section 5.2.2*). *Prana* is made up of both air and space, two of the five main causative elements (*bhuta*). In Chinese medicine, *prana* is known as *chi* (or *qi*).

Space has the same qualities as Consciousness (*cit*), which is the origin of the five elements. But space and Consciousness are not identical, because space is a material entity whereas Consciousness has soul (*atman*) and is alive.

In the body, *Prana* performs respiration, oxygenation and moves energy/cells around the body. *Prana* lights the *agni*, the sacred fire within our body. *Agni* is the light that illuminates our consciousness (*citta*). Without *agni*, there is darkness. *Agni* is what you experience when you light a candle. Physiologically, it is required for the most basic of life's processes, namely digestion, which provides fuel for our cells.

Prana is the requirement for a strong *agni* – weak *agni* results in a weak body. When there is poor digestion, the body is not receiving enough nutrients to build strength and vitality. A strong and healthy *agni* results in a long, healthy life. Agni brings longevity to the body in a similar way that a baked clay pot lasts longer than an unbaked one. It also destroys old, worn cells in order for new ones to be born.

6.5.2. The five *prana*

The five *prana* are the differentiated parts of the universal *Prana,* and each is prefixed with the word *vayu*, which means air. But *vayu* is more than air: the word encompasses movement that is symbolic of life:

Feel your *prana vayu* with:

ardha chandrasana

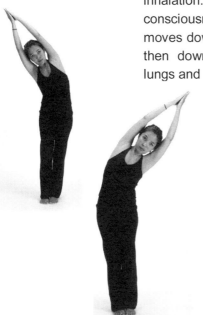

Prana vayu

From *Prana* comes *prana vayu* (or simply known as 'prana'). *Prana* moves thoughts, feelings and emotions. It lives in the head, moving downwards and inwards into the body. It is responsible for all inhalation. When *prana* stills, awareness illuminates consciousness. *Prana vayu* starts from the head and moves downwards and inwards. It moves in the head, then downwards and inwards to the throat, heart, lungs and diaphragm.

Yogasana that stimulate *prana vayu* include:

ardha chandrasana

(standing lateral bends)

....

Feel your *apana vayu* with:

malasana

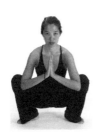

Apana vayu

Apana vayu is found in the abdominal cavity and the sex organs. It is a force that moves downwards and outwards, and stimulates urination, defecation, flatulence, menstruation and childbirth. It nourishes the bones. In pregnancy, *apana vayu* nourishes the fetus.

Yogasana that stimulate *apana vayu* include:

- *malasana*
- *tadasana*
- *anjaneyasana*

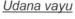

Feel your *udana vayu* with:

ustrasana

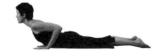

<u>Udana vayu</u>

Udana vayu starts in the diaphragm and is the energy that is responsible for upward movement, for example, speech, vomit and exhalation of carbon dioxide.

From the diaphragm, it moves up via the lungs, bronchus and throat, up to the brain where it stimulates memory.

Yogasana that stimulate *udana vayu* include:
* *ustrasana*
* *sarvangasana*
* *bhujangasana*

Feel your *samana vayu* with:

urdhva dharunasana

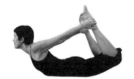

<u>Samana vayu</u>

Samana vayu is found in the navel and small intestines, where it stimulates the production of gastric juices. *Samana vayu* is therefore about *agni*. The movement of *samana vayu* is linear, like peristalsis, as it drives the body to eat, digest and absorb food.

Yogasana that stimulate *samana vayu* include:
* *urdhva dharunasana*
* *marichyasana C & D*
* *apanasana* (wind-relieving pose)

Feel your *vyana vayu* with:

bhujangasana

<u>Vyana vayu</u>

Vyana vayu moves in a circular motion. *Vyana vayu* has the important function of maintaining cardiac activity, circulation (hence oxygenation and nutrition of tissues) and reflex action. It is found in the heart.

Yogasana that stimulate *vyana vayu* include:
* *bhujangasana*
* *salambhasana*

6.5.3. Experiencing the five *prana*

Stand with your feet approximately six to eight inches apart. Focus on the sensations beneath your feet. Feel the ground beneath you. Make the full connection between your feet and the earth. Breathe deeply, drawing in the energy from the earth up your body with each inhale. With each exhale, release slowly into the earth. Surrender to gravity.

Repeat this conscious breathing for several cycles. When you can feel your breath moving in your body, begin with connecting to your *prana vayu* and *apana vayu*.

As you inhale, move your arms to upwards with your breath, palms facing skywards. At the top of your inhale, your hands should be at the level of your upper lungs. This is your body filling up with *prana vayu*. *Prana vayu* starts in the head and moves downwards and inwards. Experience its movement. Hold your breath and still your hands: this is when you experience Pure Consciousness, when *prana vayu* stills.

Now, slowly exhale. Turn your palm earthwards, and move them downwards with your exhalation. Connect with your *apana vayu*, your grounding force. At the end of your exhale, your hands should be straight by your side, a few inches away from your body. Your whole body is relaxed as you let the tension go. Hold still for a heartbeat. Repeat this *prana-apana* cycle for a minute or two.

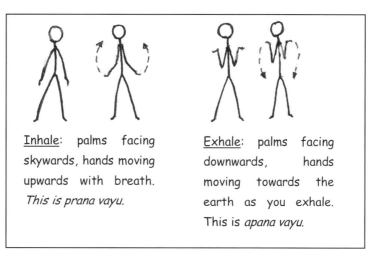

<u>Inhale</u>: palms facing skywards, hands moving upwards with breath. *This is prana vayu.*

<u>Exhale</u>: palms facing downwards, hands moving towards the earth as you exhale. This is *apana vayu*.

Now, experience your *vyana vayu* and *samana vayu*. Bring your hands to the level of your navel, palms facing each other, as if cupping a large invisible ball in front of you. As you inhale, feel your *vyana vayu* expanding in you, filling your heart, lighting your *agni*. Begin moving your hands outwards as if the ball you are holding in front of you is expanding with your breath. At your maximum inhalation, hold the posture gracefully.

Then begin the exhalation, drawing your hands inwards back into your core. This is your *samana vayu*. Draw the energy into your core to intensify your *agni*. Continue to feel your *vyana* and *samana vayu*. Bring your focus inward, shutting out the external world.

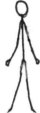 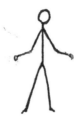 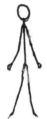

Stand with palms facing each other, slightly bent at the elbows, with hands at the level of your navel.	Inhale: palms facing still facing each other, move your hands outwards, focusing on expanding the heart center. This is *vyana*	Exhale: bring palms back towards the navel, attention focusing on the core. This is *samana vayu*.

To close, express your *udana vayu* by performing the dynamic *bhujangasana*. Start with your third eye (forehead) resting on the earth. As you inhale, lift yourself up into *bhujangasana*, chanting OM. Hold the pose at the top of the inhale. As you exhale, gently lower your forehead back towards the earth.

6.6. Energy conduits of the body

6.6.1. Movement of energy in the body

Even the smallest living entity moves. Without movement, there is no life. With each inhalation, we are connecting our individual *prana* with the *Universal Prana*, lengthening the thread of life. With each exhalation, we reaffirm our existence. Our breath is our link with immortality. Within our body, it is *prana* that moves our thoughts, feelings, sensations and consciousness. It moves the intelligence from cell to cell so that the body as a whole becomes alive.

There is no word for *prana* in the language of modern Western physiology. It is the amalgamation of these words: blood pressure, osmosis, action potential, nerve impulse, chemical messenger. In yogic anatomy, this force that gives life to the body is simply known as *prana*.

6.6.2. *Merudanda* and *sushumna*

From the Upanishads written in the 7th-8th century BCE (*Chapter 2: Philosophy, Ethics & Lifestyle*), comes one of the earliest descriptions of yogic anatomy.

The yogic anatomy's equivalent to the spinal cord is the *merudanda*, which is a column beginning from the base of the skull to the coccyx. Within the *merudanda* lies the *sushumna*, which is the main energy pathway in our body. From the *sushumna*, energy courses around the body in fine channels called *nadi (section 6.3.3).*

6.6.3. *Nadi*

According to the Upanishads, *prana* is carried around the body from the *sushumna* in miniscule tubes that criss-cross our body like rivers. These tubes are called *nadi*, or energy channels. According to yogic anatomy, there are 72,000 *nadi* in the body, ranging from subtle to gross. For comparative purposes, the *nadi* system vaguely resembles the body's circulatory system of arteries, capillaries and veins in modern Western anatomy (*section 4.2.7*).

6.6.4. *Ida* and *Pingala*

The human body is symmetrical bilaterally – there is a left side and its corresponding right side. The right side of the body is under the control of the left brain, and similarly, the left side of the body is influenced by the right brain (*section 5.3.2*).

The right side is the solar side, the male side; the left is female, lunar. The male and female here do not refer to gender, but rather to the nature of the energy: that is to say, male energy is hot, energizing, active, while the female energy is cool, restorative and relaxing. This is analogous to the sympathetic and parasympathetic nervous systems respectively: the sympathetic NS (male) stimulates or accelerates while the parasympathetic NS (female) inhibits autonomic functions (*Chapter 4: Physiology*).

The *ida* and *pingala* channels correlate with left and right single nostril breathing respectively (Telles, 2005). When we breathe through the right nostril, we are more awake, fired up and logical (because breathing through the right nostril activates the left brain). Conversely, when we breathe through the left nostril, we become more relaxed and calm (Brown and Gerbarg, 2005).

Prana bridges the masculine and feminine energies through respiration (*section 5.4.6*). The large *nadi*, *ida*, begins from the right side of the coccyx and terminates at the left nostril. The opposite number to *ida* is the *pingala*, which begins on the left side of the coccyx and terminates at the right nostril. These two main channels weave around the *sushumna* approximately five to eight times; wherever they intersect, a wheel of energy, called chakra, is located. The chakra is one of the main areas of study in yogic anatomy.

6.6.5. *Chakra*

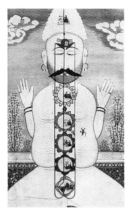

Chakra are the spinning wheels of energy, from which many *nadi* originate (the word *chakra* comes from the Sanskrit word for wheel or disc).

Much of the original information on *chakra* comes from the Upanishads and is believed to have been passed down orally for a thousand years before being written down for the first time between 1200–900 BCE.

Diagram 6.7. Yogin with seven chakras. Painting. Kangra school. Late 18th century A.D.

There are seven main *chakra* in the body, which are aligned along the *sushumna*. Each *chakra* spins at a different frequency in ascending order (from slow at the base of the spine to fast at the crown of the head), and consciousness and energy move from one frequency to the next in a spiralling fashion. They function as pumps or valves, regulating the flow of energy through our energy system.

The aim of yoga is to awaken the latent Shakti energy asleep at the *mooladhara chakra* at the base of our spine (commonly referred to as the Kundalini energy) and raise it up the *sushumna*, to merge with the Shiva energy in the crown. This is when a person experiences oneness with Universal Consciousness.

Each chakra is linked to its specific sound, light and color (*section 6.7*). Chakra can be spinning too fast or too slow. They can be broken or tarnished. *Chakra* imbalance manifests in physical, mental and emotional illnesses. In a healthy individual, all the *chakra* in his body are in optimum health. *Chakra* can be healed through several holistic methods, such as color therapy, crystal healing, *chakra*-balancing, meditation and so forth.

Although these bioenergetic vortices are not visible to the human eye (or any medical imaging instrument), their locality and functionality corresponds to the main endocrine plexus of Western anatomy (*Table 6.2, Diagram 6.8*).

Table 6.1. *Chakra*, location, correspondence with the endocrine plexus and organs innervated.

Chakra	Region, *location on spine*	Endocrine plexus	Organs innervated
Mooladhara	Root (genital), *S4*	Gonads	Testes
Svadisthana	Sacrum, *L1*	Adrenal	Ovaries, intestines
Manipura	Solar plexus, *T8*	Pancreas	Diaphragm
Anahata	Heart, *T1*	Thymus	Heart
Visuddha	Throat, *C3*	Thyroid	Throat
Ajna	Brow, *C1*	Pituitary	Brain
Sahasrara	Crown	Pineal	None

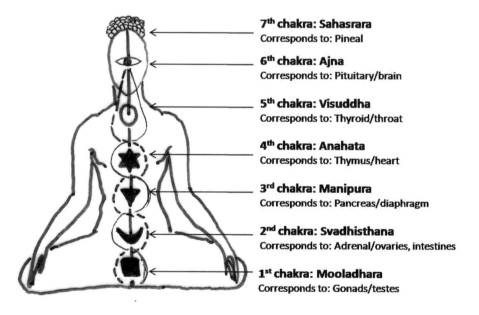

7th chakra: Sahasrara
Corresponds to: Pineal

6th chakra: Ajna
Corresponds to: Pituitary/brain

5th chakra: Visuddha
Corresponds to: Thyroid/throat

4th chakra: Anahata
Corresponds to: Thymus/heart

3rd chakra: Manipura
Corresponds to: Pancreas/diaphragm

2nd chakra: Svadhisthana
Corresponds to: Adrenal/ovaries, intestines

1st chakra: Mooladhara
Corresponds to: Gonads/testes

Diagram 6.8. **The main *chakra* and the endocrine system.**

201

6.7. The chakra system

6.7.1. *Mooladhara*: the earth *chakra* (dark red)

Mooladhara chakra is the beginning of life. Made of earth elements, this *chakra* is the home of the latent Kundalini energy.

Physiologically, it governs the excretory and reproductive systems. The gonad glands are the ovaries in women and testes in men. They produce the sex hormones such as oestrogen and progesterone, and androgens such as testosterone, which are responsible for sexual reproduction and sexual behavior.

Oestrogen and testosterone are produced in both men and women, but in different proportions. As women do not have testes, they produce low amounts of testosterone in the adrenal cortex. Therefore, because of its relationship with the reproductive organs, the *mooladhara chakra* is governed by and in turn governs the sexual attitudes and survival instincts in a person.

6.7.2. *Svadisthana*: the creative *chakra* (deep orange)

Svadisthana chakra is the *chakra* of procreation. This is the *chakra* of self identity ("me") and power. It connects us to our inner source of inspiration and gives rise to the expression of beauty in our being, generating our creative energies.

The second *chakra* is located on the L1 vertebra on the spine. The adrenal gland which sits on top of each kidney plays a very important role in governing our body's response to stress and emergency situations through the secretion of hormones which affect other organs. The organs that this *chakra* innervates are the ovaries and intestines.

6.7.3. *Manipura*: the feelings *chakra* (bright yellow)

Manipura chakra, 'the jewelled city', is the home of our sense of contentment, or *santosa*.

This *chakra* also innervates the diaphragm, which is one of the main organs of respiration. As our breath is our emotional signature, the *manipura chakra* is very much about feelings. The imbalanced manifestation gives rise to anxiety and worry, which in turn, affects respiration.

6.7.4. *Anahata*: the love *chakra* (intense green)

It is in the *Anahata chakra* that our Spirit, Self, *Atma*, resides. This *chakra* is the bridge between the lower three and the upper three *chakra*.

Love that is expressed in this *chakra* is not colored by sexuality, but by purity, innocence and is beyond sex. When the Kundalini energy flows from the lower *chakra* to this one, the "me" is transformed into pure love for humanity, or *bhakti*.

Physiologically, this *chakra* is located in the heart area. The thymus gland is located behind the heart, and its only purpose is as the warehouse for storing the T-cells used in the body's immune function.

6.7.5. *Visuddha*: the truth *chakra* (cool blue)

Visuddha chakra is the *chakra* of sound. With sound comes our relationship with others as we communicate. This is the "truth" *chakra*, because it is in our throat that we find our faculty of speech. If grief and sadness are not expressed, they will affect thyroid function.

As voice can be used to heal, it can also wound. "Words are mightier than a sword" is a common English saying. In yoga (in particular, Kundalini Yoga), we move towards Conscious Communication, where we communicate only if it makes for a better tomorrow.

This *chakra* also innervates the thyroid gland, which is situated at the base of the throat. The hormones of the thyroid regulate growth and metabolism.

6.7.6. *Ajna*: the knowing *chakra* (midnight blue)

The pituitary gland is often called the master gland, because the hormones it secretes control the functions of other glands (it is itself controlled by hormonal secretions from the hypothalamus).

Ajna chakra innervates the brain, the seat of consciousness in the human body. This is the *chakra* of intuition, where we move away from the rational mind into deeper consciousness and realms of intuition. It is related to the act of seeing, both physically and intuitively. As such, with yoga, meditation and appropriate lifestyle, the *Ajna chakra* opens our psychic faculties and our understanding of archetypal levels: as our physical eyes see the present, our third eye sees into the future.

6.7.7. *Sahasrara*: the angel *chakra* (violet)

Sahasrara is the "knowing" *chakra*, the thousand petal lotus. This *chakra* brings us knowledge, wisdom, understanding, spiritual connection and bliss.

The *Sahasrara chakra* is the meeting place of the Kundalini Shakti and Shiva. When Shakti rises from her dormant state in the *Mooladhara chakra* and merges with Shiva at the *Sahasrara*, the illusion of separateness is dissolved.

Physiologically, this *chakra* corresponds to the pineal gland, which is located deep in the brain. The pineal gland releases melatonin, an anti-depressant.

6.8. The subtle bodies

[REFER TO *section 2.1.3*]

6.8.1. The five *kosha*

The practice of yoga is for the purpose of yoking the mind, body and soul. It is also for the yoking, too, of our unit consciousness with Universal Consciousness (*section 5.6.2*), that is to say, merging the true Self in each and every one of us with the Universe. Others know it as Universal Truth, Absolute Reality, Consciousness, Light, *Brahma* or God.

But what, or who, is the Self in us that is constantly referred to in yoga and other spiritual disciplines? It has been said that the Self is indescribable, and to know the Self is the aim of meditation, Advaita Vedanta, and Tantra practices. The Self in us (which we are trying to find in our yoga practices) is part of the Self that is everything, from the smallest atom to the largest universe. It is the eternal center of Consciousness. If the Self in us is the light of a candle, then the Universal Self is the fire from which all candlelight originates from and returns to. In our world (the world our physical body lives in), the Self is shrouded with layers called *kosha*, or sheaths. We have five layers of *kosha (panda kosha)*:

1. *Annamaya kosha* - physical
2. *Pranamaya kosha* – breath/energy
3. *Manomaya kosha* – mental
4. *Vijnamaya kosha* – wisdom
5. *Anandamaya kosha* - bliss

Diagram 6.9. **The five *kosha***

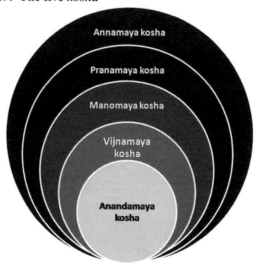

Annamaya kosha

The first *kosha* is our physical body. *Anna* actually means food, which builds the frame. Thus, the first layer of our sheath is built and nourished by food and is made up of the five *bhuta*. This is the layer of needs and wants, the grossest layer.

Go beyond this sheath with: yogasana & kriya, diet and relaxation.

Pranamaya kosha

Prana is energy (or life force), which we harness through our breath. In most – if not all – spiritual practices, the practitioner learns how to work with *prana*. *Prana* allows the Self to animate the external; it is the thread linking us to Consciousness. We also need a healthy pranamaya kosha for a healthy physical body, which is nourished by prana. In this layer, you will find the nadi, the channels in which the life force flows to every cell in the body.

Go beyond this sheath with: pranayama

Manomaya kosha

Manas means mind. This is the layer of thoughts, emotions, and memories. Conflict arising from this layer – tension, anxiety, etc - is called *Awadhi*, or stress. If one is not the master of one's mind, then one becomes a slave to the senses. The mind is able to generate illusions, which drive us to chase fools' gold.

Therefore, the important spiritual practice of yoga starts here – we have to understand *manas*, to train it, so that it is driven by the self within, rather than the illusory world outside.

Go beyond this sheath with: meditation and devotional sessions (kirtan and satsang).

Vijnamaya kosha

Vijna comes from *jnana,* which means means knowing. It is the level that 'knows'. This is a powerful level; it is our 'conscience', or small voice inside that challenges us to choose the righteous path. But if *vijnamaya kosha* gets taken over by *manas*, it loses its potency. Spiritual practice would involve lifting this sheath and separating it from the *manas*, so that the knowing is clear, untainted.

Go beyond this sheath with: spiritual retreat

Anandamaya kosha

Ananda is bliss. Bliss can be experienced by the mind (we experience bliss when we are soaking in a spa), but *ananda* at the fifth sheath level is actually a sense of being that is beyond mind. It is the joy, peace, love and serenity that are felt in the absence of external stimulus. It is just <u>being</u>. It is the feeling that suffuses you from resting in bliss. Even this layer has to be discarded in meditation. Letting go of bliss, to journey onward to the true centre, where the Self lies.

Go beyond this sheath with: karma yoga and practicing joy in all aspects of your life.

This concept of the five layers of Self has been propagated as far back as the Upanishads, and is also held by other schools of thought, including the Hellenistic Hermetic and Neoplatonic. Life is but the journey of the soul, and with Death, the layers are discarded so that only the soul remains…and the journey continues.

6.8.2. The Ten Bodies

Almost all of us are living at the grossest level of existence – we identify only with the gross elements that we can touch, smell, feel, see and hear. We think of ourselves primarily in the physical terms, and we are aware only of our physical body. But even at the simplest definition, there is more to you than your physical body which you use to touch, smell, feel, see and hear. Take the phrase "human being" for example. There is the "human" part of you, and there is the "being" part, too, which is more subtle but no less real (if not more real!). Even the word "human" can be broken down further, to "hu", which means light, and "man" which means "mind" (Bhajan, 2003). As mentioned at the beginning of this chapter, the yogic equivalent to modern Western anatomy is the anatomy of light, and light is the sum of subtle energies from which all things are created.

Like the *chakra* system and the five *kosha*, the Ten Bodies are a further refinement of the way in which your energy manifests itself on the physical plane. Each of the Ten Bodies has its own quality. According to Yogi Bhajan, Master of Kundalini Yoga (Bhajan, 2003), the root of all diseases exists first in one of these spiritual or energy bodies before it manifests outwardly. Therefore, understanding and keeping all Ten Bodies healthy plays an important role in our overall wellbeing.

Table 6.2. **The Ten Bodies**

Order	Body	Description	To balance
First	Soul	This is the first body, and it links you to your inner infinity. This is your essence. *When it is out of balance:* Unable to access the beauty within.	Open the heart and raise the Kundalini with Kundalini Yoga.
Second	Negative (Protective Mind)	This is the protective element that gives shape and form to the Soul Body. *When it is out of balance:* Clingy. No perception of danger.	Practice discipline, commitment, integrity. Have faith.
Third	Positive (Expansive Mind)	This is the source of your bountifulness, expansiveness. *When it is out of balance:* Paralyzed by negative mind.	Strengthen navel point. Choose a positive affirmation and repeat it.
Fourth	Neutral (Meditative Mind)	This is your mind working in a balanced way that sees reality and experiences win-win negotiations. *When it is out of balance:* Indecisiveness. Unable to have a broader perspective of a situation.	Meditate.
Fifth	Physical	Your soul's earthly vehicle; temple of your spirit. Those with strong physical presence teach, bringing the abstract into the physical world. *When it is out of balance:* Inner and outer realities out of balance. Greedy, ambitious, jealous.	Exercise regularly.
Sixth	Arc line	This is your halo, your radiance. It's your integrity on display: all your past actions are written here. *When it is out of balance:* Mood swings, unable to focus. Vulnerable and easily influenced.	Awaken the third eye.

Order	Body	Description	To balance
Seventh	Auric	This body envelops your physical body like a glove of electromagnetic energy. It is your protection; when bright, it inspires others. *When it is out of balance:* Vulnerable to diseases. Paranoid and lack self trust.	Meditate. Wear white clothing to project aura.
Eighth	Pranic	This is the circulation system of your Ten Bodies and *chakra* system. It allows you to transform energy from the universe into more subtle vibrations, thoughts, actions, and creativity. *When it is out of balance:* Chronic fatigue and suffering from omnipresent anxiety. Low energy, fearful and defensive (overly sensitive).	All *pranayama*.
Ninth	Subtle	This body surrounds your soul and gives you the experience of detail and perception in the subtle realm. It gives you the opportunity to understand and master the subtlety in life. *When it is out of balance:* Naïve and read people wrongly. Crude in speech and behavior.	Do any meditation or *kriya* for 100 days.
Tenth	Radiant	This is the body that gives you radiance, courage and spiritual royalty. You glow when this body is healthy and strong. *When it is out of balance:* Wallflower syndrome: afraid of conflict and attention. Ineffective and nondescript.	Commitment. Do not cut hair.

The Eleventh Embodiment: sum of all Ten Bodies. It is the sound current from which all mantra originate.

6.9. The yogic way to good health

6.9.1. Do everything in balance

The yogic way is all about balance, rather than the absence of the "bad". For example, from the section on the Ten Bodies (*6.8.2, Table 6.3*), we see that having a Negative Body is actually a good thing, because it gives us the inbuilt protective instincts. Children, whose Ten Bodies are not fully developed yet, are often unaware of dangers.

Tamas, the attribute (*guna*) of heaviness, inertia and dullness, has a positive role to play in our wellbeing too, despite the negative connotations that the words associated with it conjure up. Without any *tamas* present (or too little), a person is fickle, lacking in commitment and unstable. Physically, the individual would have fluctuations in his weight, difficulty in digesting food and excreting waste products, and may have light, brittle bones. As in yoga philosophy, in Ayurvĕda, the physicians' efforts are focused on maintaining the balance between the three *dosha*. It is also about keeping the *agni*, *dhatu* and other elements in good working order so that every component of the body functions in harmony with each other and their surroundings.

6.9.2. Eat a balanced diet

A yogic diet is lacto-vegetarian. It is important for a vegetarian to choose his food carefully to ensure that there is enough food from each category to provide for all the needs of the body: leafy greens, dark fruits / vegetables, nuts, grains and pulses.

Fasting for prolonged periods is not conducive to good health, as the *agni* needs fuel to burn. Without *agni*, life's processes slowly come to a shutdown, and a weak *agni* is often the cause of many diseases. Cultivating good eating habits includes eating sensibly, not over-eating due to emotional hunger and not eating after sunset.

6.9.3. Live a balanced life

Excessive work, excessive exercise or excessive anything are not good for the body in the long run because they over-tax the body's systems. Keeping irregular hours, skipping meals and disturbed sleep all add additional stress to the systems of the body.

Sex in excess can be detrimental, too. Although celibacy is no longer prescribed for yogis, being addicted to sex can rob the act of its true meaning, namely, a meaningful union between two people where love is expressed in its purest form. Sex merely for the sake of the sensory experience it brings is no different from the mindless coupling of animals and provides little in terms of deep emotional bliss.

6.9.4. Cultivate balanced relationships (stay away from destructive ones)

Human beings are created incomplete, so that we seek completion with a Higher Self (the basis of religion). It is a very common mistake in relationships when two people seek completion with each other. The need aspect obscures pure love: you should be with someone because you love them, not because you need them. Neediness creates dependency, which in turn creates fear of losing the beloved.

Although it may be tempting to seek a partner who needs you or is one you need, this polarity between two people is rarely healthy. You have to be whole first before seeking to extend yourself to another.

6.9.5. The Ayurvĕdic way

In the Ayurvĕdic way, good health is not merely by the absence of disease. Good health is when everything is in balance and in harmony.

The current state of a person's dosha is called the *vikruti. Vikruti* is affected by lifestyle, diet, emotional state and other factors. Good health is when the *vikruti* is in balance with the *prakriti*.

An Ayurvĕdic physician never treats a symptom or disease directly without first establishing a global view of the patient – from his history, to his physical, mental and emotional state, to his lifestyle. Ayurvĕda believes in treating the whole person, not mending discrete body parts.

As such, an Ayurvĕdic physician, after taking a detailed history, making observation and rationalizing the data, would prescribe and make recommendations on how to bring the patient's body (and mind and soul) back into balance.

Central to Ayurvĕda's beliefs is that good health can be restored through following a proper diet (which includes eating the right foods cooked in the correct way), making lifestyle changes and having a healthy attitude towards life. Ayurvĕda's way is an integrated approach to health in which the patient takes personal responsibility for his own well-being. This methodology has proven to be very effective over the centuries and is gaining a resurgence of popularity in the modern world.

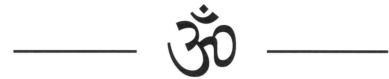

References

Balachandran, P., & Govindarajan, R.(2005). Cancer--an ayurvedic perspective. *Pharmacol Res*. 2005 Jan;51(1):19-30.

Bhajan, Y (2003). *The Aquarian Teacher: KRI International Kundalini Yoga Teacher Training Level 1*. USA: Kundalini research Institute (KRI).

Brown, R.P., & Gerbarg, P.L. (2005). Sudarshan Kriya yogic breathing in the treatment of stress, anxiety, and depression: part I-neurophysiologic model. *J Altern Complement Med*. 2005 Feb;11(1):189-201

Fischer, J.E. (2005). On the uniqueness of surgery. *Am J Surg*. 2005 Mar;189(3):259-63.

Gogtay, N.J., Bhatt, H.A., Dalvi, S.S., & Kshirsagar, N.A. (2002). The use and safety of non-allopathic Indian medicines. *Drug Saf*. 2002;25(14):1005-19.

Satow, Y.E., Kumar, P.D., Burke, A., & Inciardi, J.F. (2008). Exploring the prevalence of Ayurveda use among Asian Indians. *J Altern Complement Med*. 2008 Dec;14(10):1249-53.

Sharma, H., Chandola, H.M., Singh, G., & Basisht, G. (2007). Utilization of Ayurveda in health care: an approach for prevention, health promotion, and treatment of disease. Part 1--Ayurvĕda, the science of life. *J Altern Complement Med*. 2007 Nov;13(9):1011-9.

Subhose, V., Srinivas, P., & Narayana, A. (2005). Basic principles of pharmaceutical science in Ayurvĕda. *Bull Indian Inst Hist Med Hyderabad*. 2005 Jul-Dec;35(2):83-92.

Telles, S. (2005). Oriental approaches to masculine and feminine subtle energy principles. *Percept Mot Skills*. 2005 Apr;100(2):292-4.

CHAPTER SEVEN

Techniques

OVERVIEW OF THE CHAPTER

7.1   The yoga universe

7.2   Practicing *yogasana*

7.3   YogaSense™: The Seven Core Principles

7.4   *Drishti*

7.5   *Bandha*

7.6   Meditation

7.7   *Pranayama*

7.8   Relaxation and visualization

7.9   Sanskrit chants

7.1. The yoga universe

7.1.1. Introduction

Although there are as many varieties of yoga, all traditional yoga practices guide the practitioner toward union of the mind, body and spirit. It is in the Yoga Sutras of Sri Patanjali that the foundations of yoga can be found. (*Chapter 2: Philosophy, Ethics & Lifestyle*). In his book, the yoga path is comprehensively written down in detail. The role of all yoga teachers is to introduce their students to the Yoga Sutras of Sri Patanjali.

"Techniques" in the context of yoga refers to the steps and methodology that a practitioner has to undertake to achieve the state of yoga. The techniques covered in this book are the proprietary YogaSense™ principles and methodology developed by the authors.

7.1.2. The main schools of yoga

Although the classical schools of yoga share the same basic philosophy, the approach and methodology vary widely. Overall, there are four major forms of yoga:

Raja Yoga *The highest form of yoga*
Brahma Kumari

Hatha Yoga *Self realization through the physical body*
Ashtanga Vinyasa, Iyengar, Sivananda

Karma Yoga *Yoga of action*
Sahaja Yoga

Bhakti Yoga *Yoga of devotion*
Hare Krishna

Kundalini Yoga has elements of all schools of yoga listed above.

214

The most popular approach is the Hatha way, as the majority of yoga schools start with *asana*, the third limb, rather than the first. This is because it is easier to open a new student's body than to open his mind: it is through opening the physical body, releasing past experiences and breaking set patterns that a teacher opens his student's mind to new ideas and new ways of being.

One of the most recognizable names in yoga today is Ashtanga, which is popularly associated with the school of yoga founded by Shri K. Pattabhi Jois. Ashtanga Yoga is now practiced by thousands of people in all corners of the world, following set practices prescribed by Shri K. Pattabhi Jois. However, this school is more accurately known as Ashtanga Vinyasa Yoga, as "ashtanga" is a generic term for a core yoga philosophy. This generic term means 'eight limbs' and is the foundation on which most traditional and classical yoga schools are founded. According to Ashtanga Yoga, there are eight pathways in the study of yoga (*Chapter 2: Philosophy, Ethics & Lifestyle*). These are briefly summarized in Table 7.1:

Table 7.1. Ashtanga yoga: **the eight limbs of yoga**

Limb	Abbreviated meaning	Type of yoga
Yama	The great vow (*mahavratam*)	Karma yoga – yoga of action
Niyama	Personal observances	Karma yoga – yoga of action
Asana	"Being comfortable" (often taken to mean 'postures')	Karma yoga – yoga of action
Pranayama	Breathing consciously	Jnâna yoga – yoga of knowledge
Pratyhara	Withdrawal from the world of senses	Jnâna yoga – yoga of knowledge
Dharana	One-pointed concentration	Jnâna yoga – yoga of knowledge
Dhyana	Meditation	Bhakti yoga – yoga of devotion
Samadhi	Bliss, self-realization	Bhakti yoga – yoga of devotion

7.2. Practicing *yogasana*

7.2.1. Introduction to *yogasana*

Yoga is most widely associated with flexibility. *Yogasana* does indeed emphasize stretching, which promotes flexibility, but *yogasana* is more than the 'flexibility' which many bystanders associate it with.

Stretching is about peace. Take yourself back to your high school physics class. You will remember learning that for a given quantity of gaseous molecules, pressure is higher if the volume that holds the gas is small; that is to say, pressure is the inverse of volume. Translate that to the body, and note how a tense, stressed out person's body looks like – taut muscles, bunched shoulders, hunkered down frame, closing down.

Apart from releasing tension, stretching is about creating new spaces within the body. And through the other limbs of yoga, you fill the new spaces with love, compassion and equanimity. This is what yoga is about and this is why many students say they feel calm and at peace after a yoga class, often without knowing why.

7.2.2. Scope of this book

This book does not set out to teach you the yoga postures, because there is only one way to learn how to do *yogasana* properly, and that is under the guidance of a suitably qualified yoga teacher.

Books on *yogasana* – however comprehensive and well-written - are no substitute to learning from a teacher, especially learning the basics. Neither are instructional CDs and DVDs, which are useful tools to supplement your yoga practice. A teacher is invaluable in correcting your alignment and guiding your inner path. There is also much benefit to be gained from group practice.

This book therefore assumes that you are familiar with *yogasana*. Its aim is to take your *yogasana* to another level so that you can begin the process of self-inquiry. As you deepen your practice it will enable you to teach with greater clarity and wisdom.

7.2.3. How many postures are there?

According to Dharma Mittra, who compiled the seminal work, "908 postures of Hatha yoga", there are an infinite number of postures. In Ashtanga Vinyasa Yoga, the postures are as described in Shri K. Pattabhi Jois's in the Series, and should be practiced as prescribed. In Kundalini Yoga, individual postures are put together to make up a *kriya*, or a set of actions with a defined end-goal.

Prefixes can be used on any pose to explain a variation:
- *Ardha* means half
- *Supta* means reclining
- *Adho* means downward
- *Pavritta* means revolved or twisted
- *Urdhva* means upward
- *Utthita* means extended

Many yoga teachers come up with new postures. If you are compelled to develop new postures, make sure that you adhere to the three key points:

1. the posture serves a purpose (for instance, facilitating a deeper stretch);

2. the posture is congruent with classical yoga;

3. the posture is not detrimental to your body (that is to say, causing strain and compression).

The YogaSense™ way, as developed by the authors, is a comprehensive and scientifically driven methodology of practicing and teaching *yogasana*. It fosters development in multiple areas to promote overall wellness of all the systems in the body.

YogaSense™: it makes sense physiologically☺.

7.3. YogaSense™: The Seven Core Principles

7.3.1. *YogaSense™ Core Principle One*: Respect your body

Yogasana when done according to the core YogaSense™ principles will nurture the body. To achieve YogaSense™'s first principle – *Respect the body* – requires awareness of the body types, limitations and tendencies. Acknowledgement of past injuries and an appreciation for vulnerable areas of the body will help the practitioner to "do no harm".

Work intelligently for your body type
For those with a lot of flexibility, an effort is made to pull in strength with the pose. In a forward bend, if someone has a lot of flexibility and bends all the way to the floor the pose is lost if no effort is made to engage the muscles.

On the other hand, if the stiff body rounds the thoracic spine to make up for the lack of bend from the hips then the essence of the pose is also lost.

Injury occurs if the body goes too far into a pose without muscle engagement or compensation when the body fails to perform the desired movement.

Vulnerable Areas of the Body
Vulnerable areas are found in some joints where two bones that join together do not stay aligned or may be found in tears of the muscles and tendons. There are some joints and muscles that are more vulnerable to injury than others. The shoulder joint with its mobility in multiple directions is vulnerable to injury during weight bearing *yogasana*. If a person cannot control the movement while weight bearing, modifications should be made so that the movement in and out of the pose is controlled.

Chaturanga dandasana is a classic example. The body weight plus the pull of gravity requires considerable strength to lower down into the pose. Try the modification of placing the knees down to reduce the weight on the shoulders or practicing on the wall to learn the alignment to protect the shoulders.

Table 7.2. **Weaknesses of the body**

Body area	Weakness	Postures for concern
Ankle	Turning Ankle	Balance poses
Knees and elbows	Hyperextension	Standing and balancing poses
Lower Back	Overstretching of SI ligament. Creating outward pressure on the disc.(posteriorly)	Forward bends – especially seated forward bends
Neck	Closing off circulation to brain, pinching nerves in neck	Back bend with head extension – *ustrasana*
Shoulder	Tearing of capsular ligaments	*Chaturanga dandasana*
Hamstrings	Tear in muscle or tendon.	Standing hamstring stretches
Groin	Ligaments or adductor muscles are torn.	Wide legged forward bend

7.3.2. *YogaSense™ Core Principle Two*: Starting the fire

The body must be warmed up adequately before any stretching is undertaken to prevent muscle damage. There is the mistaken belief that stretching is a form of warm-up, but in actual fact, warming up requires a group of actions that warms the muscles up. Inadequately warmed up muscles are like cold steel. Over-stretching cold muscles leads to tears of the muscle fibers, and more seriously, to tears in the tendons and ligaments (which take longer to mend as there is less blood circulation).

The fire has to be started from within. The fire cannot be started from the outside: no teacher can take you to enlightenment. The fire cannot be started from the head: you cannot "think" your way through yoga, that is to say, you cannot achieve the end-goal by read about it. As Shri K. Pattabhi Jois (*section 1.5.3*) so profoundly said, yoga is "1% inspiration, 99% perspiration". The first step of yoga is doing, hence the focus on personal practice.

In a yoga class, practitioners are often impatient with the warm-up routine, impatient to get to the "real" yoga part of the class. This is a good opportunity to invite students to embrace the teachings of the Yoga Sutra. Consider the word *abhyasa*. *Asa* means to sit or to abide in (as in *asana*). *Abhy* means intensely focusing on the goal. *Abhyasa* is made up of devotion and dedication. A true yogi would show devotion and dedication to all aspects of his practice, instead of being motivated only by the "exciting" parts. Through putting sufficient effort, enthusiasm and mindfulness into this part of the practice, we learn the importance lessons of patience and being in the moment.

7.3.3. *YogaSense™ Core Principle Three*: Optimal alignment

Alignment is a fundamental component in nature, yet it is only human beings who are challenged by alignment: we are upright on two feet and are mobile. Thus, we face a constant struggle to maintain our relationship with gravity. As Vanda Scaravelli (*1.6.1*) memorably said, "Don't let gravity kill a posture". Alignment allows for grace and ease of movement. When alignment is at its optimal, energy will flow effortlessly. Thus, a practitioner must not lose sight of the alignment (or lines of his body) in *yogasana*: alignment should be his premier consideration, not how far he can go in a posture. It introduces mindfulness to the practice. The rounding of shoulders in forward bend in the ambitious fight to stretch further is a classic example of the violation of optimal alignment. Here, substance is sacrificed for form.

Alignment requires the right amount of strength and flexibility to achieve. It takes both strength and flexibility to overcome gravity. A balanced state for the body structure is one of optimal alignment. When the body is in this state, minimal energy is required to overcome gravity and to move. Example: when the vertebrae of the back are rounded (as seen in kyphosis) it takes more energy to keep the shoulders lined up and to walk.

7.3.4. *YogaSense™ Core Principle Four*: Balancing opposing forces

The trunk is the body's anchor for the movement of the extremities: movements occur because the trunk is engaged as a stabilizer while the limbs are allowed freedom of movement.

Every muscle has an origin and an insertion, and the pull is between the two: one stabilizes while the other either lengthens or shortens depending on the muscle contraction (in isometric, it stays the same length). The underlying principle is that tension is being created between the two points.

Tadasana is a bigger version of all this principle. The trunk is the anchor. Within the trunk, the separation occurs at the lower hip, where everything below this line belongs to gravity, while anything above it rises upwards. Your feet and pelvis are engaged to the ground as you lift your trunk upwards, lifting up to the crown of your head.

Balancing opposing forces is about grounding and lifting; it is the movement in two opposite directions. The spine is elongated for the most favorable energy flow, and optimal spinal alignment is best obtained through mindfulness.

7.3.5. *YogaSense™ Core Principle Five:* Opening like a flower

One of the most common features demonstrated by practitioners, especially new ones, is the collapsing of the chest in forward bends. Due to stiffness in the lower back and tightness in the hamstrings, there is a tendency to compensate for the lack of bending from the hips, resulting in the rounding of the thoracic spine during the effort to go down further. This kyphotic structure could cause a lot of pressure at the lower back; it accentuates an area that is already weak (extension of the thoracic spine) and it reduces the efficiency of respiration because the ribs are pressed into the lungs in this kyphotic position. Many people adopt this position frequently, resulting in an over-stretching of those tissues (posterior ligaments and muscles of the spine) and weaknesses in back extensors. Alignment-wise, the energy doesn't flow optimally.

Breathe in consciously and deeply to open the chest and to fire the flame of life (this is the second of the seven YogaSense™ Core Principles). Let go and allow for opening the way a flower opens to the sun.

7.3.6. *YogaSense™ Core Principle Six:* **Nurturing**

The body has an inbuilt ability to heal and grow. Thus all physical yoga practice should lead to the nurturing of the body, mind and soul. If it does not, you have to reassess what you are doing, because this is (or should be) the ultimate aim of a physical *yogasana* practice. Yoga allows for self-awareness, namely, understanding your strengths and weaknesses whether in your mind and body. Your practice should be dsigned for rebalancing and nurturing.

The definition of nurture and restoration differs between different bodies: an overworked or sick person requires a practice that slows his body down to allow for healing, whereas a person who is overweight or depressed has to start her fire with a more vigorous practice.

All *yogasana* classes should include a period of relaxation. This is because body intelligence works in a different way from mental intelligence. Your body needs time to rationalize and to absorb the movements you performed during *yogasana*, and this process takes time. If you had rushed off immediately after class without giving your practice time to sink into your body's memory system, you would have lost the nuances and the subtleties of your *yogasana*. In yoga, there should be no rush. And as you practice, you will gain insight into your daily life and can readjust your path as needed.

7.3.7. *YogaSense™ Core Principle Seven:* **Live it!**

The highest purpose of yoga is *samadhi*. But yoga also has a more practical purpose, and that purpose is for us to learn to be happier with ourselves and to be able to share that with our family and others. It is about taking the lessons we learn on the yoga mat and extending them to our daily lives. "Do no damage", awareness, mindfulness and peace are among the *yogasana* philosophies that are scalable to "real life". This is the real gem of yoga. According to the words of Yogi Bhajan, Master of Kundalini Yoga, "Happiness is your birthright".

7.4. Drishti

7.4.1. Focus, clarity and alignment

Training the eyes at specific gazing points during *yogasana* brings the focus inwards and moves *asana* practice up the higher rungs of the Ashtanga Yoga ladder, namely, *pratyhara*, *dharana* and *dhyana*. It also brings clarity of the moment to the practitioner. On the physical side, *drishti* assists the body into proper alignment.

A *yogasana* is built up of *asana*, breath, *bandha* and *drishti,* though it is common that *drishti* is overlooked, especially by new practitioners who are often overwhelmed by the physical aspects of a *yogasana*. However, it is important to bring practitioners' attention to this component of *yogasana*.

The nine *drishti* are*:*
1. *Nasagrai* = tip of the nose
2. *Angusta ma dyai* = the thumbs
3. *Broomadhya* = the third eye
4. *Nabhi chakra* = the navel
5. *Urdhva* = up to the sky
6. *Hastagrai* = the hand
7. *Padhayoragrai* = the toes
8. *Parsva* = the far left
9. *Parsva* = the far right

Practice being conscious of your *drishti* during *yogasana*, and slowly, consciously, make the gazing point an integral part of each and every *yogasana*. Preliminary *drishti* practices are to be found in *section 8.4.*

7.5. Bandha

7.5.1. Sending the energy upwards

Bandha are like energy valves along a length of vertical pipe: the pressure from shutting those valves off in a controlled and sequential manner sends the water upwards against gravity. Similarly, when applied to the body, conscious contraction of *bandha* has the effect of moving energy up from the base to the crown.

There are different *bandha* for different regulation of pranic flow in the body, but the four main ones are:

1. *moolabandha* – the root lock
2. *uddiyanabandha* – the diaphragm lock
3. *jalandharabandha* – the neck lock
4. *mahabandha* – the great lock (combination of all three)

All *bandha* can be contracted at the end of inhalation or at the end of exhalation. In *yogasana*, *bandha* (especially *moolabandha*) create lightness and fluidity to movements. Awareness and subsequently mastery of *bandha* start with the gross and move inwards to the subtle.

7.5.2. *Moolabandha*

Location of the male *moolabandha*

This is to be found in the space about one inch above the perineum. The perineal space is domed and is drawn inwards and upwards, creating an empty space for the front of the pubic bone and sacrum to move toward each other.

Location of the female *moolabandha*

It is located in the same location as the male *moolabandha*, except that the center of the action occurs at the cervix where it is drawn up and in. *Aswini*, *vajroli* and *sthula basti* are preparatory *kriya* to get us in touch with the often ignored and stagnant energies in the base and second chakra areas. The first step is cultivating awareness in the area, moving from the coarse to the subtle, and finally, the inner energy dynamics.

Anatomy of the *moolabandha*

In the area of the *moolabandha*, there are at least twelve independent muscles in ten muscle groups that connect at the sacrum and run across the ileum, ischium, the back, to the legs, the pubis, and to the tailbone.

On the posterior surface of the sacrum are attached the iliocostalis, longissimus, multifidus, erector spinae, latissimus dorsi, longus and brevis rotatores.

On the lateral surface of the sacrum, the gluteus maximus attaches, while at the anterior surface of the sacrum we find the levator ani group, piriformis, and coccygeal groups. It is valuable to note that the latissimus attaches all the way up into the upper arm.

Therefore, the relationship of the moolabandha is with the whole body, with the spine as the conduit.

Getting in touch with the *moolabandha*

An effective way to bring awareness into this area is to focus all your awareness there, visualize it and touch it with your senses. When you are as familiar with the area as you are with the neighborhood you live in, imagine a fine thread running in and out of the muscles, like random stitching. By playing with the thread in your mind, pulling and loosening at whim, you can consciously feel the effect in the locality.

Learning how to engage the *moolabandha*

This is a four stage-process:

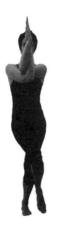

Moolabandha: finding yours with *garudasana*

1. Contract your anus – pull your anal sphincter inwards and upwards;

2. Contract your perineum by engaging your pelvic floor muscles. A good way of practicing this is starting and stopping urine flow;

3. Lift your pelvic diaphragm by contracting the levator ani (engaging the transverse abdominis): draw your belly button inwards towards your spine;

4. Isolate the previous three actions and work on refining each muscle group.

With better control of the *moolabandha*, we hold the energy within the body instead of letting it leach out. It also binds the senses inwards, taking us to *pratyhara*. Thus, from learning the *moolabandha*, we learn how to refine our senses, taking our journey inwards from the gross to the subtle, from unconscious to enlightenment.

7.5.3. *Uddiyanabandha*

Uddiyanabandha protects your lower back, keeping the spine long and preventing against too much backward bending in the lower back.

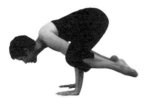

Uddiyanabandha: sending energy upwards

It is known as the flying upward energy lock and works on the second *chakra*. This lock moves the energy upwards from the earth, water and fire centers into the air region of the heart. *Uddiyanabandha* is created when a vacuum is formed as the lower abdomen is sucked in.

Learning how to engage the *uddiyanabandha*

Place your hands on your knees, bending forward slightly at the hips. Exhale completely, squeezing every last bit of air out from your lungs.

When your lungs are empty, close your throat. With your throat closed, create a vacuum by expanding your chest. This sucks the abdomen inwards and upwards. Note that there is no muscular engagement needed for this *bandha*, only the vacuum from locking out the breath and expanding the thoracic cavity. Hold the *bandha*. To release *uddiyanabandha*, swallow and release from the belly.

Initially, *uddiyanabandha* may be awkward to engage, but with frequent practice (such as when waiting in queues!) it will become second nature. And with the mastery of this *bandha*, you will fly higher!

Intensifying the experience

You will experience this *bandha* strongly at the end of an exhalation. To experience this, perform the Surya Namaskar and stop at *adho mukha svanasana*, where you will stay for five breaths.

Exhale fully without clenching your lower abdomen, keeping this area soft. As you inhale, bring your breath towards the back of your body and chest, keeping the softness. Remember to keep the neck free of compression and the throat relaxed. Release this *bandha* before any signs of strains.

7.5.4. Jalandharabandha

This is the throat energy valve. It is named thus because of the rich network of arteries and veins that innervate this area.

Jalandharabandha: securing the neck and opening the throat

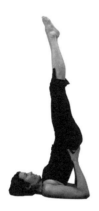

Jalandharabandha connects the head with the heart and opens the throat chakra. It is a lock especially for *pranayama*, where it helps pump the energy through the throat chakra into the crown and keeps the energy that has risen to the crown, third eye, and talu chakras from sinking down, leaking, or being dissipated, so it may continue to circulate in the chakra system. It also prevents the build-up of pressure in the head during breath retention.

How to engage the *jalandharabandha*

In *jalandharabandha*, the throat softens as it curves softly, as the neck elongates. The chin drops inwards and downwards towards the sternum. It is important to keep shoulders straight and not hunched. Gently bring your neck into a lock position.

Do not perform *jalandharabandha* if you are suffering from whiplash.

7.5.5. Mahabandha

This lock is also known as *tribandha* or *trayabandha*, and is composed of *moolabandha, uddiyanabandha*, and *jalandharabandha* applied in a sequential order.

Classically *moolabandha* is performed first, followed by the *uddiyanabandha*, and lastly, the *jalandharabandha*. To release, the *jalandharabandha* is released first and *moolabandha* last (the reverse order of application).

7.6. Meditation

7.6.1. Meditation: a simple explanation

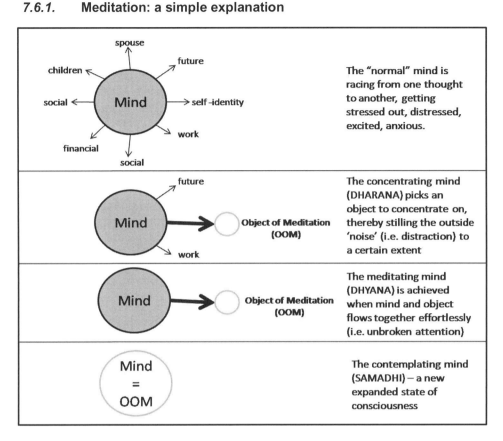

	The "normal" mind is racing from one thought to another, getting stressed out, distressed, excited, anxious.
	The concentrating mind (DHARANA) picks an object to concentrate on, thereby stilling the outside 'noise' (i.e. distraction) to a certain extent
	The meditating mind (DHYANA) is achieved when mind and object flows together effortlessly (i.e. unbroken attention)
	The contemplating mind (SAMADHI) – a new expanded state of consciousness

Diagram 7.1. **Stages of the mind**

7.6.2. The Yoga Sutra and meditation

In a sense, asana and *pranayama* are practices of *dharana* (concentration) to rein in the *vritti* so that *pratyhara* (withdrawal of the senses) is facilitated. As one moves deeper into *pratyhara* and *dharana*, one reaches the realms of *dhyana* (meditation).

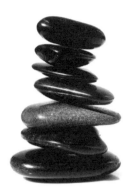

The last three stages of *ashtanga yoga* - namely *dharana, dhyana* and *samadhi* - are *samyama*. This is the state of meditation when the withdrawal of the *cit-prana* from the torment of the senses and the chattering mind is complete, and the energy flows inwards. In human beings, this has to be cultivated (as in following the path of *ashtanga yoga* or other practices) except in cases where the individual has fortunate past life (*karma*).

desa bandhas cittasya dharana [Sutra 1, Pada III]

Dharana (concentration) binds the mind in one place.

tatra pratyaya-ekatanata dhyanam [*Sutra 2, Pada* III]

Dhyana (meditation) is when the mind is focused in one place, then dissolved, and awareness flows. When the mind and *prana* are gathered and dissolved, all boundaries are dissolved and we are free to merge with the Ultimate Reality, a state described as *samadhi*. Together, *dharana, dhyana* and *samadhi* form *samyama*:

trayam ekatra samyamah [Sutra 4, Pada III]

Samyama is introduced in Chapter 3 of Patanjali's Yoga Sutra, in a chapter called Vibhuti Pada. There have been many books written and many schools founded to help those seeking *samadhi*. Patanjali's system is simple – becoming free of the *vritti* that keep us in our ignorance. This means letting go of the over-active analytical mind, *samskara, klesha, karma, vasana* and other activities which allows the *vrtti* to flourish.

When we have mastered *samyama*, wisdom shines (*prajna alokah*):

taj-jayat prajna-alokah [Sutra 5, Pada III]

When this light shines, we see the Universal Light reflected in all. In the words of Yogi Bhajan, Master of Kundalini Yoga, "If you can't see God in all, you can't see God at all".

7.7. *Pranayama*

7.7.1. Spirit of *pranayama*

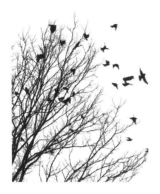

"As long as there is breath in the body, there is life. When breath departs, so too does life. Therefore, regulate the breath."
- Hatha Yoga Pradipika, Ch.2:S.3

"Controlling the breath, and thus calming the nerves, is the pre-requisite to controlling the mind and the body."
- Swami Rama, Science of Breath

Pranayama is the science of breathing consciously. In Eastern traditions and monasteries, there are those who have spent entire decades devoted entirely to studying the breath.

A serious teacher of *pranayama* would take pulse readings and make note of other vital signs to identify ailments of the body, and then prescribes a course of *pranayama* to eliminate the ailments. *Prana* lights the *agni,* or the sacred fire within (*section 6.5*). As agni is responsible for most of the important bodily processes such as metabolism and tissue-creation, a weak *prana* in the body would lead to ill health.

Take the focus off *asana* for its own sake – *asana* alone is not yoga. Yogis of the highest order are so completely absorbed into their yoga that *asana* burst forth from within, with the breath guiding and molding their bodies according to divine alignment. This is the highest union between the body and breath.

7.7.2. Definition of *pranayama*

Prana with the small 'p' is individual *prana*, whereas *Prana* with the capital 'P" is universal.

Classically:
Prana – life-force (*pra*, first unit; *na*, energy)
Ayama – control (expansion, manifestation)

However, I do not like this literal translation. We do not control the breath, nor seek to control it. It is not a beast to be controlled and tamed. Our breath is us; it is our Divinity. We should move towards being at one with our breath instead of fighting for supremacy. *Pranayama* is thus the movement of life's energy, the *prana*, through breathing consciously.

7.7.3. Benefits of *pranayama*

> **"The purpose of *Pranayama* is to make the respiratory system function at its best. The respiratory system is the gateway to purifying the body, mind and intellect. The key to this is *Pranayama*"**
> -   *BKS Iyengar*

During normal inhalation, an average person takes in about 500 cubic centimetres of air; during deep inhalation the intake is about six times as great, amounting to almost 3000 cubic centimetres. (The capacity of individuals varies according to constitution, but the practice of *pranayama* increases lung capacity and allows the lungs to achieve maximum ventilation).

Multiple scientific researches linking *pranayama* with measured health benefits have emerged in recent decades. Diaphragmatic breathing had been shown to have a potential as a therapeutic tool in dealing with anxiety-states and several other unrelated abnormalities.

Essential hypertension (high blood pressure of unknown causes) has been shown to respond favourably to a daily regime of diaphragmatic breathing (Funderburk, 1977). Even short-term training in yogic breathing techniques have been shown in a pilot study to bring about favorable respiratory changes in patients with chronic obstructive pulmonary disease (Pomidori, Campigotto, Amatya, Bernardi, and Cogo, 2009).

On a daily level, research by Joshi and Telles (2008) showed that an immediate effect is observed in verbal and spatial scores with alternate nostril breathing.

___

7.7.4. Key features of *pranayama*

> If you are struggling with your practice, whether it is because you get out of breath or find it difficult to get into a certain *yogasana*, always go back to first principles and focus on *pranayama*.
>
> Breathing incorrectly is often the reason for the difficulties encountered in a *yogasana* practice.

Stretching from within

With *yogasana*, you are stretching your body from the outside; with *pranayama*, you are stretching your body from the inside. Therefore you need both to grow in your yoga practice.

If you are struggling into a challenging position, such as a backbend, ask yourself why. *Is your breath constricted as you force your body further back? Are your muscles not at ease in the position you are trying to achieve?* Approach the posture from a different angle: find a position you are at ease in, *sukha*, let your breath flow, let go of your attachment to attain this asana, surrender to the breath, take time out and enjoy….this is yoga.

The breath initiates the move into *yogasana*

Central to any yogasana is the breath. The breath is your teacher. The body movement is the breath movement, and the breath movement is the body movement. The attainment of *yogasana* is not for its own sake; we practice *yogasana* to facilitate breath and *pranayama*.

Breath is Consciousness

Pranayama is moving the life force through conscious breathing. It is not merely about moving air in and out of our body, but our connection with the whole cosmos. There is *prana* in the air that we breathe in, which we incorporate into matter. When we chant or do something positive with good intentions, we return the *prana* to the Source, or transfer it. The plants, the skies, the clouds – that's all *prana* – and we are constantly inter-exchanging it with the cosmos.

7.7.5. Anatomy of *pranayama*: Western view

1. Nose
2. Ribs, intercostals muscles, diaphragm
3. Collarbone, sternum, abdominals

Breathing involves the following:
1. Movement of the abdomen
2. Movement of the pelvic floor
3. Movement of the sacrum, coccyx and lumbar spine
4. Movement of the spinal column
5. Movement of the hips
6. Movement of the shoulder girdle and arms

Primary muscles for *pranayama:*
1. Intercostals
2. Diaphragm
3. Abdominals (4 layers)

Secondary muscles for *pranayama*
1. Scalenes
2. Sternocleidomastoid
3. Trapezius
4. Pectoralis minor

7.7.6. Yogic anatomy of *pranayama*

The sound, smoothness and balance of the breath is a reflection of the state of mind and a *sadakh*'s practice. In *pranayama*, we aim for balance, ease and equanimity.

Inhalation (*puraka*): lengthens the spine, expands the ribcage and is facilitated by backbends and limbs moving away from the trunk.

Exhalation (*rechaka*): movement from the base of the body to lift the diaphragm to expel, which relates to calming and releasing postures (forward bends and twists).

From the chapter on Yogic Anatomy & Ayurvĕda (*Chapter 6*), the features of *prana* conduits in the body are:

- *Pingala* (right, *surya*)
- Ida (left, *chandra*)
- *Sushumna* (central channel, when both nostrils flow freely without obstruction)
- All three major *nadi* originate from the base of the spine and travel upwards (total of 72,000 *nadi*)
- *Ida* and *pingala* also travels up along the *sushumna*, and terminate at the left and right nostrils respectively
- The intersection between the *sushumna, ida* and *pingala* are the *chakra*
- Other *nadi* also extend from the *chakra* like the spokes of a wheel.

There are five components of *prana* within the body (*Diagram 7.2*). In a healthy body, all the five work together in harmony: *prana* brings in the fuel, *samana* converts this fuel to energy, *vyana* circulates the energy to the various work sites. *Apana* releases the waste materials or byproducts of the conversion process. *Udana* governs the positive energy created in the process and determines the work that the machine is able to do. Merging the *prana* with the *apana* also creates a pressure that raises the Kundalini.

udana-jayat-jala-panka-kantaka-adishuasanga utkrantis-ca [*Sutra* 40, *Pada* III]

When one masters *udana vayu*, one is no longer touched by obstacles such as water, mud and thorns, and rises above them [*Sutra* 40, *Pada* III].

samana-jayaj jvalanam [*Sutra* 41, *Pada* III]

Through mastery of *samana vayu*, we radiate light.

To experience the components of *prana*, refer to *section 6.5.2*.

Diagram 7.2. The five prana of the body

PRANA VAYU

This is the basic force that drives us in life, which sets things in motion.
It flows upwards and inwards into empty spaces, and governs important functions such as breathing, eating, drinking and receiving sensory inputs.

UDANA VAYU

This is the upward moving force that governs things that go upwards, such as growth, ability to stand, speech and vomit.
This force is about our enthusiasm for life!

VYANA VAYU

Moving from core to outside, this is the force that governs circulation: food, water and oxygen throughout the body, and keeps our emotions and thoughts circulating in the mind, imparting movement and providing strength.
This is the force that supports the work of Other prana.

SAMANA VAYU

This is 'churning air', a force that moves from the outside to the core. It governs digestion at all level, from digestion of food to oxygen to emotional, mental and sensory experiences.

APANA VAYU

A rooting force that moves downwards and outwards, governing the elimination of urine stool and menstrual blood, ejaculation and childbirth.
It also governs 'letting go' of negative emotional, mental and sensory experiences.

7.7.7. Learning *Pranayama*

Pranayama should only be studied under a suitably trained yoga teacher or one who is trained in the appropriate arts. Therefore, this book does not intend to teach its readers the techniques of *pranayama,* and urges readers to seek instructions prior to developing self-practice and teaching *pranayama.*

7.7.8. Summary of basic *pranayama* techniques

Many of the more obscure *pranayama* have been lost to the world, performed only by a few yogis who practice them in distant places. As a yoga teacher, your first task is teaching your students how to breathe again.

The *pranayama* described here are no more than basic notes into this deep and complex science, which you should have studied under the guidance of an appropriately qualified teacher for a length of time (and supplemented with personal practice) before attempting to teach others.

Yogic breath (diaphragmatic breathing)
This is the first exploration of the yogic breathing. It addresses the common issue of 'grasping' in this modern, head-led society, where most people suck in their breath, i.e. contracting the abdominal muscles to force the breath into the body.

Inhalation should be a passive process, so with diaphragmatic breathing we are teaching people to relax the abdominal muscles to allow the breath to flow in passively. Surrender, instead of grab.

Diaphragmatic breathing relaxes the autonomic nervous system and is essential preparation for deep meditation. Ensure that students take their breath down to their lower abdomens (putting a hand there helps).

Deerga swasam (three-part breath)
- The three parts are abdominal, chest and upper chest.

- Breathing slowly, concentrating on each of the three parts mentioned above in turn (from abdomen up), you actually take in seven times more air than you would if you breathe shallowly.
- This is very invigorating and calming, and you can feel the effect even with a minimal numbers of rounds.

Anuloma viloma / nadi sodhana (alternate nostril breathing)

- The hand that closes the nostrils is always the right hand in Vishnu Mudra.
- The general pattern is you inhale through one nostril, retain the breath, and exhale through the other nostril in a ratio of 2:8:4
- This is a wonderfully balancing breath that equilibrates both hemispheres of the brain.

Kapalabhati

the pranayama that makes the forehead and entire face lustrous

- It is a *panchakarma*, cleansing through all the chakra
- *Kapalabhati* is known as the yogic cup of coffee because of its invigorating effect.
- This breath is not to be done by pregnant and menstruating women, and those with slipped disc (heavy abdominal movement may aggravate the problems)
- To teach, sit next to the student. Ask her to put both hands on her abdomen, and as she forcefully exhales, feel the abdominal muscles contracting to expel the air. Do one exhalation at a time. The focus is on the exhale only, exhaling through the nose.
- Students new to this breathing technique may complain of giddiness and nausea – this is due to a high volume of oxygen delivered to the brain – but there is nothing to be concerned about.

Bhastrika

- This is the "bellows breath", so with this *pranayama*, open your lungs like bellows, with fast inhalation and fast exhalation.
- Strong use of abdominal muscles as in Kapalabhati.
- Equal focus on inhale and exhale
- Finish by inhaling through right nostril and performing *kumbhaka* with bandha and exhaling through left nostril.

Brahmari

- Humming bee breath, wonderfully focusing and suitable for entering into a meditative state. Children love it!
- Cover your ears with your thumbs, and cover your eyes with the rest of your fingers.
- Hum with your inhale and exhale, keeping your breath regular, so that your pitch is smooth.

Sitali

- This is the "tongue-hissing" breath, where the tongue is curled into a "straw" and the breath is sipped through the straw.
- Inhale through curled tongue, exhale through the nose.
- As it is a cooling breath, the tongue may taste bitter because of the toxins excreted.

Sitkari

- Open your lips as if you are smiling, the lower row of your teeth touching the upper row. Inhale through teeth (making a hissing sound) and exhale through the nose.
- This is a cleansing breath which boosts glandular function.

Ujayyi

"Victorious breath"

- This is the main *pranayama* of Ashtanga Vinyasa Yoga.
- It helps you to use the whole capacity of your body.
- The sound of this breath brings meditative quality to your practice.
- It enhances ventilation of the lungs, removes phlegm, calms the nerves and fills the whole body with vitality.
- *Ujayyi breathing* is not that easy to get a hang of. Always practiced with mouth closed, but to learn, whisper "ahhhhh" with mouth open (inhale and exhale through the mouth), focusing on the throaty sound at the back of your throat, which should sound free and surrendered, not constricted.

Last word on *pranayama*: you really need to learn this from an experienced teacher.

7.7.9. *Pranayama* and the Yoga Sutra

Firstly, it is important to recognise that *prana* refers to life force, not just the breath alone. Therefore, observation of the breath is but a means of getting our physical self in touch with the subtle energy to reach higher awareness as well as to reap the benefits of breathing properly.

sthira sukham asanam [*Sutra* 46, *Pada* II]

prayatna saithilya ananta samapattibhyam [*Sutra* 47, *Pada* II]

tatah dvanda anabhighatah [*Sutra* 48, *Pada* II]

tasmin sati svasa-prasvasayor gati-vicchedah pranayamah
[*Sutra* 49, *Pada* II]

The practice of yogasana should be balanced and comfortable [*Sutra* 46, *Pada* II]. This state of balance is achieved when the effort to perform the yogasana is relaxed (*prayatna saithilya*). With the letting go of effort, we are merging (*samapattibhyam*) with Infinity (*ananta*) [*Sutra* 47, *Pada* II]. In this state, duality ceases to exist [*Sutra* 48, *Pada* II].

tasmin sati svasa-prasvasayor gati-vicchedah pranayamah – I always tell my yoga students that this simply means, "practice your *yogasana* well and *pranayama* comes naturally".

Svasa-prasvasayoh means inhalation and exhalation. *Gati* is the movement and *viccedah* is cessation. Therefore, *Sutra* 49 could be taken to mean that upon accomplishing the states described in Sutras *46*, *47* and *48* (mastery of yogasana, merging with Infinity and destruction of duality), the movement of inhalation / exhalation ceases, and *pranayama* follows as surely as night follows day.

7.7.10. Living *Pranayama*

Pranayama is a subtle practice in awareness and observation, nothing at all to do with control, though "*ayama*" is often translated as control.

239

As we become more comfortable in our yogasana, our attention turns inward and moves from the gross to the subtle. This is when we become of our energy, the life force that circulates in our body (*prana*) and its relationship with the universal life force (*Prana*).

> The best way of advancing your own *pranayama* practice is to check in with your breath throughout the day (*section 7.4.2*).

The merging of *prana* with *Prana* is the state of yoga. Yoga is not a linear science, but something that is more complex, beautiful and interconnected. Ease in *yogasana* leads to breathing consciously, but similarly, if a student is encountering obstacles in his practice of *yogasana*, he should return to *pranayama* and work on this. Breathing incorrectly causes many of the problems one commonly encounters in *yogasana*.

The practice of *pranayama* contains these three components: *puraka* (inhalation), *rechaka* (exhalation) and *kumbhaka* (breath-retention). When we are breathing normally (subconsciously), this is karmic breathing. By practicing *pranayama*, we are disrupting established patterns, which disrupt the *vritti*. In an advanced practice, *pranayama* also moves us into a "karma-free" zone in which healing can take place.

Within the confines of a typical yoga class, *pranayama* is invaluable in that it elevates an ordinary posture into a *yogasana*. It gives practitioners an entrée into *dhyana* and *samadhi*. *Samapattibhyam* is a necessary component – *samapattibhyam* means merging or aligning with Infinity. As discussed at the beginning of this section on *pranayama*, our breath is our link to Infinity.

7.8. Relaxation and visualization

REFER TO BOOK 3: YOGASENSE™ (under the Guided Relaxation section).

7.8.1. Go within and heal

True relaxation occurs when the body and mind expend very little or no energy. It is Nature's way of regrouping the body's resources to channel inwards for maintenance and healing. *Yogasana* are the physical technique for retraining the muscles to be able to relax. However, some practitioners may find it difficult to let go.

Visualization and guided meditation can be used to aid relaxation. They also are a practice of *dharana*, where one gathers one's thoughts and focus it in a certain direction or on a particular object.

For a deeper relaxation, do Yoga Nidra or "sleep of the yogis". This is a state of conscious deep sleep for extreme relaxation and subtler spiritual exploration, and can be experienced under the guidance of a yoga teacher or CD.

7.9. Sanskrit chants

7.9.1. AUM (OM)

OM is the universal sound. When I teach children yoga, I tell them it is the sound of the Universe breathing.

In the book of the Upanishads, it is said that "Om is the one eternal syllable of which all that exists is but the development. The past, the present, and the future are all included in this one sound, and all that exists beyond the three forms of time is also implied in it".

You can break down the sound into four components, and enjoy, assimilate and honor each component:

- A = sound of the infinite expanding energy of the Universe, the light of Consciousness and Divine Love
- U = that energy manifesting and materializing into our waking reality
- M = we integrate the energy into our being
- Silence after the AUM.

In the silence that follows, we give our humble thanks and allow the sacred sound AUM to vibrate within us.

This is what AUM looks like in Devanigri script, which you can type in Microsoft word (backslash\ in the Wingdings font): ॐ

There are a lot of intellectual meanings attached to AUM relating to the various waking states. Your first approach to experiencing AUM is to embrace and feel the power of the word: with the 'A' sound, spread your arms wide to your side, as if to embrace the Universe. With the 'U' sound, bring your arms above your head in a prayer pose, and with the 'M' sound, bring the prayer pose to your heart, integrating the energy into your being. Repeat several times, bringing *prana* and joy into your body, until you hear AUM singing in your soul.

7.9.2. Gâyatrî Mantra

Aum Bhur Bhuva Svah
Tat Savitur Varenyam
Bhargo Devasya Dhimahi
Dhiyo Yo Naha Prachodayat

Translation:
We meditate on the glory of the Creator;
Who has created the Universe;
Who is worthy of Worship;
Who is the embodiment of Knowledge and Light;
Who is the remover of all Sin and Ignorance;
May He enlighten our Intellect.
(translation by Swâmi Sivânanda)

Written around 2,500-3,500 years ago in the Rig Veda (iii, 62, 10), the Gâyatrî Mantra is probably the most widely known *mantra*. Chant for 108 cycles.

7.9.3. Asatho Maa

Om Om Om
Asatho Maa Sath Gamaya
Thamaso Maa Jyothir Gamaya
Mruthyor Maa Amrutham Gamaya
Om Shanti. Shanti. Shanti.

Translation:
Om Om Om
Lead me from unreal to Real
Lead me from darkness to Light
Lead me from death to Immortality.
(Peace, peace, peace be to all.)

7.9.4. *Mantra* of Ashtanga Vinyasa Yoga

Opening Mantra
OM, Vande Gurunam charanaravinde
Sandarshita svatmasukhavabodhe
Nishreyase jangalikayamane
Samsara halahala mohashantyai
Abahu Purushakaram
Shankhacakrsi dharinam
Sahasra sirasam svetam
Pranamami patanjalim OM

Translation:

OM, I pray to the lotus feet of the supreme guru

Who teaches knowledge, awakening the great happiness of the Self revealed

Who acts like the jungle physician

Able to remove the delusion from the poison of conditioned existence

To Patanjali, an incarnation of Adisesa, white in color with

A thousand radiant heads (in his form as the divine serpent, Ananta),

Human in form below the shoulders, holding the sword of discrimination,

A wheel of fire representing infinite time and the conch representing divine

sound to him I prostrate. OM

Closing mantra

OM, Swasthi-praja bhyah pari pala yantam

Nya-yena margena mahi-mahishaha

Go-bramanebhyaha-shuhamastu-niyam

Lokaa-samastha sukhino-bhavanthu. OM.

Translation:

OM, May prosperity be glorified

May administrators rule the world with law and justice

May all things that are sacred be protected

And may people of the world be happy and prosperous. OM

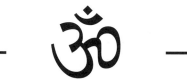

References

Funderburk, J. (1977). Science Studies Yoga. Honesdale, PA, USA: Himalayan Institute

Joshi, M., & Telles, S. (2008). Immediate effects of right and left nostril breathing on verbal and spatial scores. *Indian J Physiol Pharmacol*. 2008 Apr-Jun;52(2):197-200.

Pomidori, L., Campigotto, F., Amatya, T.M., Bernardi, L., & Cogo A. (2009). Efficacy and tolerability of yoga breathing in patients with chronic obstructive pulmonary disease: a pilot study. *J Cardiopulm Rehabil* Prev. 2009 Mar-Apr;29(2):133-7

CHAPTER EIGHT
Teaching Methodology

OVERVIEW OF THE CHAPTER

8.1   Ethics of a yoga teacher
8.2   The teacher-student relationship
8.3   Teaching yoga as a yogi: the *yama*
8.4   Teaching *drishti*
8.5   Teaching *bandha*
8.6   Teaching meditation
8.7   Teaching *pranayama*
8.8   Teaching relaxation and visualization
8.9.   Teaching YogaSense™
8.10   Teaching *padmasana*
8.11   Teaching safely
8.12   Structuring a yoga class

8.1. Ethics of a yoga teacher

8.1.1. "Sat Nam" – teach truthfully

Yoga is like a multi-faceted diamond: it means different things to different practitioners. For some, it is merely a system of physical exercise, weight management or stress relief. For others, it is a spiritual path handed down for centuries to help us make sense of the world today. And for some practitioners, yoga is simply a way of life. Whatever your students' motivation, you as their teacher should honor the trust they placed in you.

As a teacher, your task is to lead your students to their inner teacher, so that he may find his own yoga. You are merely a facilitator, passing down the centuries-old teaching like a conduit, but you are never the master. The moment a teacher sees himself as a master rather than a facilitator is the moment the ego stops the teacher from fulfilling his role as a teacher. The greatness of a teacher comes from his humility, not his self-promotion.

The innate knowledge and inner wisdom already lie within each and every one of us. Your job is to guide your students to this space without the colorings of your own ego.

8.1.2. Be firmly rooted in your practice

It is common that as a yoga teacher becomes more popular and takes on more classes, he finds less time for his personal practice.

Without a strong personal practice, the teacher within will not blossom and thus, you will not be able to reach out to your students from your own core. Without that deep connection, your teaching will be mechanical and devoid of any real heart.

You need to keep your connection with your own yoga strong before you can teach with passion, fire and deep emotional connection. At Sun Yoga, it is a set practice that our teachers become full-time students at intervals during their teaching career *.

At Sun Yoga, our philosophy for those training to be yoga teachers is "You will not become a yoga teacher from what you learn here; you become a teacher from your personal practice".

8.1.3. Teach with integrity

Asteya, or non-stealing, is part of *yama*, which is a *mahavratam* or the Great Universal Vow (*Chapter 2: Philosophy, Ethics & Lifestyle)*.

The worst a teacher could do is to steal another's teachings for his own glory. Attending a workshop and then teaching the same thing the next day without feeling and assimilating the new knowledge is equivalent to pirating a CD – you are mass-producing another person's originality dishonorably. Teachings and knowledge are often imparted with generosity of spirit and pure intent, so honor those who teach you.

Grow with what you learned from your teachers, assimilate their teachings into your practice, live with those teachings for a while and only then teach from within*.

* All Sun Yoga's teacher training courses are taught only by those who played a role in developing those courses. They are never taught by those who pay a fee to learn how to deliver those courses.

8.1.4. Be a <u>real</u> teacher, not a false prophet

Because of the *ahamkara, manas* and *buddhi (section 5.6.5)*, it is all too easy for one to believe in one's own greatness. A yoga teacher, especially one with charisma and who is prepared to travel to far-flung outposts, will have students clamoring at her feet for her teachings, even though she may be new to yoga herself.

As a new teacher's student base grows, she must diligently practice the eight limbs of yoga herself to ensure that she is not beset with a sense of false grandeur, or *asmita* (*section* 5.6.7). If teaching from the ego perspective, one's teachings will be impure and corrupt.

A teacher should always remember that central to the yoga path is the letting go of one's identity (the ego); thus all teachers should be equal in the absence of the ego*.

* At Sun Yoga, all teachers earn the same basic rate for teaching regular classes, and new teachers are given equal billing as more experienced ones.

8.1.5. "I am a teacher"

Life in the real world is such that teachings are not given free of charge – a yoga teacher needs to earn her living. However, a more important benefit for paying for a yoga class is that this transaction makes clear the relationship between a yoga teacher and her students.

Even if you are teaching your relatives, you should charge for your teachings. Even if you are not interested in making money, you should still charge for your teachings. Then give the money away to charity.

Charging for a yoga class clarifies the situation in the mind of all. And most of all, for you, the yoga teacher, it sets forth your obligations as a teacher (*section 8.2*).

8.1.6. Let your students go with grace

One of the lesser known philosophies of yoga is that when a student is ready, the teacher will come. Similarly, as your students outgrow you, they will leave you. If you are too focused on teaching instead of growing in your own practice, your students will definitely outgrow you and reach the point where they need a new teacher to guide them to their next level. Also, according to the Yoga Sutra, whether one achieves enlightenment or not is dependent on *karma*, so it may be that those students will outgrow you anyway.

Practice *vairagya*, or non-attachment and *aparigraha*, which is non-grasping. It is the opposite of *raga*, which is greediness and grabbing. If you are not attached to your students and to the material benefits of being a 'successful' teacher, you are on your path to self-liberation. This is when your teaching takes on a new dimension. Therefore, let your students go with grace.

8.1.7. Teach an empty class

As teachers, we are often disappointed when we turn up to teach a class and find that there are only one or two students there. Apart from the financial factor and a waste of your time to teach a class of one, the disappointment is built by what we think of as "lack of group energy".

Well, you are the yoga teacher. You have to infuse your teaching with passion, whether it is to a class of one or one hundred.

Also, an empty class is a wonderful opportunity to do a self-review on whether you truly love teaching yoga or if you are merely teaching for the sake of the money and glory.

8.2. The teacher-student relationship

8.2.1. Stay within your scope of practice

As the boundaries of the esoteric arts are somewhat blurred, it is easy to stray beyond our scope of practice. For example, a yoga teacher can all too often get carried away when talking about the yogic diet and morph into the role of a dietician, something that he is not qualified to do without the appropriate training (in the UK, a degree in Nutrition typically takes three years of studying to obtain).

A good way of remembering what the boundaries are is to ask yourself "How does this piece of advice that I am giving relate to my student's yoga practice?" Always go back to yoga and the Yoga Sutra as your starting point.

Example of staying within and going beyond your scope of practice
Student: Do I need to be a vegetarian to be a yogi?

✓ Teacher: Classically, yogis are vegetarians because killing animals contravenes ahimsa, which is the principle of non-violence.

X *Teacher*: Oh yes! You have to stop eating meat! You don't need meat anyway, and meat gives you cancer...you can buy supplements from me to make sure you get enough nutrients.

8.2.2. Sexual misconduct

There have occasionally been allegations of sexual misconduct directed at yoga teachers. Of course, there are a few unscrupulous teachers out there who take advantage of their students, which is a breach of professional trust of the highest degree. To protect yourself from these allegations, ensure that your actions are not open to misinterpretation. For example, always ask for permission before performing a manual adjustment on a student, especially a new student (*section 8.2.3*). Do not use inappropriate dialogue or make comments of a personal nature to a student.

Dating your yoga student is never a good idea because it changes the dynamics of a class.

Note: see section on *brahmacharya* (*section 8.3.4*).

8.2.3. Respect boundaries

Cultural differences and personal perspectives create differences in what a person would or would not perceive as a violation.

Mentioning a student by name could be perceived as getting too personal. "Debra, you are doing so well this week" could be deemed unacceptable by some students who value their anonymity in class.

However, most serious breaches are encountered when a teacher performs a manual adjustment on her students. In some yoga schools, such as Kundalini Yoga, a teacher never adjusts a student physically. This is based on the philosophy that as teachers, we should respect where our students are today in their practice, and that ultimately their inner wisdom will guide them there.

But for the Ashtanga and Hatha Yoga teachers, manual adjustments prove invaluable in guiding our students to exploring and deepening their *yogasana* practice.

249

These are the key guidelines to manual adjustments:

<u>Avoid large area of skin-to-skin contact</u>
If you intend to adjust your students manually, respect their modesty. For example, if you and your student are both bare-skinned (as per the typical Ashtanga practice wear), it would be a good idea to use a towel to avoid large area of skin-to-skin contact.

<u>Where never to touch!</u>
Touching a student in the crotch is definitely a taboo, even if only to illustrate the *moolabandha*!

<u>Ask for permission first</u>
It is also a good idea to ask for permission, especially from new students.

Example of a good dialogue
> "I am going to adjust you in three ways. First, I am going to adjust you visually: I will show you a posture, and you follow what I do. Second, I am going to adjust you orally: I will tell you what to do. Third, I will adjust you manually, which means I am going to be touching you to help you get into postures. If you are not comfortable with manual adjustments, just let me know before I adjust you".

<u>Never use your feet</u>
Feet are often considered unclean in some cultures. The only universally acceptable use of feet in adjustment is using your feet to adjust your students' feet, as in angling the back foot in *trikonasana* and so forth.

You should never put your foot on your student's head to get him to relax the neck muscles in *adho mukha svanasana*! Instead, use the oral cue "Let your head drift to the ground like a drop of molten wax". If you have a small class, massage your student's neck to illustrate the need to totally relax the back in this *yogasana*.

8.2.4. Respect your students' rights

Never photograph or video your students without their written consent. In many countries, it is against the law to publish (even in newsletters and websites) a person's photograph without a signed release form.

8.2.5. Socializing with students

When your students become your friends (as it does in the case of long-term loyal students), the boundaries are, of course, blurred.

As with most things in life, there is no clear-cut answer. Act, speak, think and live the way of the Yoga Sutra, in particular the *niyama* (*Chapter 2: Philosophy, Ethics & Lifestyle*) which always stands one in good stead.

8.3. Teaching yoga as a yogi: the *yama*

8.3.1. *Ahimsa* – non-violence

On the mat, teach your students how to practice non-injury towards their own bodies. This should be the first lesson. All too often, we see ambitious students going too far beyond the capabilities of their bodies instead of respecting where they are today in their practice. This is the source of most injuries sustained in a yoga class. Moreover, yoga is not about how far you can go in a *yogasana*, but the alignment of your body as you bring the *yogasana* deeper mindfully. It should be emphasized that in *yogasana,* substance always takes precedence over form, or external appearance.

Once *ahimsa* has been mastered on the mat and embraced wholly by the practitioner, it will suffuse his inner being. With *ahimsa*, a person can then subdue the *Pasu-Svabhava* (bestial nature) that exists within him. We need to practice non-violence in ourselves before we can extend it to the external world. In the words of Sri Swami Sivananda, non-injury requires a harmless mind, mouth, and hand.

8.3.2. *Satya* – truthfulness

Teach truthfully. Do not abandon your personal practice in search of fame and adulation as a yoga teacher, because it is through your personal practice that you evolve as a teacher of yoga.

Be truthful to yourself about your own capabilities. If you are not truthful to yourself, how can you be truthful to others? Your personal practice is the ideal way of getting to know yourself, and facing up to your limitations, issues and boundaries. Be truthful to your students about where you are today as a teacher.

Teach within your capabilities. If you have never been trained as an Ashtanga teacher, do not advertise yourself as one. If you have never attended a teacher training course but still teach yoga, be upfront to your students and let them know that you are here to share your experience and love of yoga with them from the vantage point of a passionate practitioner. It is from practicing *satya* at this gross level that the words, deeds and wisdom materialize to take us closer to the Ultimate Truth.

8.3.3. *Asteya* – non-stealing

In recent years, there has been a proliferation of 'Hot Yoga' classes, almost all of which are copied directly from the Bikram system. While yoga should never be patented because the wisdom belongs to all, profiting blatantly from someone else's hard work without acknowledging the source is a form of stealing.

Duplicating CDs without the copyright holder's permission, photocopying complete books and using your students' photographs without prior consent are three other obvious forms of stealing.

But *steya,* stealing, exists in subtler forms. One common example is short-circuiting your practice by moving on to advanced postures before putting in the months and years of hard work to get there. By wanting less and by expecting nothing, we move away from the need to steal. Enjoy your practice and feel blessed by what you have.

8.3.4.   *Brahmacharya* – focused and committed

Brahmacharya is popularly taken to mean celibacy and sexual continence. Thus, in this context, a breach of this vow occurs when the teacher has a sexual relationship with a student (or several students!).

But meditating on the deeper meaning of the word, *Brahma* (God) and *acharya* (guide) lead us to the notion of being devoted and pure in our actions and thoughts. It speaks of self-discipline. For the yoga teacher to embrace *brahmacharya* into his code of conduct would be as simple as being faithful to his yoga path: being committed to self-practice and practicing the eight limbs of Ashtanga Yoga (*Chapter 2: Philosophy, Ethics & Lifestyle*) in his daily life.

8.3.5.   *Aparigraha* – non-grasping

[REFER TO *section 8.1.6*]

8.4.   Teaching *Drishti*

[REFER TO *section 7.5*]

8.4.1. Focus and adjustment from within

Incorporating *drishti* into a yoga class need not be complicated. Make it part of a *yogasana* instructional dialogue in an organic way. To start with, introduce a few basic ones. For example (in *bhujangasana*): as you lift your torso, focus on the lateral expansion of your chest and your heart. Now, roll your eyeballs upwards so that you are looking into the space between your eyebrows. This is the *broomadhya drishti*.

8.4.2. The yoga eye exercise

Sit in *padmasana* or easy pose. Curl up the four fingers of your right hand into a fist with your thumb facing upwards. Position your thumb directly in front of your eyes with your arm straight.

Relax your eyes and softly gaze straight ahead. Now elevate your arm as illustrated in *Diagram 8.1*. Without moving your head, lift your eyeballs up towards your thumb. Focus your gaze on the fingernail of your thumb. From this 12 o'clock position, move your thumb to the 1 o'clock position. With your head kept absolutely still, follow the movement of your thumb with your eyes only. Focus your gaze on your thumbnail. Keep your gaze in this position for a few breaths.

Move your thumb around all the twelve positions of the clock's face, pausing at each position to focus your eyes and holding the gaze at each position for a few breaths before moving on to the next.

To finish, stare at your thumb in neutral position (*Diagram 8.1*), then look into the distance, Relax and repeat. Cup your hands over your eyes for 30 seconds and relax.

Diagram 8.1. **Yoga eye exercise**

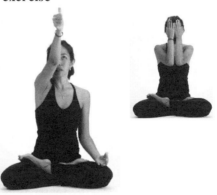

A simpler version of the yoga eye exercise is moving the eyes around an imaginary clock. This allows the focus to be on the eye movement if holding the arm up is difficult. Finish with the hands over eyes.

8.4.3. Using the mind's eye: disappearing objects (beginner)

Place two objects in front of your eyes, about 12 inches between each other. Focus on the space between the two objects. Look intensely at the space. Then with your mind's eye, make the two objects disappear so that you are gazing at the endless stretch of empty space.

8.4.4. Using the mind's eye: mountain and rock (intermediate)

With your eyes wide open, imagine a tiny rock as a big mountain. See the big rock right in front of you, as if it is really there. Stretch your eyes as wide as you can so that you can wrap your gaze around the perimeter of your mountain. Hold your gaze there.

Now slowly bring your field of vision inward as your big mountain morphs into a small rock. Keep the form, texture and nuances of the mountain intact as it shrinks into the small rock – continue to see its fine features clearly in front of you. Squeeze your mountain into a smaller and smaller rock, maintaining the clarity and fine details at all time. See as if the rock is really in front of your eyes. Relax and repeat. Cup your hands over your eyes for 30 seconds and relax.

8.5. Teaching *bandha*

[REFER TO *section 7.5*]

8.5.1. Getting in touch with the energy locks

Firstly, *bandha* is not just about squeezing muscles, as is commonly believed and taught by many yoga teachers.

Bandha is a lot more subtle and complicated than that, and there has been some debate as to whether *bandha* should be taught to new practitioners, who are perhaps not yet aware of the subtleties of their bodies.

However, without *bandha*, a yoga practice is like a building without strong foundations. The *bandha* is important for the correct positioning of *yogasana*, and conversely, *yogasana* refines *bandha*. An Ashtanga yogi would appreciate how *bandha* elevates (literally!) his practice, especially in the forward jump from *ardho mukha svanasana* to *uttanasana*.

To teach bandha, preparation or groundwork has to be undertaken first. This involves getting to know each of the main *bandha* areas.

_____

8.5.2. *Moolabandha* – root lock

How to teach the *moolabandha*

Yoga teachers sometimes find it embarrassing and awkward to teach the *moolabandha* because of its location (no manual adjustments permitted in this area!). The best way to teach students how to engage this very important lock is by first giving them an overview of the location and how this *bandha* works:

Moolabandha takes place low in the perineum and depends upon the energetic relationship between the sacrum/tailbone complex and the pubic bone. It simultaneously draws the pelvis down from the torso and spine while the pelvic diaphragm domes upward.

Moolabandha roots the body by creating a foundation with the pelvis and the spine. The sacrum moves away from the occiput, and the spine becomes long. *Moolabandha* should be present in most, if not all, *yogasana* (except *savasana*).

Start with relaxing the perineum as the first step to get in touch with the *moolabandha*. Then bring awareness into the area. Gently bring movement to the muscles. From section 7.6.2, the four stages of engaging the *moolabandha* are:

5. Contract your anus – pull your anal sphincter inwards and upwards;

6. Contract your perineum by engaging your pelvic floor muscles. A good way of practicing this is starting and stopping urine flow;

7. Lift your pelvic diaphragm by contracting the levator ani (engaging the transverse abdominis): draw your belly button towards your spine;

8. Isolate the previous three actions and work on refining each muscle group.

8.5.3. Uddiyanabandha

After students have had some experience of the *moolabandha*, introduce them to the *uddiyanabandha,* which is the second lock in the sequence.

How to teach the *uddiyanabandha*
Teach *uddiyanabandha* according to the techniques described in *section 7.6.3*:

Place your hands on your knees, bending forward slightly at the hips. Exhale completely, squeezing every last bit of air out from your lungs.

When your lungs are empty, close your throat. With your throat closed, create a vacuum by expanding your chest. This sucks the abdomen inward and upward. Note that there is no muscular engagement needed for this *bandha*, only the vacuum from locking out the breath and expanding the thoracic cavity. Hold the *bandha*. To release *uddiyanabandha*, swallow and release from the belly.

Further practice of this *bandha* can be experienced according to instructions detailed in *section 7.5.3* under the section heading *Intensifying the experience.*

8.5.4. Jalandharabandha

The important thing to remember when teaching this *bandha* is that it is not to be performed by students suffering from whiplash.

How to teach the *jalandharabandha*
A simple way of teaching this *bandha* is instructing students to place an orange, tennis ball or sock under their chins and holding the objects there gently whilst keeping the neck long and the throat soft. Check that shoulders are not hunched.

8.5.5. *Mahabandha*

<u>How to teach the *mahabandha*</u>
When instructing students, it may be effective if students perform the *maha mudra* first. This is done by pressing the anus with the left heel. Place the right foot upon the left thigh. Slowly draw the *apana vayu* upwards through the lock.

To begin the practice, instruct students that on exhalation, apply *moolabandha, uddiyanabandha* and *jalandharabandha* sequentially. Hold the breath out, keeping the throat soft.

> The rule of thumb is to apply the *bandha* from the bottom up, and release them from the top down.

Release *jalandharabandha,* followed by *uddiyanabandha* and finally *moolabandha:* as you inhale, draw air into the lower abdomen by passively relaxing the diaphragm down (the classic mistake is to suck the breath in).

For beginners, repeat this sequence 10 times.

Mahabandha is applied in *pranayama, pratyhara, dharana, mudra* and meditation practice. Exhort students to try doing all the *bandha* during the day while walking, sitting, and working.

> Intense *bandha* practice should not be undertaken by practitioners who suffer from:
>
> 1. Whiplash injuries (contra-indicated for *jalandharabandha*)
> 2. Low Blood Pressure
> 3. Heart Diseases
> 4. Hernia
> 5. Stomach or Intestinal Ulcer
> 6. Visceral Ailments

8.6. Teaching meditation

8.6.1. Meditation via concentration

You cannot teach meditation: you can only teach concentration, which leads your students to a meditative state of mind. If concentration is the drops of oil being poured from one container to another in drips, then meditation is when the oil's flow ceases to be in drop-by drop form but flows smoothly in one steady stream.

Meditation is not only sitting still in lotus position chanting OM, but can take various formats: choose one that is most relevant for your age group/students' maturity.

8.6.2. Some common types of meditation

One of the main barriers to meditation is students' inability to sit comfortably. The classical position for meditation is *padmasana*, but few could sit in this position for any length of time.

Thus, for new students, ensure that they are sitting with a straight spine and are sitting comfortably (use props such as cushion beneath the knees or sit against a wall).

Observing the Breath (for beginners: 3 - 7 minutes)
"Sit comfortably. Close your eyes. Breathe deeply. Take the breath deep into your body. Enjoy being in your body. Feel your breath moving in your body; follow that movement. Feel your breath, hear your breath and enjoy your breath."

Note: to take this meditation deeper (i.e. 11 minutes), ask students to concentrate on sounds furthest away from them, and then slowly bring their attention to sounds that are closer, and then into nothingness.

Visualization (beginner to intermediate level)
By staring at the gross features of an object, students are led inwards into the object until they are completely immersed in the subtle features of the object of meditation and finally, absorbed totally into it.

<u>Advanced level meditation: Tratakam</u>
This is a meditation that focuses the *prana* and heightens concentration. This is often done by gazing at an object with eyes 9/10th closed, and losing yourself into the object of your meditation. Because of the intensity of this practice, I would not advise Tratakam meditation for beginner students or those who are suffering from mental health conditions.

8.6.3. Methods for leading meditation

<u>Visualization</u>
Ask students to visualise themselves lying on a beach on a sunny day, feeling the sand beneath their bodies and sunshine on the faces. Can they hear the sound of the sea beating against the shore? Imagine there are breadcrumbs on their outstretched palms; they have to lie still enough for the seagulls to come and pick those crumbs up......

Use beautiful inspiring music and instruct your students to immerse themselves in it.

<u>Contemplation on self-discovery</u>
"*What's in it for me*?" Explain to students the benefits of meditation and how it can affect their lives positively. Talk about the calming effect, or that how some meditations can energize you, or how it can leave you rested as a nights sleep.

<u>Using objects of meditation</u>

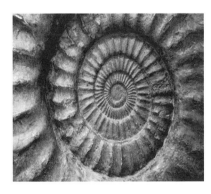

Give your class something beautiful to contemplate (rock crystals, fruits, stones, anything of beauty).

Divide the class into groups of three or four, with each group given an object to meditate on. Guide the class into a short meditation by visualization.

8.6.4. Moving meditation

Do the Surya Namaskar, first by focusing on the breath, then on chanting the *mantra* and finally focusing on each *chakra* as you take the students through the sequence (*Table 8.1*):

Table 8.1. Surya Namaskar meditation

Breath/Asana	Mantra	Chakra
Inhale, arms overhead	Om Mitraaya Namaha *Salutations to the Friend of All*	Anahata
Exhale, forward bend	Om Ravaye Namaha *Salutations to the Shining One*	Vishuddhi
Inhale, step back into lunge	Om Suryaaya Namaha *Salutations to the Source of Creation*	Svadishtana
Exhale, downward dog	Om Bhaanve Namaha *Salutations to He who illumines*	Ajna
Inhale, plank pose	Om khagaaya Namaha *Salutations to One who moves through the sky*	Vishuddhi
Exhale, chaturanga	Om Pooshney Namaha *Salutations to the Giver of strength and nourishment*	Manipura
Inhale, upward dog or cobra	Om Hiranayagarbhaaya Namah *Salutations to the Golden Womb*	Svadishtana
Exhale, downward dog	Om Mareechibhyoh Namaha *Salutations to the Rays of the Sun*	Vishuddhi
Inhale, step forward into Lunge	Om Adityaaya Namaha *Salutations to the Infinite Cosmic Mother*	Ajna
Exhale, forward bend	Om Savitre Namaha *Salutations to the rising sun*	Svadishtana
Inhale, come to standing, arms overhead	Om Arkaaya Namaha *Salutations to the Source of Life Energy*	Vishuddhi
Exhale, back to centre	Om Bhaaskaraaya Namah *Salutations to the one who leads to enlightenment*	Anahata

To perform Surya Namaskar on a quicker flow, use the *bij* (seed) *mantra*:

1. Om Hram
2. Om Hrim
3. Om Hroom
4. Om Hraim
5. Om Hraum
6. Om Hrah

Repeat these six *mantra* for the remaining six *asana* of the Surya Namaskar sequence. Perform this for several cycles.

8.6.5. Meditation in motion

Incorporating *mantra* to *vinyasa* greatly enhances the meditative effect of the *yogasana*. It also enhances the awakening of the mind, body and soul. Often, in meditation, the lesson is teaching students to let go – first physically, and then mentally (of the thinking mind). The YogaSense™ meditative flow is given in Part 3 of this book.

8.7. Teaching *pranayama*

[REFER TO *section 7.8*: Pranayama]

8.7.1. Explaining *pranayama*

Pranayama is the window of the Self. That is why it is called the great austerity (*maha tapas*) and the true knowledge of the Self (*Brahmavidya*).

A soul was asked by God to return to Earth. She said, "Oh no, please, I am happy here by your side. I don't want to leave your side."

And God said to the soul, "Go, but remember this: when you need to talk to me, use your breath."

8.7.2. *Pranayama* within a class setting

Within the context of a yoga class, *pranayama* is practiced either at the beginning or at the end of a yoga class. It is very much the poor relation of *asana* – though it is one of the eight limbs of *ashtanga yoga* (as is *asana*), the practice of *pranayama* very rarely exceeds 20% of total class time.

The prevailing reason for this lack of focus on *pranayama* is largely market forces –most students attend yoga for the workout, and view sitting still watching their breath as a waste of money. There are incidences, too, when students mistake *pranayama* for a religious practice.

8.7.3. The technical points

1. In *pranayama*, there is less attention to the body and more focus on the subtleties of the inner being.

2. The breath envelops the body movement. Breath starts slightly before and finishes slightly after the movement. Remember, the breath always initiates the movement into the *yogasana*.

3. Generally, inhalation is associated with postures that are upward-facing and stretches (such as *urdhva mukha svanasana*) while exhalation is associated with forward bends and grounding postures (such as *adho mukha svanasana*).

8.7.4. *Pranayama* basics

<u>Sitting comfortably</u>
Full description in Bhagavad-Gita (VI, 10-15):
- Use cushions to ensure that kneecaps are lower than hip socket
- Beginners may sit against a wall
- OK to sit on chair or lie flat on the ground. In both cases, both feet must remain flatly planted on the ground
- Relax face, the brain feels light as if floating
- Ears must be alert to the sound of breathing
- Pay particular attention to the eyes, ears and lungs

Starting from the basics

Breathe normally. How long is the duration of the inhalations and exhalations? Consciously slow down your breathing rhythm. Deepen this exploration: lie on your back and breathe into your abdomen, chest and upper chest.

Breath and Body

Start with *yogasana* that easily establishes the principles of the body/breath relationship: perform *Surya Namaskar*, paying special attention to the breath.

8.7.5. Teaching *pranayama*

The five exercises presented in this section will give your students an experience of *pranayama*:

1. Do the Sun Breath as an example of how to move *prana* around your body.
2. Chant long OMs for 5-15 minutes, each person chanting at his /her own pace. This is brings lots of fresh *prana* into the body. Then say Peace, followed by Shanti, hands in prayer pose, bowing to each and every person in the class (if it's a small class).
3. Give your students the experience of *pranayama* - namely of receiving *prana* from the universe. Ask them to lie in *savasana*, but with palms facing downwards and toes pointing inward. Stay in this position for several breaths. Then turn your palms upward to face the sky, rotating from your shoulders outward. Turn your toes outward, too. Breathe, and feel the difference.
4. To use *pranayama* to cultivate inner awareness, do this exercise: with eyes softly closed, breathe deeply, focus on your Third Eye, and let the union of Shiva and Shakti play as you consciously move your breath around your body, focusing on these elements and bringing them into harmony:

Male	Female
Exhale	Inhale
Below	Above
Right	Left
Back	Front
Inner	Outer
Light	Dark
Heat	Cool

5. Experience baby breath, breath with your whole body! If you do not know how to do the baby breath, just observe how a baby breathes! Start by exaggerating the movements of your ribcage as you inhale, filling your cheeks with air, feeling yourself almost lifted off the ground with the inhale. As you exhale, feel the grounding force rooting you to the ground; exhale noisily. Then, slowly quieten down by allowing your soles and palms to breathe for you.

8.7.6. **Developing your students' breath capacity**

> **"regular practice of breath awareness and breathing exercises.....the result is an awakening of a whole part of oneself that he did not know was there before; a completely new aspect of his being, his life and his living to which his eyes before had been closed."**
> - *Swami Rama*

1. Even and comfortable inhalation (*puraka*) and exhalation (*rechaka*)
2. Extend exhalation
3. Introduce retention (*kumbhaka*) after exhalation
4. Extend inhalation
5. Introduce retention after inhalation

8.7.7. **Teaching *pranayama***

Pranayama is a subtle and complex science that requires years of practice to master. Therefore, do not teach *pranayama* unless you have gained competence in the type of *pranayama* you intend to teach. The best way of advancing your own *pranayama* practice is to check in with your breath throughout the day *(section 7.4.2)*.

List of *pranayama* that should be in every classical yoga teacher's toolbox:
1. Yogic breath (diaphragmatic breathing)
2. *Deerga swasam* (three-part breath)
3. *Anuloma viloma / nadi sodhana* (alternate nostril breathing)
4. *Kapalabathi*
5. *Sitari*
6. *Sitkari*
7. *Ujayyi* (for Ashtanga Vinyasa Yoga)

8.8. Teaching relaxation and visualization

REFER TO BOOK 3: YOGASENSE™ (under section on Guided Relaxation).

8.8.1. How to teach

Teaching relaxation is often difficult, as students do not fully appreciate the benefits of relaxation. Therefore, the most effective route in this case would be to relate relaxation to body parts:

1. In the *savasana* position with eyes closed, tense all the muscles of the face (or "make an angry face") – tightening the forehead, cheeks, mouth and upper neck, screwing your face into a grimace or an angry expression. Then release totally.
2. Now tighten the shoulders by pulling them upwards and forwards. Release.
3. Tense your arms, clenching your fists, taking that tensing deep into the arms, not only the surface. Release.
4. Tense up your chest and abdomen, while maintaining even breath. Release.
5. Clench your buttocks and tighten your hips. Take this tension down to your legs and feet. Release.
6. Curl up your toes. Point them inward and then release everything, flopping the toes so that they point outward.
7. Let your attention drift back up your body, and feel a warm, soothing wave in its wake.
8. Take this wave up to your face.
9. Smile.

8.9. Teaching YogaSense™

This section is based on the YogaSense™ Seven Guiding Principles (7.3).

> There are 3 reasons why a practitioner who is free from any medical conditions or disability is unable to achieve a certain *yogasana*, no matter how much effort is invested. The 3 fundamental limitations are:
>
> 1. Limitations of the muscles and joints
> 2. Structural limitations (skeletal structure)
> 3. Limitations of the mind.

Different diseases and conditions will alter this benchmark. The YogaSense™ Guiding Principles discussed below still hold, though the applications will vary according to an individual's needs. This is discussed in Yoga Therapy (*Book 2*).

8.9.1. Finding your own way
YogaSense™ Guiding Principle #7: Live it!

One of the comments a teacher may frequently experience is "But my yoga teacher does it another way, different from what you are teaching me".

Each yoga teacher has his or her own way. The practice of yoga is to internalize and to explore, because YOU are your own teacher. The person standing in front of you is merely a guide to guide the teacher inside you to finding your way. Yoga is not painting-by-numbers – you have to do some thinking, too, and a lot of self-exploration (self practice!). You don't just obey instructions like performing monkeys in a zoo.

There is no right way or wrong way, only safe or unsafe way, and these are the guidelines to instructing *yogasana* safely (though there are general rules attached to classical yoga postures):

8.9.2. Foundations of teaching asana

<u>Personal space</u>
YogaSense™ Guiding Principle #1: Respect your body
Ask, before you manually adjust a new student. Respect where your students' bodies are in their practice today.

<u>Never lock knees (hyper-extension)</u>
YogaSense™ Guiding Principle #3: Optimal alignment.
Hyper-extension increases knee stability but it has a detrimental effect. In the hyper-extended position, you are using the posterior ligaments of the knee joint for stability instead of your muscles. Those ligaments are going to end up over-stretched especially if you are already hyper-extended in the knee.

Optimal alignment is when the two bones are stacked one on top of each other and when both the flexors and extensors co-contract. Pushing the knee into the hyper-extended position could push the bones out of alignment, putting undue pressure on the ligaments from weight-bearing.

<u>Focus on the feet and work upwards</u>
YogaSense™ Guiding Principle #4: Balancing opposing forces.
The foundations must always be strong and firm. It is not a bad idea to start a class by bringing awareness to the feet.

And then lift, and lengthen, bringing the two opposing forces into perfect equilibrium.

<u>Always lift and lengthen</u>
YogaSense™ Guiding Principle #3: Optimal alignment.
Yoga is about trying to create new spaces within your body. It is about extending your personal boundaries. In all yogasana, always lift and lengthen before a twist, forward bend, backbend, everything!

<u>Stabilize the core</u>
YogaSense™ Guiding Principle #4: Balancing opposing forces.
In all inversions, take time to stabilise the core. If this is not practised, the spine will collapse out of alignment and the extremities will have no stable anchor - the weight will end up on the vulnerable parts of the

body, that is to say, either on the neck (in headstands) or wrists (in handstands).

Substance, not form

YogaSense™ Guiding Principle #5: Opening like a flower.

Yogasana comes from within. It starts from the heart and emanates outwards as an expression of the breath. To experience this, bring your focus inwards. Feel your *yogasana*; do not twist your body into what you want it to be:

i.   In seated forward bends, always aim to bring heart to earth, not the head. This ensures that the posture is soft and surrendered, not forced with the chest collapsing;

ii. In standing forward bends, bend from the lower hip, not the waist. Tilt your weight to your back ("put your backlights on"!), and bend from lower hip. This also applies to sideways bending, such as *utthita trikonasana*;

iii. Lift and lengthen. Ensure that the chest is open at all times.

Check alignment

YogaSense™ Guiding Principle #3: Optimal alignment.

But in the memorable words of Vanda Scaravelli, do not let gravity kill a posture. Always start with the first principle of grounding, followed by lifting and lengthening before moving consciously into a posture.

Some of the common markers (though it may vary according to teachers and schools) are:

i.   The distance of the feet of *trikonasana*-based yogasana (such as the warrior poses) is one leg-width apart;

ii. The distance of the feet of *parsvakonasana*-based yogasana (such as the *prasaritta padottanasana* family) is the distance of your wrists you when you stretch your arms at shoulder height.

Modifications may be introduced for non-generic practitioners, but should ideally embrace the principles of classical yogasana blended with body intelligence.

Go back to the breath
YogaSense™ Guiding Principle #6: Nurturing.
If a student is having difficulty in a *yogasana*, go back to *pranayama*. This brings the attention inwards, and where attention goes, consciousness and the breath follow.

Adequate Warm-ups
YogaSense™ Guiding Principle #2: Starting the fire.
Cold muscles are more prone to injury. Ensure that the muscles are warm and fluid before intense stretching poses. It is always good discipline to take a class through a warm-up routine which includes Surya Namaskar.

Move consciously
YogaSense™ Guiding Principle #6: Nurturing.
It is equally important to engage the mind to prepare your muscles to be ready for what you are going to ask those muscles to do. The mind and the muscles work as one to safeguard the body's wellbeing. Injuries are sustained when practitioners get into a pose too quickly, before the mind has time to self-align the muscles.

8.10. Teaching *padmasana*

8.10.1. Why the lotus?

"What is the ultimate posture in *yogasana*?" The most popular answer by far is *sirsana* but according to classical texts, all our *yogasana* work is in preparation for *padmasana*, the lotus pose. Indeed, the purpose of *yogasana* is to prepare the body for meditation.

In Hatha Yoga Pradipika, the classic text of Hatha Yoga, there is a long discourse into how one should sit for meditation.

Sitting correctly – hence, comfortably – for long meditation requires two things:
(i) strong back muscles to hold up the trunk and the head in an upright position;

(ii) hips that are opened enough to get into and remain in the cross-legged position. It is particularly important that the knees are below the hip socket, so that the lower vertebrae are not crunched and strained.

Sitting in *padmasana* is not as easy as it looks. Even if you can, you should still continue to work on opening up your hips and building your back strength, to enable you to sit for long periods in this *yogasana*.

I still remember the suffering I went through when I was training to be a yoga teacher, as I had to sit in *padmasana* throughout the theory part of the training – no slouching, no leaning against walls, and certainly no lounging on the yoga mat as if it was a beach mat!

8.10.2. Preparing for *padmasana*

Getting into *padmasana* is hindered by tightness in the muscles and ligaments of the hips, and to a lesser extent, the leg muscles.

Forcing legs into this position is a common cause of injury, as the muscles and ligaments in this area can be easily strained.

If there is no physical limitation, sitting in *padmasana* automatically places the kneecaps below the hip joints, which facilitates a straight spine. Additionally, the position of the legs forms a Figure 8, which closes the energy circuit of the body, so that there is no leakage especially during long meditation.

Beginner students often sit in *sukhasana*, or easy pose. In this pose, the legs are arranged in casually in some semblance of the lotus pose. Personally, I would prefer my students to sit in half-lotus, or *ardha padmasana*, where the ankle of the left leg sits on top of the knee of the right leg and vice versa. It's all too easy to sit in *sukhasana* and not endeavor to progress, whereas the *ardha padmasana* one is always conscious that this is but a transition pose.

However, for some categories of students, such as prenatal and senior citizens, it might be a bit too harsh to set *ardha padmasana* as the base for sitting poses. In these cases, in addition to encouraging your students to sit in whatever position that they find comfortable, you may suggest that they sit against the wall, or use cushions to elevate their hips. Students should be encouraged to do **YogaSense™ Supported Hip & Hamstring Opening Routine** sequence at home.

8.11. Teaching safely

[REFER TO Chapter 4: Physiology under the High risk categories (section *4.4*) for a thorough presentation of the subject]

8.11.1. Before you start

- Yoga is a system of wellness – students in an open class must be in good general health. Anyone under medication for ailments such as high blood pressure should seek medical advice before starting yoga. Even then, it should be in a small class with an experienced teacher who is familiar with the ailment and knows what to avoid.

- Students with slipped discs should not come for an open class – forward bends (which happens a lot in a typical class) should not be done by those with slipped discs.

- Students with any weakness or history of pain in the neck area should not do headstands. This applies to those who do not have a regular spine, too.

- Active infections and fever
- Recent fractures
- Recent surgical procedures
- Uncontrolled seizures

For all regular students, the following rules should always be observed:

- No inversion during menstruation
- Do not put pressure on knees – no to grabbing knees and clutching them.

Pregnant students should be referred to an appropriate prenatal yoga class.

8.11.2. Importance of warming up

It is a known fact that cold muscles are more prone to injury. Muscles are like metal when it comes to flexibility: when they are warm, they are more malleable.

The standard yoga warm-up is Surya Namaskar; it is said that Sun Salutations warm up every single muscle in your body needed for *yogasana*. However, if you are intending to lead your students into *yogasana* that involve intense stretching (such as *hanumansana*), it is prudent to ensure that your students do more than Sun Salutations before going into full stretch.

You may wish to focus on more stretching in addition to Surya Namaskar, or schedule the more intense *yogasana* for later on in the class when muscles are more malleable. Some students, especially senior citizens, those recovering from injury or those with exceptionally tight muscles, may find it difficult to begin with Sun Salutations. In these cases, you may wish to start the *yogasana* with a gentler warm-up:

<u>In seated position</u>
i. Neck rotation
ii. Shoulder shrugs
iii. Sufi grind (circling motions of the upper trunk, the head drawing an imaginary circle)
iv. Spinal rock (grabbing the ankles with both hands, inhaling torso forward and exhaling back)
v. Half twists
vi. Lateral stretches
vii. Dynamic *baddha konasana* (knees moving up and down simulating butterfly wings)

<u>On all fours</u>
i. cat-cow
ii. drawing large circles with your hips

<u>In standing position</u>
i. Sun Yoga Breath [**Book 3: YogaSense™Sun Breath**]
ii. Surya Namaskar (or a gentle version)

8.12.   Structuring a yoga class

8.12.1. What to teach?

If you are teaching Ashtanga Vinyasa Yoga, teach your students as you have been taught by your teacher. With Ashtanga, especially if you have a consistent practice (daily, except on moon days) you should find that teaching is an extension of your personal practice. The beauty of Ashtanga Vinyasa Yoga is that you are following the template set by the master, thereby reducing the margins of error.

The same also applies to Kundalini Yoga: you teach *pranayama*, *kriya* and meditation as you have been taught to teach during your teacher training course. A Kundalini Yoga teacher also has access to the large collection of *kriya* designed by Yogi Bhajan.

For those wishing to teach a hybrid-form of yoga, which is commonly known as "flow", "*vinyasa*" or even "power yoga", then considerable effort needs to be invested (especially in the early stages of your teaching career) to ensure that you are moving your students forward with each class, and moving in the light of yoga.

8.12.2. Components of a yoga class

A typical Hatha yoga class should contain these elements, roughly in this order:

1.   Tuning-in
2.   *Pranayama*
3.   *Yogasana*
4.   Cooling down
5.   Relaxation / Meditation /Visualization
6.   Close

Appropriate music is sometimes used as background music, and though the use of music can enhance the ambience of a class, it could prove to be distracting, too, especially if it is too loud and has lyrics.

8.12.3. Designing a *vinyasa*

This is a huge topic that lies outside the scope of this book. To ensure that your students have a balanced *yogasana* class, the first rule of thumb is to create a class that has roughly the equal amount of postures from the following main categories:

1.   Forward bends
2.   Backbends
3.   Standing balancing & strengthening
4.   Seated postures
5.   Inversions
6.   Restorative/nurturing

The simplest way for a beginner teacher to plan her class is to sit down with a piece of paper and create a table with the above-mentioned headings. Fill in the table with the postures (classical and modified versions/variations), and then string these postures together into a *yoga mala*, the way one would string beads together to make a necklace.

The most beautiful and inspiring classes come from the hearts of teachers who live their yoga. You have to live your yoga and to be dedicated to your personal practice to be able to inspire and lift others. It is only through personal practice that you discover the little nuances that lift what you do to another level. Otherwise, however good you are with your postures, your class would be merely technical and devoid of yogic soul.

8.12.4. Tuning-in

The purpose of tuning in is practical: to make the mental separation between the outside world and the world of yoga that your students are now entering into and will remain in for the next hour or hour and a half. This mental cue is important, as your students may have been driving around in a traffic jam, circulating the block looking for parking and feeling frazzled by the pressures of getting to your class that they are carrying a lot of tension when they first settle on their mats, their concentration still angled at the world outside.

Once your students are settled comfortably on their mats, you could invite them to chant OM or just sit quietly for a few minutes, observing their breaths.

8.12.5. Duration of a yoga class

Typically, a yoga class lasts either an hour or 90 minutes. If you teach in a gym, more often than not, the expectation is an hour long class.

A classical yoga class in a *shala* or a yoga studio generally lasts 90 minutes. 90 minutes is an appropriate duration to give practitioners the opportunity to experience the yoga microcosm: tuning-in, *pranayama, yogasana*, cooling down and relaxation, meditation or visualisation.

Typical time allocation for a 90 minute class:
* Tuning-in: 5 minutes
* *Pranayama*: 15 minutes
* *Yogasana*: 45-60 minutes
* Relaxation: 10 – 15 minutes
* Meditation / Visualization: 5-10 minutes

In the Kundalini Yoga tradition, a teacher sometimes brings yogi tea for students to share after class. This sharing makes the class special, and also serves to build group consciousness. It provides a good opportunity for the teacher to address any issues and to answer questions that students may have about their practice.

8.12.6 "How many times a week?"

Most people attend yoga class once a week, others up to three times. Personally, I am not that concerned over how many times a student attends class – I am more focused on getting my students to build a strong and consistent personal practice that they can do on their own. This is something I drum into students who walk into my *shala* from Day One.

In yoga, it is not the once or even twice a week class that will progress a student ultimately, but what she is inspired to her own to find her own way. A teacher is merely a guide, not the path.

My focus as a yoga teacher is, first and foremost, to teach yoga accurately to students to enable them to practice at home and to inspire them sufficiently to develop a personal practice. And from this, the YogaSense™ way (*section 7.3*) is born. Yoga is about you and your Self – it is not mindlessly following your teacher's movements in the quest for a good workout and losing a few pounds.

In the Ashtanga Vinyasa Yoga schools, students attend standard classes, which are supplemented with Mysore practice. Mysore practice is more like a personal practice session supported by a teacher. You just go in there, do your Primary Series in your own time. There is no one leading the class but when you need help, a teacher will step into your space to help. You stop where and when you reach your limit for the session.

Many practitioners find Mysore sessions useful as it gives them time to work on the postures that they find challenging, and to be able to devote time to challenging postures under the guidance of a teacher. Mysore session is one of the most important aspects of the Ashtanga Vinyasa Yoga path, and one of the most valuable for its practitioners. Posture clinics are Sun Yoga's way of working with students on an individual and deeper level.

Book 2
Yoga Therapy

CHAPTER ONE

Introduction: The Spirit of Yoga Therapy

OVERVIEW OF THE CHAPTER

1.1   What is Yoga Therapy?

1.2   Key elements

1.3   Key yoga tools

1.4   Physical benefits of *yogasana*

1.5   Emotional benefits of *yogasana*

1.6   Scope of practice

1.7   Limitations

1.8   Yoga props

1.9   Gong

1.10   Caregiver

1.1. What is Yoga Therapy?

1.1.1. The art and science of self-healing

Yoga Therapy is the modification of classical yoga practice to meet the medical needs of an individual while honoring the core principles of yoga. In Yoga Therapy, the yoga teacher (or other health professional) uses the tools of yoga to guide the practitioner toward self healing.

In the next few chapters, yoga for a variety of disabilities is presented and discussed. The chapters are not meant to be a recipe but rather a guide to the direction and spirit of Yoga Therapy.

> *Yoga Therapy Intention:*
> **Find your inner wisdom and**
> **heal from within.**
>
> ∞∞

1.1.2. Holistic approach

Yoga Therapy offers a holistic approach for illnesses by addressing the mind, body and spirit in the healing process.

The body cannot heal if the mind and spirit are broken.
The mind cannot heal if the body and spirit are broken.
The spirit cannot heal if the body and mind are broken.

1.2. Key elements

1.2.1. Essential principles

There are a few principles that should never be compromised. These are essential to yoga and to Yoga Therapy. They are as follows:

- **Use of the breath**. The breath is an integral part of each movement. There should be continuous attention to the breath in, out and during a pose.

- **Alignment of the body**. Maintaining proper alignment of the body means that we are working with the body in a way that is most efficient. With proper alignment, the muscles, skeletal structure and internal organs are in optimal position. Props may be used to assist in achieving optimal alignment.

- **Honoring the body:** Listening to the body allows for the mind and body to be in sync with its potential as well as its limitations. Proper modifications ensure that no injury occurs with the yoga practice. A focused daily practice will lead us to fulfilling our potential.

  [REFER TO *Book 1, Section 7.3:* YogaSense™: The Seven Core Principles]

1.2.2. Mindfulness

Mindfulness is an essential part of Yoga Therapy. By being aware of how we move, what we eat and how we breathe, we can correct our posture, move with better alignment and maintain a steady breath throughout the day. Mindfulness is the first step towards making healthy choices. Repetition of healthy choices over time leads to the formation of healthy habits.

> **Without mindfulness we lack awareness to make choices.**
>
> ∞∞
>
> **Mindfulness allows us to make healthy choices.**

1.3. Key yoga tools

1.3.1. *Yogasana*

Yogasana are the yoga poses. There are seven major categories of *yogasana* – standing poses, balance poses, inversions, forward bends, backbends, twists and restorative poses.

In Yoga Therapy, *yogasana* is assigned and modified based on individual needs to achieve health benefits for the practitioner.

In a typical yoga class, the intention is to teach classical yoga and the correct form.

The intention of Yoga Therapy is to promote self healing. *Yogasana* is modified to meet the needs of the practitioner.

1.3.2. Restorative Yoga

Restorative Yoga is a form of *yogasana*. In these poses, the body is positioned in supported positions and is allowed to rest. This is of great benefit for those whose immune system is compromised. Additionally, in a pilot study, Restorative Yoga has been found to be beneficial to overweight adults with metabolic syndrome (Cohen, Chang, Grady and Kanaya AM, 2008).

Savasana, a relaxation posture, is given at the end of a yoga practice to allow the body time to absorb the benefits of the practice.

1.3.3. Yoga Nidra

Yoga Nidra is known as yogic sleep. In Yoga Nidra, the practitioner is guided to a state of awakened deep sleep: the practitioner is led through body-mapping, breath awareness and creation of a resolution. After 30 to 60 minutes, the practitioner is awakened to feel rejuvenated.

During yogic sleep, mind and body conflicts are resolved. The resolution or *sankalpa* that is formed and repeated during Yoga Nidra facilitates release of conflict and formation of a new pattern of thinking. Yoga Nidra impacts the subconscious mind and is a powerful tool for promoting healing.

1.3.4. *Pranayama*

Pranayama is yoga breathing exercises. The breath is our life force and is essential for good health. The nutrient oxygen is delivered to the lungs with the inhale, and toxins are removed from the body with the exhale. Full breaths maximize the body's ability to heal.

The breath is also our direct link to our nervous system. Regulating our nervous system with the breath occurs naturally. For example, we take a big sigh when relieved or a gasp when surprised. *Pranayama* is a learned form of breath control which aids in keeping the nervous system balanced. In Yoga Therapy, there are four main categories of *pranayama*:

1. Cooling Breath
2. Energizing Breath
3. Relaxing Breath
4. Balancing Breath

When selecting a specific *pranayama*, the state of the practitioner's nervous system and intention of the Yoga Therapy should be considered. Someone with high blood pressure will benefit from a relaxing breath exercise. A person with a slow metabolism will benefit from an energizing breath. A full description of how physiology is affected by the breath is given in Book 1, Section *4.2.2*: The nervous system.

[REFER ALSO TO *Book 1, Section 7.8: Pranayama*]

1.3.5. Meditation

A calm and positive mind is essential in the healing process. Meditation is a simple tool that can be practiced by anyone.

A common technique is to focus on the breath or a single word. Scientific studies (Davidson *et al*, 2003) have shown that with meditation practice, the brain shifts from using the right prefrontal cortex to the left frontal cortex. The left prefrontal cortex is dominant in individuals with a more positive outlook and a stronger immune system whereas the right prefrontal cortex is dominant in depression and negative thinking. The influence of the amygdala is also reduced with meditation. The amygdala is a more primitive part of the brain which registers our immediate emotional response to situations (*Book 1, Section 5.3.5.* The limbic system).

[REFER TO *Book 1, Section 7.7:* Meditation]

1.3.6. Positive Affirmation

During Yoga Therapy, positive affirmation may be chanted, repeated out loud or silently. A positive affirmation helps to emphasize the intention of the Yoga Therapy session. For someone working to build strength and confidence, "I am strong" is an excellent positive affirmation. For someone feeling stressed, "I am calm" repeated silently with the breath will reinforce relaxation. A positive affirmation can also be created by the practitioner who will personalize and make the affirmation more effective.

1.3.7. Guided Relaxation

During relaxation, a yoga teacher may choose to verbally guide the practitioner through the relaxation process: the practitioner is made aware of the different parts of her body as each part is systematically identified verbally by the teacher. By naming the different body parts, the mind consciously brings awareness to the state of the body.

The intention for the guided relaxation will vary depending upon the issues of the practitioner. For example, for those with tense muscles, the focus is on releasing with the exhale as each body part is named. For individuals with a brain injury whose sensation is impaired, the focus can be on body awareness. For those whose coordination is impaired, the focus can be on visualizing a task being performed successfully.

Guided relaxation can last between 10 and 20 minutes. It is done sitting in a chair or lying in a comfortable position. Although the body is relaxed, the mind is conscious, staying focused on visualizing the instruction.

1.4. Physical benefits of *yogasana*

[REFER TO *Book 1, Section 7.2:* Practicing *Yogasana*]

1.4.1. Flexibility

Flexibility without strength leads to instability.

Yoga is best known for stretching and improving flexibility. During *yogasana*, muscles and soft tissues of the body are allowed to lengthen. Combining the categories of *yogasana* – back bends, forward bends, twists and standing postures, we have a comprehensive stretching of all of the major muscle groups. Each muscle and joint has an optimal range of motion. Yoga Therapy strives for working within the normal range.

1.4.2. Strength

Standing and holding poses are known for strengthening the body. By using the combination of body weight and gravity, sufficient tension can be generated in the muscles to build strength.

1.4.3. Posture

Yoga acts to improve body posture by bringing awareness to the structure and positioning of the body and by correcting imbalances which cause poor posture.

Yogasana is practiced to strengthen or stretch the muscles that interfere with the maintenance of good posture. For example, a practitioner with rounded back and shoulders would practice *yogasana* to open the anterior chest and then follow up with a different *yogasana* to strengthen the back extensor.

285

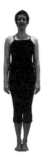 *Tadasana,* can be described as standing with relaxed attention. It is an excellent *yogasana* for bringing awareness to our posture.

1.4.4. Balance

Balance is improved through the practice of balancing poses and by improving overall flexibility, core strength and body awareness.

1.4.5. Cardiovascular system

The cardiovascular system benefits when physical exertion is maintained, allowing the muscles to work aerobically. By creating a *vinyasa* (flow of yoga postures), we are able to create an increased demand on our cardiovascular system. A practice of *vinyasa* yoga 5 days a week for at least 30 minutes is recommended for cardiovascular fitness.

Research has shown that yoga practice incorporating sun salutation postures exceeding a minimum period of 10 minutes may contribute to an improvement in cardio-respiratory fitness in unfit or sedentary individuals (Hagins, Moore and Rundle, 2007).

1.4.6. Pulmonary function

In human beings, having a healthy pulmonary function means that, on the most generic level, one is free from the debilitating effect of breathlessness and susceptibility to lung-related illnesses.

Yoga improves efficiency of breathing by increasing mobility of the chest, strengthening the diaphragm (the primary muscle for inspiration) and improving breath awareness.

In patients with chronic obstructive pulmonary disease (COPD), yoga-derived breathing exercises have been shown to be well-tolerated and induces favorable respiratory changes (Pomidori, L., Campigotto, F., Amatya, T.M., Bernardi, L., & Cogo, A., 2009).

1.4.7. Nervous system

[REFER TO *Book 1*, Section *4.2.2*: The nervous system]

The peripheral nervous system is divided into the parasympathetic and sympathetic system. The parasympathetic system is responsible for the calming of the nervous system while the sympathetic system is responsible for the flight, fright and fight response. The two systems work like a balanced scale. When one goes up, the other goes down, and vice versa. Today's hectic lifestyle tips the balance towards the sympathetic system. Unfortunately, when the sympathetic system is dominant, the results are the symptoms associated with chronic stress.

Yoga's greatest gift to the human body is its effectiveness in reducing the influence of the sympathetic system.

1.4.8. Immune system

[REFER TO *Book 1, Section 4.2.3.* The immune system]

With consistent and prolonged practice of yoga, the immune system is boosted and thus improves the body's ability to recover and fight off infections.

The field of psychoneuroimmunology has defined the role of stress in reducing effectiveness of the immune system in combating infection and growth of malignant tumors. The article by Coker (Coker, 1999) explains the development of meditation practice and explores the indications that the practice of meditation is effective in reducing the harmful effects of stress. In addition, there are encouraging reports of studies citing the influence of melatonin on breast and prostate tumors. A preliminary study finds an association between meditation practice and levels of melatonin produced by the pineal gland.

1.4.9. Sensory system

The major senses are hearing, sight, taste, smell, touch, vestibular and proprioception. Yoga eye exercises are used to improve our visual sense. Chanting is good for the auditory system. The proprioceptive and vestibular systems are integrated with *yogasana*.

1.5. Emotional benefits of *yogasana*

1.5.1. Inner strength

Using the yogic tools of breath, movement and meditation, the practitioner gradually becomes more mindful. This is a key element for healthy living. A doctor may tell someone lose weight or stop smoking, but the person needs inner strength to follow through in changing a habit.

As a practitioner becomes more mindful of his or her own patterns of thinking and behavior, he or she will begin to understand their root causes. Transformation to a healthy life style occurs, starting with inner changes.

1.5.2. Inner peace

Sometimes an illness occurs and we wonder "why me?" Elisabeth Kübler-Ross described the five phases of death – denial, anger, bargaining, depression, and acceptance – in her book on death and dying (Kübler-Ross, 1997). Yoga can assist a person in moving through these phases and not getting stuck in one phase. Whether it is a parent mourning an illness of a child or dealing with her own illness, acceptance and letting go will allow the energy to be expended in healing.

1.6. Scope of practice

1.6.1. Credentials

While there are many courses for yoga instructors' training, there is no standard licensing or regulation to determine who may teach Yoga Therapy or call themselves yoga therapists. The key element of a yoga teacher is honesty. This includes being honest with regard to their own credentials, experience and abilities.

Some yoga teachers have dual professions. There are physicians and therapists who combine yoga with their primary profession and can practice beyond the scope of a yoga therapist. A yoga teacher without additional credentials is obliged to stay within the scope of a yoga practice, namely teaching yoga as a system of wellness.

1.7. Limitations

1.7.1. Not a miracle cure

Yoga does a lot of good things, but it does not cure everything. Often an illness requires medical intervention. It is important that the idea "yoga will cure it" does not interfere with a proper plan of medical care.

Yoga does have something to offer everyone. Breathing exercises, restorative poses and mediation can be very beneficial for serious illnesses or for those with limited capabilities though they are not the magic cure.

1.7.2. Adjunct to Medical Care

Yoga therapy is best viewed as an adjunct to medical care. The medical profession is best equipped to diagnose an illness. The physician and patient then jointly devise with a plan of care best suited for the individual. Deciding not to take medication or follow the recommended medical intervention should be an informed decision between the medical doctor and patient.

1.8. **Yoga props**

1.8.1. **Blankets**

Natural fiber blankets are needed to assist and support the practitioner in the best alignment for a particular *yogasana*. Most often the blanket is folded to provide support in sitting poses or in restorative poses.

The blanket is also used to provide a covering so that the body maintains a steady temperature during relaxation.

1.8.2. **Blocks, stools and chairs**

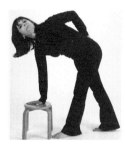

Yoga blocks provide an extension for the arm when weight bearing onto the hands. For example, when reaching towards the floor in a standing forward bend, the block allows a practitioner to reach the floor and maintain good alignment if she otherwise could not touch the floor. It is better to use blocks and maintain good alignment than to compromise the alignment without the blocks.

A stool can provide the same benefits as a block. Practitioners with less flexibility or balance can find a stool more stable than blocks. The wedge is an option for weight bearing on the hands for practitioners with wrist pain or limited range of motion.

1.8.3. **Straps or ties**

A strap is used to close the chain during a *yogasana* and is particularly helpful when there is limited flexibility. The strap is also used to support the body in better alignment in restorative poses.

1.8.4. **Chairs or table or bed**

For some practitioners, it is difficult to get onto the floor. In this case, the yoga can be done on a bed, a massage table, a chair or a wheelchair.

1.8.5. Beanbags, cushions and bolsters

Beanbags are a good alternative for sitting if the practitioner is not able to get down onto the floor. Bolsters and beanbags are also useful in positioning the practitioner in supportive restorative poses.

1.8.6. Wall, counter or desk

The wall, counter or a desk may be used to give support and to aid balance. These items are easily accessed in daily routines at home or work.

1.8.7. Ball

The ball is used to assist a practitioner in increasing her range for backbends and building strength for the *yogasana*.

1.9. Gong

1.9.1. Gong and vibration

The gong is often played in Kundalini Yoga. When the gong is played, energy is created in the form of sound vibrations. These vibrations enter the body and assist in realigning the body at a cellular level. The body can go into a deeper relaxation when the gong is played during *savasana*.

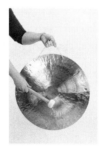

1.10. Caregivers

1.10.1. Taking care of the caregivers

Whether you are a parent taking care of a child or a child taking of your parent or other loved one, the role of caretaker is stressful and demanding. It takes strength, stamina and patience. Yoga for the caretaker is as valuable as for the patient. The statistics for divorce of parents with a child with a disability are staggering.

A regular yoga practice provides caretakers the tools for managing stress and the ability to approach situations with a neutral mind.

References

Cohen, B.E., Chang, A.A., Grady, D. & Kanaya, A.M. (2008). Restorative yoga in adults with metabolic syndrome: a randomized, controlled pilot trial. *Metab Syndr Relat Disord.* 2008 Fall;6(3):223-9.

Coker, K.H.(1999). Meditation and prostate cancer: integrating a mind/body intervention with traditional therapies. *Semin Urol Oncol.* 1999 May;17(2):111-8.

Davidson, R.J., Kabat-Zinn, J., Schumacher, J., Rosenkranz, M., Muller, D., Santorelli, S.F., Urbanowski, F., Harrington, A., Bonus, K. & Sheridan, J.F. (2003). Alterations in Brain and Immune Function Produced by Mindfulness Meditation. *Psychosomatic Medicine* 65:564-570 (2003)

Hagins, M., Moore, W., & Rundle, A. (2007). Does practicing hatha yoga satisfy recommendations for intensity of physical activity which improves and maintains health and cardiovascular fitness? *BMC Complement Altern Med.* 2007 Nov 30;7:40.

Kübler-Ross, E (1997). *On death and dying.* USA, Scribner.

Pomidori, L., Campigotto, F., Amatya, T.M., Bernardi, L., & Cogo, A. (2009). Efficacy and tolerability of yoga breathing in patients with chronic obstructive pulmonary disease: a pilot study. *J Cardiopulm Rehabil Prev.* 2009 Mar-Apr;29(2):133-7

CHAPTER TWO

Neurology

OVERVIEW OF THE CHAPTER

2.1   Yoga for neurological conditions
2.2   Parkinson's Disease
2.3   Multiple Sclerosis
2.4   Cerebral Vascular Accident
2.5   Traumatic Brain Injury
2.6   Alzheimer's
2.7   Vestibular Disorder
2.8   Peripheral Neuropathy

2.1. **Yoga for Neurological Conditions**

2.1.1. **Nervous system**

[REFER TO *Book 1*, *section 4.2.2*: The nervous system]

The nervous system is made up of the central nervous system and the peripheral nervous system. The brain and spinal cord make up the central nervous system. The nerve roots and the nerves outside the outside the spinal cord makes up the peripheral nervous system.

Illnesses of the nervous system can in part be understood by the location of the lesions. In Parkinson's, a disorder of the central nervous system, the cerebellum is affected. The cerebellum is responsible for coordination of movement, and this is why Parkinson's is sometimes known as a movement disorder. In Carpal Tunnel, the peripheral nerves of the wrist are damaged, and the symptoms are localized to the hand and wrist.

Disorders of the central nervous system which affect the brain and spinal cord include the following:
*   Parkinson's Disease
*   Multiple Sclerosis
*   Cerebral Vascular Accidents
*   Traumatic Brain Injuries
*   Alzheimer's

Disorders of the peripheral nervous system, known as peripheral neuropathy, occur when there is damage to the nerves outside the spinal cord. Common causes of Peripheral Neuropathy are toxins, infection, autoimmune response or trauma. Examples of peripheral neuropathies include the following:

*   Vestibular Disorders
*   Sciatica
*   Diabetic Neuropathy
*   Guillain-Barré Syndrome
*   Carpal Tunnel

When considering yoga for neurological disorders, symptoms and issues can vary widely within the same diagnosis and between different diagnoses. Recommended yoga for neurological disorders is generalized for commonly seen issues. The practitioner and the yoga therapist must tailor the yoga to the needs of the individual for the Yoga Therapy to be effective and safe.

2.1.2. Muscle tone

Muscle tone is controlled by the brain. Ideally, the signal from the brain to the muscle is just the right amount so that the muscles are ready when needed. When the muscle tone is low, it is called hypotonia and is often described as floppy. Hypertonia is when the muscle tone is increased, and is often described as stiffness. The amount of hypertonia will vary from minimal to severe. Rigidity is when stiffness exists throughout the range to the point of stopping the movement. If the tone is fluctuating and the movement writhe-like, it is known as athetoid.

In cases where there is low tone, *yogasana* for strengthening is recommended. Standing poses and weight bearing poses are good for strengthening. In cases where there is high tone, yoga done in supported positions with a focus on the release of tension during exhalation is recommended.

2.1.3. Sensation

The peripheral nervous system picks information up from the body and sends the information back to the brain to be processed. There are tracks of fibers to carry information regarding pain, touch, temperature and vibration.

In cases where the nervous system is compromised, there can be an abnormal registering of sensation. The problem may come from the peripheral nerves such as in a neuropathy or from the central nervous system as seen in brain injuries.

Yogasana and guided relaxation techniques can be used to calm irritated, oversensitive nerves and to stimulate undersensitive nerves.

2.1.4. **Postural control, balance reactions, protective reactions**

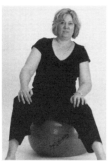

Postural control, balance and protective reactions occur at a sub-cortical level. These reflexes develop early in life and remain present throughout our lives.

Postural control is about the body's ability to maintain core stability as we move. When we tip to one side, the body "rights" itself automatically so that the eyes line up horizontally.

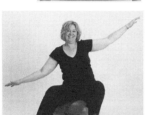

When the body's loss of balance requires the counterbalance of the extremities, it translates into the balance reactions that assist in regaining our balance. The legs or arms or both may come into play when we "catch our balance".

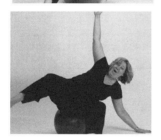

And when all is lost and we are going to fall, the protective reactions respond. Protective reactions includes extending of the arms or legs used to break a fall.

Lesions occurring in the central nervous system can compromise these "automatic" reactions.

2.2. Parkinson's Disease

2.2.1. **Description and pathology**

Parkinson's disease is a chronic progressive degeneration of the brain that affects motor function. In Parkinson's there is insufficient quantity of the chemical dopamine, which is responsible for sending messages to the motor cortex of the brain. Onset of Parkinson's is seen most often after 50 years of age. Progression of the disease generally continues at a slow rate. There is no cure.

2.2.2. Presentation

Parkinson's presents with stooped posture, mask-like face, shuffling gait and tremors while at rest. The body feels stiff and movements are slow. Initiating movement to roll over or to get up is difficult. Loss of postural control puts the person at risk of falls. Impairment of the throat muscles lead to low voice production and difficulty swallowing. Emotionally, depression and sleep disturbance may be present. Mental functions may also be affected.

2.2.3. Yoga intention

Keep the yoga dynamic to counteract Parkinson's.

2.2.4. Key problems and recommended *yogasana*

Problem	Recommended *yogasana*
Shuffling Gait: small step size, difficulty getting started and turning, forward propulsion of gait.	**Supported Strengthening Sequence:** *Yogasana* with a wide stance and controlled flowing movements is recommended to counteract the narrow stance. Warrior Poses and *trikonasana* using a wall or chair for support is recommended.
Stooped posture: rounded back and shoulders, flexion at the hips and knees.	**Sun Breath** **Hip & Hamstring Opening Exercise**
Tremors: occur at rest and when under stress, and decrease with movement. Seen in hand; can be described as "pill-rolling"; also seen in foot and head.	**Guided Relaxation**
Decreased voice production	Chanting *(p. 243)*

Problem	Recommended *yogasana*
Rigidity: stiffness to movement throughout range of motion. Cog wheel or clasp knife effect where the tension is released after initial resistance.	**Sun Breath** **Hip & Hamstring Opening Exercise**
Loss of postural balance reaction: The body loses its ability to spontaneously restore the balance or to use the extremities to assist in restoring the balance.	**Balance Sequence**
Mask-like face	*Simhasana* reduces the tightness of the face muscle, opens the jaw and increases vocalization.
Reduced breath	**Sun Breath**
Bradykinesia: slow movement	Increase and vary the speed of yoga movements in **Pawanmuktasana Sequence** and **Sun Breath**

2.2.5. Common muscle imbalances

As a result of the abnormal gait and characteristic postures, the following muscles imbalances are common in Parkinson's.

Tight	Weak	Recommended *yogasana*
<u>Pectoralis</u>: muscles across front of chest and shoulders cause rounded shoulders and stooped posture.	<u>Spinal Extensors</u>: these muscles are needed to pull shoulder back to keep the spine straight.	**Sun Breath**
<u>Hip Flexors</u>: muscles across front of hip joint tighten as the result of stooped posture, shuffling gait and increased time sitting.	<u>Hip Extensors</u>: The opposing muscles to the tight hip flexors are the gluteus maximus and hamstrings.	*Setu bandhasana*: stretches hip flexors and strengthens hip extensors. *Virabhadrasana III*: Strengthens hip extensors for back leg.
	Weak Core	**Core Strengthening Exercise**
Hamstrings Gastrocnemius Soleus		**Hip & Hamstring Opening Exercise**

2.2.6. Safety and special consideration

Ability to move and balance will vary greatly during the day and from day to day. Take care to give support with standing balance *yogasana*.

2.3. Multiple Sclerosis

2.3.1. Description and pathology

Multiple Sclerosis (MS) is an autoimmune disease which attacks the myelin covering of the nerves of the central nervous system. The myelin is a fatty insulation that allows nerve impulses to be transmitted with speed and efficiency. In MS, the myelin is destroyed and replaced with sclerotic scar tissue. When nerves lose their myelin, the tissues that are innervated no longer receive and send information for proper functioning.

It is most often diagnosed between the ages 20 and 50. There are different forms of MS. MS may follow the pattern of relapse/remittance or be a continuous progressive. There is no cure for MS.

2.3.2. Presentation

Common presentations for MS include decreased balance, decreased coordination, numbness to the extremities, dizziness and visual disturbances. Muscle weakness and fatigue is common. Additional symptoms include bowel and bladder dysfunction, and depression.

2.3.3. Yoga intention
Strengthen the immune system for self healing.

2.3.4. Muscle imbalances

Tight	Weak	Recommended *yogasana*
Hip Adductors	Hip Abductors	Baddha Konasana
Hamstrings	Lower leg muscles	*Adho Mukha Savasana*
Low back extensors, hip flexors, anterior chest	Core	**Core Strengthening Exercise**

2.3.5. Key problems and recommended *yogasana*

Problem	Recommended *yogasana*
Fatigue	**Restorative Yoga**
Muscle weakness - generalized	**Core Strengthening Exercise** **Supported Strengthening Exercises**
Muscle spasticity in lower extremities	**Hip & Hamstring Opening Exercise**
Vertigo and loss of balance	**Balance Sequence**
Bowel and bladder	**Pelvic Floor Routine** **Gastrointestinal Sequence** Bandha *(p. 225)*
Numbness in feet and hands	**Guided Relaxation** **Pawanmuktasana Sequence**
Blurred vision	**Yoga Eye Exercise *(p.256)***

2.3.6. Safety and special commentary

Practitioners must take care not to fatigue or work out in a heated room. Heat and fatigue will exacerbate the symptoms of MS.

2.4. Cerebral Vascular Accidents

2.4.1. Description and pathology

The brain needs constant, fresh, oxygenated blood to survive. Cerebral Vascular Accidents (CVA), better known as stroke, occur when the brain's blood flow is stopped, thus creating ischemia in the brain. The ischemia can be due to a bleed (hemorrhage) or clot (thrombosis). Where ever the ischemia occurs, brain damage is the outcome.

2.4.2. Presentation

[REFER TO *Book 1*, *Section 5.3*: Anatomy and physiology of the brain]

The stroke will present differently based on where the brain damage has occurred:

Right hemisphere damage: will affect the left side of the body and impact language center.
Left hemisphere damage: will affect the right side of the body, reasoning and judgment.
Cerebellum: will impact the coordination and balance.
Brainstem: will affect the survival centers.

Muscle function and sensations will be reduced in the affected area. Muscle tone will be abnormal in the extremities (increased or decreased) and core strength reduced. The severity of the brain damage will determine the level of functional limitation and the degree of yoga modifications required.

2.4.3. Yoga intention
Strengthen and restore function in the affected area of the body.

2.4.4. Key problems and recommended *yogasana*

Problem	Recommended *yogasana*
Loss of postural control and balance reaction	**Balance Sequence**
Weakness to opposite side of body from side of brain injury	**Supported Strengthening Sequence**
Loss of sensation and body awareness	**Guided Relaxation** with focus on sending the breath to the unresponsive area(s)
Loss of postural control and balance reaction	**Balance Sequence**
Spasticity in affected muscles	**Hip & Hamstring Opening Exercise** **Sun Breath**
Wheelchair-dependent	**Wheelchair / Chair Yoga**

2.4.5. Safety and special commentary

Weakness and subluxation of the shoulder joint is not uncommon in CVA. Yoga poses that are too demanding can damage the weakened shoulder joint and result in pain or further subluxation.

Weakness and abnormal tone in the foot may cause instability of the ankle joint in standing poses. If the joint is unstable a brace and shoes will need to remain on during standing yoga activities. Alternatively, opt for lying and seated yoga.

Be sure that the heart and blood pressure are stable, and monitor the practitioner for signs of stress. Practitioners with compromised cardiovascular systems should avoid inversion and over-exertion.

2.5. Traumatic Brain Injury

2.5.1. Description and pathology

Traumatic brain injury (TBI) occurs when there is a blow to the head that results in damage to the brain. TBI is classified as mild, moderate or severe. Common causes of TBI are motor vehicle accidents, falls, firearms and for soldiers in combat, bomb blasts.

Any area of the brain damaged and suffering from anoxia will result in death of that area of the brain. Though similar to a CVA, the damage tends to result in more global injuries.

2.5.2. Presentation

How a person with TBI presents will vary widely based on the severity of the injury. It is common to see personality changes, emotional instability, difficulty with focus and thinking, lack of motor coordination and dizziness.

2.5.3. Yoga Intention
Ground, organize and focus the mind.

2.5.4. Key problems and recommended *yogasana*

Problem	Recommended *yogasana*
Poor focus and organization	**Brain Organizing & Grounding Meditation**
Lack of coordination and loss of balance	**Supported Strengthening Sequence** **Balance Sequence**

2.5.5. Safety and special commentary

Personality changes can occur with TBI. Be aware of possible emotional instability, social/behavior problems and possible history of seizures. Refer to appropriate professionals to address coexisting issues.

2.6. Alzheimer's

2.6.1. Description and Pathology

Alzheimer's is a form of dementia that usually occurs in people over 60 years of age. There is a slow loss of brain cells in the cerebral cortex, namely, the thinking part of the brain.

2.6.2. Presentation

People with Alzheimer's have decreased memory and slowly lose the ability to take care of themselves.

2.6.3. Yoga Intention

Stimulate the mind and body.

2.6.4. Key problems and recommended *yogasana*

Problem	Recommended *yogasana*
Decreased cognitive skills and memory	Consistency with yoga routines and instructions. Add a challenge with a slight variation once a routine is established.

Problem	Recommended *yogasana*
Loss of balance	**Balance Sequence**
Generalized weakness	**Chair / Wheelchair Yoga**
Loss of speech	Chanting *(p. 243)*

2.6.5. Muscle imbalances

Imbalance is primarily due to increased time in wheelchair and decreased walking.

Tight	Weak	Recommended *yogasana*
Hip Flexors	Hip Extensors	*Setu bandhasana*
Hamstrings	Generalized lower leg weakness	*Uttanasana* *Padangusthanasana*

2.6.6. Safety and special commentary

Supervise practitioner closely due to increased risk for falls. Keep instructions simple and establish routines to reduce confusion.

2.7. Vestibular Disorders

2.7.1. Description and pathology

The vestibular system is a small organ the size of a thumbnail. It is part of the inner ear and is responsible for registering head movement. This system enables us to know where the body is in space. Spatial information is sent from the vestibular system to the brain through the 8th cranial nerve. Inflammation results in dizziness, loss of balance, ringing in the ear and nausea. Damage to the nerve may occur due to toxins or a virus.

2.7.2. Presentation

In episodes of vertigo, a person may be dizzy and have blurred vision, which may result in nausea. Onset can be sudden in acute cases or can manifest as a chronic problem.

2.7.3. Yoga Intention

Recalibrate the vestibular system and restore balance.

2.7.4. Key problems and recommended *yogasana*

Problem	Recommended *yogasana*
Ringing in ear	
Nausea	
Loss of balance	**Vestibular Rebalancing Exercise**
Decreased neck mobility	
Blurred vision	

2.7.5. Muscle imbalances

Fear of movement due to resulting dizziness may lead to general decreased mobility of the neck and trunk.

2.7.6 Safety and special commentary

In vestibular disorders, a person may respond to changes in head position with the feeling of nausea, dizziness or loss of balance. Medical clearance should be pursued to determine the cause of vertigo.

2.8. **Peripheral Neuropathy**

2.8.1. Description and pathology

In peripheral neuropathy, the peripheral nerves of the body are damaged. The peripheral nerves provide the communication from the spinal cord and brain (central nervous system) to and from the muscles, skin, joints and organs of the body. When communication is disrupted, the motor, sensory and organ functions are disrupted.

Neuropathy can be systemic with multiple nerves involved or mononeuropathy with a single nerve involvement. Polyneuropathy is seen in Guillain-Barré syndrome, which is an autoimmune disease, or diabetic neuropathy. Mononeuropathy is commonly seen in trauma or compression injuries to a single nerve. When the nerves of the autonomic nervous system are involved, organ and gland functions are impaired.

2.8.2. Causes of neuropathy

Cause	Examples
Compression/Entrapment	Pressure to spinal root – low back or neck pain Carpal Tunnel
Infection	Lyme Disease Herpes Zoster (Shingles) Leprosy HIV
Autoimmune	Guillain-Barré Lupus
Metabolic	Diabetic
Toxins	Alcoholism

2.8.3. Common nerves involved in neuropathy

Neuropathy (body part)	Nerve
Bell's Palsy (face paralysis)	Cranial VII
Carpal Tunnel (wrist)	Median
Erbs Duchenne (shoulder)	Brachial Plexus
Foot Drop (foot)	Peroneal
Sciatica (lumbar disc)	Sciatic
Radiculopathy	Spinal
Winged Scapula	Long Thoracic

2.8.4. Presentation

Depending on the nerves or multiple nerves involved, there may be loss of sensation, loss of motor function and pain to the area those nerves innervate. When the sensory nerves are involved, the symptoms may be numbness, tingling, sharp shooting or burning sensations.

When the autonomic nerves innervating organs and glands are involved, the symptoms may include urinary incontinence, sexual dysfunction and constipation or diarrhea. In addition, dizziness can result when the muscles of the blood vessels are slow to respond when the body changes positions.

2.8.5. Yoga intention
Calm the nerves and promote healing to area involved.

2.8.6. Key Problems and recommended *yogasana*

Problem	Recommended *yogasana*
<u>Paresthesia</u>: Loss of sensation	**Guided Relaxation**
Pain	**Restorative Yoga** Meditation: release of pain with the exhale
Loss of strength in the involved areas	Gentle *yogasana* **Pawanmuktasana Sequence**
Autonomic nerve involvement: system and organ dysfunction: 1. Bowel and bladder 2. Dizziness 3. Sexual dysfunction	 1. **Pelvic Floor and GI Routines** 2. **Vestibular Rebalancing Exercise** 3. **Tantra Yoga**

2.8.7. Safety and special commentary

Care should be given not to damage the joints in poses where the individual is not aware of the stress occurring due to loss of sensation.

Modified *yogasana* are recommended based on individual limitations.

CHAPTER THREE

Medical Conditions

OVERVIEW OF THE CHAPTER

3.1   Introduction
3.2   Diabetes
3.3   Obesity
3.4   Irritable Bowel Syndrome and Gastroesophageal
        Reflux
3.5   Coronary Artery Disease
3.6   Pulmonary Disease
3.7   Cancer
3.8   Infectious Diseases: HIV/AIDS

3.1. Introduction

3.1.1. Benefit of yoga for medical conditions

Medical conditions are categorized by the organs or systems involved. Yoga is an effective adjunct therapy to allopathic medical treatments. The major benefits of yoga in medical conditions are as follows:

- Yoga offers a boost to the immune system. When stress is reduced, the body is then able to utilize its own fighting system effectively.

- Yoga calms the nervous system. Reducing the influence of the sympathetic nervous system on the body and increasing the parasympathetic system input allows the body to use its energy internally for healing instead of using it for "fight, flight and fright".

- Yoga fosters a positive perspective. Keeping a positive outlook is an important part of healing and staying healthy.

- Yoga improves circulation. Gentle stretching in *yogasana* helps to bring fresh nutrients to tissues in need of healing and to assist in the removal of toxins through the venous and lymphatic systems.

3.1.2. Systems and Organs

[REFER TO *Book 1*, *Section 4.2*: Main systems of the body]

Endocrine System
The endocrine system is a communication system for the body. The system includes the glands of the body as well as the hormones these glands secrete. The hormones are chemical messages sent into the blood system to go to specific tissues of the body for regulating functions such as metabolism, growth and development. Two common diseases of the endocrine system are diabetes and obesity.

Gastrointestinal (Digestive) System

The gastrointestinal (GI) system, more commonly known as the digestive system, is responsible for the process of ingestion, digestion and elimination. The upper GI system consists of the mouth, esophagus and stomach. The lower GI system includes the small intestines, large intestines and anus. A common disease of the lower GI is irritable bowel syndrome. Gastroesophageal reflux disease is a common disease of the upper GI system. Though each disease is different in location and presentation, both are exacerbated by stress.

Circulatory System

The circulatory system is made up of the heart, blood and the blood vessels. The circulatory system ensures that the body's tissues get fresh nutrients and oxygen. Cardiovascular disease is the broad term for diseases related to the heart and blood vessels. When the circulatory system fails, ischemia and death to tissues deprived of oxygen result. In cases where the arteries to the brain are clogged, the result is stroke (section 2.4), and in cases where the arteries to the heart are involved, the outcome is a heart attack. Coronary Heart Disease is the most common of the cardiovascular diseases and the number one killer in the United States, Canada and England. Diet, exercise and lifestyle are the most effective means of preventing coronary artery disease.

Respiratory System

The respiratory system is made up of the lungs, airways and muscles used in respiration. It is responsible for the exchange of gases which occurs in the alveolar of the lungs. The upper respiratory tract includes the nasal cavity, pharynx and larynx. The common cold is an example of illness of the upper respiratory tract. The lower respiratory tract includes the trachea, bronchi, bronchioles and alveoli. Well-known respiratory diseases include asthma, chronic obstructive pulmonary disease (COPD) and pneumonia. Diseases that affect the muscles of respiration include Amyotrophic Lateral Sclerosis (ALS) and Guillain-Barré syndrome. Other diseases include tumors and inflammation to the pleura, the lining of the lungs.

Immune System

The immune system is a network of cells, tissues and organs that work together to defend the body against harmful viruses, bacteria and parasites. It is responsible for mounting the body defenses and is found throughout the body - bone marrow, spleen, thymus, tonsils, adenoids, lung and lining of the digestive tract. When the immune system is weakened or not able to defend against an invader, disease develops. A common disease related to the breakdown of the immune system is HIV/AIDS. The immune system also helps in eliminating cells that may become cancerous. The lymphatics, part of the immune system, is the transportation system for removing toxins from the body. The stretching in yoga is excellent for facilitating lymphatic drainage.

3.2. Diabetes

3.2.1. Description and pathology

The hormone insulin which is made in the pancreas is responsible for the breaking of glucose down into a simpler form of energy that can be utilized by the body. When the body is not able to regulate the blood glucose, the person is said to have diabetes. In Type 1 Diabetes, which is also known as juvenile diabetes, the body is not able to make insulin. In Type 2 Diabetes, commonly known as adult onset diabetes, the body shows resistance to utilizing the insulin. Management of diabetes is through medication and diet. Studies have shown that yoga is an effective adjunct to diet and medication in the management of diabetes (Malhotra, Singh, Tandon and Sharma, 2005).

3.2.2. Key problems and recommended *yogasana*

Problem	Recommended *yogasana*
Peripheral Neuropathy (*2.8)*	**Pawanmuktasana Sequence**
Elevated blood sugar Diet restriction	Yogic diet (Koay, 2009)
Decreased circulation to extremities	**Foot Care Routine**
Eye	**Yoga Eye Exercises**

3.2.3. Safety and special commentary

In cases of increased eye pressure, inversion should be avoided.

In cases of peripheral neuropathy, especially in the foot, loss of strength and sensation increases risk of injury during weight-bearing *yogasana*.

3.3. Obesity

3.3.1. Description and pathology

Obesity describes an excess of adipose (fat) tissue in proportion to other tissues. It is sometimes defined as 20% above a person's ideal weight or by the Body Mass Index (BMI). Diseases associated with obesity include increased risk of diabetes, heart disease, cancer, sleep disorders, strokes and joint deterioration.

From Centers for Disease Control and Prevention (CDC) *Defining overweight and obesity* (updated 2004):

BMI:
To calculate your BMI, determine your height in inches and multiply it by itself (ex. 64 x 64 = 4096). Divide your weight in pounds by your height calculation (ex. 175 / 4096 = 0.04272); then multiply this result by 703 (ex. 0.04272 x 703 = 30).

- Underweight = <18.5
- Normal weight = 18.5-24.9
- Overweight = 25-29.9
- Obesity = BMI of 30 or greater

Waist Measurement
Fat around the waist area corresponds with increased risk of cardiovascular disease. This risk increases with a waist measurement of over 40 inches in men and over 35 inches in women.

3.3.2. Key problems and recommended *yogasana*

Problem	Recommended *yogasana*
Slower metabolism	Kapalabathi Pranayama *(p. 238)* Surya Namaskar
Imbalance of caloric intake and caloric expenditure	Yogic diet (Koay, 2009) Meditation to bring awareness of food Yoga to increase caloric expenditure

3.3.3. Safety and special commentary

Due to excess weight which results in potential stress on joints, jumping in and out of poses should be avoided.

3.4. Irritable Bowel Syndrome and Gastroesophageal Reflux

3.4.1. Description and pathology

Irritable Bowel Syndrome (IBS), or "nervous stomach", is a condition in which the colon muscles are intermittently hyperactive, causing sudden and uncontrolled emptying of the bowels. It is exacerbated by stress and certain trigger foods, in particular, alcohol, milk products, high fat foods, caffeine, coffee and carbonated drinks. IBS produces significant anxiety associated with the inability to control the bowels. The lives of sufferers of IBS can be significantly impacted by the fear of going out. Studies have shown yoga to be effective in reducing symptoms anxiety and improving functional outcomes (Javnbakht, M., Hejazi Kenari, R. and Ghasemi, M., 2009).

Gastroesophageal Reflux (GERD) is commonly known as heartburn. The lower esophageal sphincter is responsible for closing the opening to the stomach from the esophageal. When the muscles of this sphincter are weakened or stretched, the acid from the stomach goes up the esophagus, causing an unpleasant sensation recognized as heartburn. The reflux is made worse by a fatty diet, alcohol, large meals or the head in a head-down (inverted) position. People who are obese and/or have pulmonary disease are at risk of developing gastric reflux.

3.4.2. Key problems and recommended *yogasana*

Problem	Recommended *yogasana*
Irritable Bowel Syndrome	Yogic diet (Koay, 2009)
Gastroesophageal Reflux	Yogic diet (Koay, 2009) Avoid inversions
Both of the above (exacerbated by stress)	Meditation *(p. 261)* Calming Pranayama *(p. 238)* **Restorative Yoga**

3.4.3. Safety and special commentary

For GERD, avoid inversion or poses where the esophagus is lower than the stomach. Restorative poses with the head elevated are indicated.

For both GERD and IBS, avoid poses that compress the stomach.

3.5. Coronary Artery Disease

3.5.1. Description and pathology

Coronary artery disease (CAD) results when the arteries of the heart become clogged by fat. This fatty build-up in arteries is known as arteriosclerosis. Arteriosclerosis leads to a heart attack when blood supply to the heart muscle is cut off. Diabetes, obesity, high blood pressure, high cholesterol, smoking, diet high in fats, stress and a type

A personality increase a person's risk of developing heart disease. Over time, CAD will weaken the heart and lead to arrhythmia and heart failure. Various researches have shown the risk factors associated with heart disease have been reduced with a regular yoga practice (Prasad *et al*, 2008, and Innes *et al*, 2005).

3.5.2. Key problems/risk factors and recommended *yogasana*

Problem/risk factors	Recommended *yogasana*
High blood pressure	Meditation *(p. 261)*
Increase cholesterol level Diabetes Obesity	Yogic diet (Koay, 2009)
Stress	Meditation *(p. 261)* Calming Pranayama *(p. 238)*
Sedentary lifestyle	*Vinyasa* to work cardiovascular system aerobically

3.5.3. Safety and special commentary

Clearance from the physician is recommended before starting a yoga program.

Facilities for yoga classes should have personnel trained in CPR.

3.6. Pulmonary Disease

3.6.1. Description and pathology

Consideration of how effective our breathing is takes into account various factors such as strength of the muscles of respiration, flexibility of the lung tissue, airway resistance and mobility of the chest. Pulmonary diseases can be categorized as a restrictive or an obstructive lung disease.

Restrictive Lung Disease

In restrictive lung disease, the lungs are not able to fully expand and the patient experiences difficulty in taking a deep breath. The restrictive breathing pattern may come from a physical limitation of the chest to expand. This is seen in postural abnormality such as scoliosis and kyphosis. Other limitations may be due to pain arising from post operative chest surgery or weak muscles of inspiration.

Obstructive Lung Disease

Common obstructive lung diseases include asthma, emphysema, chronic bronchitis and cystic fibrosis. Obstructive lung disease is characterized by increased secretion, narrowing and obstruction of airways and destruction of the alveoli. Due to the obstruction in the airways, prolonged and forced expiration is characteristic of those with obstructive lung disease. Chronic obstruction pulmonary disease (COPD) occurs with irreversible damage to the lungs.

3.6.2. Key problems and recommended *yogasana* (common for both restrictive and obstructive lung disease)

Problem	Recommended *yogasana*
Reduced chest mobility	**Sun Breath**
Weak muscles of inspiration	Pranayama *(p. 238)*
Poor posture – rounded shoulders, forward head	**Posture Awareness Exercise**
Shortness of breath and decreased endurance	Gentle *yogasana*
Decreased strength in muscles of respiration	Kapalabathi Pranayama *(p. 238)*

Breathing Pattern Difference in Restrictive and Obstructive Lung Disease

	Breathing Pattern	**Recommended** *yogasana*
Restrictive	Difficulty with inspiration and taking deep breaths	Long Deep Breathing Pranayama for strengthening the breath
Obstructive	Trapping of air in lungs and difficulty with expiration	Pranayama working toward increasing length of exhalation and for breath control

Muscles of Respiration

[REFER TO *Book 1, section 3.10.4:* Breathing and the abdominals and *Book 1, section 4.2.8:* The respiratory system]

Muscle	**Function**
Diaphragm	Major muscle. Contracts like an upside down umbrella upon inspiration and relaxes back up upon exhalation
External Intercostals	Upon inhalation, assist in opening space between the ribs. Ribs move up and out like a bucket handle during inspiration
Scalenes, Sternocleidomastoid, Upper Trapezius	Accessory muscles for inspiration and used for labored breathing. Used during strenuous exercise or when respiratory disease is present
Abdominals	Used during forced expiration
Internal Intercostals	Depress ribs in forced expiration

3.6.3. Safety and special commentary

Avoid forced expiration breathing exercises for obstructive pulmonary disease.

Take precaution as in osteoporosis for clients who have taken long term steroids for treatment of pulmonary disease

3.7. Cancer

3.7.1. Description and pathology

Cancer is the uncontrolled growth of the body's own cells. Excess cell growth develops into a mass or tumor. Tumors can be benign or malignant. In malignant tumors cells invade surrounding tissues and can travel to other parts of the body. Cancer is named according to what kind of cell the cancer comes from and the location of the cancer. Accumulating evidence supports the beneficial impact of complementary therapies (such as acupuncture, yoga, meditation and physical activity) on physical and emotional symptoms associated with cancer treatment (Cassileth, Gubili, and Simon Yeung, 2009), though Smith and Pukal (2008) suggested that further research in this area is warranted.

[REFER TO Book 1, section *4.4.2. Cancer*]

3.7.2   Yoga intention (applicable to all medical conditions):
Boost immune system, reduce stress, improve well-being and promote healthy yogic lifestyle (Book 1, Chapter 2).

3.7.3. Key problems and recommended *yogasana*

Problem	Recommended *yogasana*
Depression/Anxiety/Fear	Meditation *(p. 261)*
Pain	Pranayama *(p. 238)*
Reduced functioning of the immune system	**Restorative Yoga**
Weakness and debilitation	Gentle *yogasana*

3.7.4. Safety and special commentary

Yoga offers a positive adjunct to cancer intervention but is not the cure for cancer. Practitioners should recognize the limitations of yoga as they embrace its many benefits.

3.8. HIV/AIDS

3.8.1. Description and pathology

Human immunodeficiency virus, HIV, is an infectious retrovirus that attacks the immune system. The virus enters the cells of the immune systems and multiplies, destroying the body's T-cells (or CD4-T cells). The T-cells are an important part of the immune system because they coordinate the immune response.

Acquired immunodeficiency syndrome, AIDS, is the name given to the later stages of an HIV infection. The Center for Disease Control's definition of AIDS is HIV positive people with a CD4-T cell count below 200 per µL of blood or when opportunistic infections occur.

3.8.2. Key problems and recommended *yogasana*

Problem	Recommended *yogasana*
HIV Weight loss Swollen lymph nodes Fever/night sweats Cough Fatigue Diarrhea Headache Flu-like symptoms	**Restorative Yoga** Meditation *(p. 261)* Pranayama *(p. 238)* Gentle *yogasana*
AIDS Development of associated infections and cancers Worsening of HIV symptoms	
Both Decreased body image Depression	Meditation with Positive Affirmation Karma Yoga (charity work)

3.8.3. Safety and special commentary

Continue practicing the universal precaution as appropriate.

In case of fever, Restorative Yoga is recommended.

Be aware of changing medical status and adjust the yoga practice accordingly.

References

Cassileth, B.R., Gubili, J., & Simon Yeung, K. (2009). Integrative medicine: complementary therapies and supplements. *Nat Rev Urol.* 2009 Apr;6(4):228-33.

Innes, K.E., Bourguignon, C., & Taylor, A.G. (2005). Risk indices associated with the insulin resistance syndrome, cardiovascular disease, and possible protection with yoga: a systematic review. *Journal of American Board of Family Practice, 18(6), 491-519.* Nov.-Dec. 2005.

Javnbakht, M., Hejazi Kenari, R. & Ghasemi, M.,(2009). Effects of yoga on depression and anxiety of women. *Complement Ther Clin Pract.* 2009 May;15(2):102-4. Epub 2009 Mar 20.

Koay, J. (2009). *Simply Yogic. Food for the mind, body and soul.* London, UK: Sun Yoga.www.sunyoga.com

Malhotra, V., Singh, S., Tandon, O.P. & Sharma, S.B. (2005). The beneficial effect of yoga in diabetes. *Nepal Medical College Journal, 7(2):145-7.* December 2005.

Prasad, K.VV., Sunita, M., Raju, P.S., Reddy, M.V., Sahay, B.K., & Murthy, K.J.Y.(2008). Impact of Pranayama and Yoga on Lipid Profile in Normal Healthy Volunteers. *Journal of Exercise Physiology Online, 9, 1-6.*

Smith, K.B., & Pukall, C.F. (2008). An evidence-based review of yoga as a complementary intervention for patients with cancer. *Psychooncology.* 2008 Sep 26. [Epub ahead of print].

CHAPTER FOUR
Orthopedic

OVERVIEW OF THE CHAPTER

4.1   Introduction

4.2   Spinal alignment and pathology

4.3   Scoliosis

4.4   Osteoporosis

4.5   Arthritis

4.6   Lower back

4.7   Neck

4.8   Upper extremities

4.9   Lower extremities

4.10   Hyperextended joints

4.1. Introduction

4.1.1. Yoga and modern orthopedic medicine

Orthopedic comes from the Greek words *orthos*, meaning straight and *pais* meaning child. Modern medicine refers to this specialty as orthopedic surgery. This specialty involves the treatment of injuries and disabilities of our bones, muscles, tendons, ligaments and innervating nerves.

Yoga is an excellent adjunct to orthopedic medicine. *Yogasana* is geared toward working these same structures and with the intention of achieving optimal function and alignment with each posture.

The orthopedist uses many treatment approaches. Non-invasive approaches often use exercise, splinting and bracing. In cases where a non-invasive approach is not effective, best practice may require an invasive or surgical intervention.

Yoga's role in orthopedics starts with prevention and continues through the healing phase once an injury has occurred. Yoga helps the body find its optimal alignment by stretching the tissues that are tight and strengthening muscles that are weak. Mindfulness helps reinforce maintaining good alignment in our daily lives.

4.1.2. Acute and chronic traumatic injury

When we experience a trauma such as a fall or car accident the musculoskeletal system is often the first to be injured. Once the acute phase has passed, yoga can be helpful in restoring function to the injured body part. Be sure to get clearance from the medical doctor or health professional before resuming yoga.

Acute: In the case of acute injury, it is important to follow recommended RICE protocol, which is an acronym for rest, ice, compression and elevation. This is because when an injury first occurs, the inflammation process causes swelling. Ice, compression, rest and elevation all work to reduce the swelling and prevent further damage to the injured area. Following our core principle DO NO

HARM, those with an acute injury should not practice active yoga to the involved area until the acute stage is over. An acute stage generally lasts 2-3 days. Resumption of activity should be gradual. Medical assessment should be pursued if in doubt about the severity of an injury.

Chronic: In a chronic injury, yoga can be of great assistance in the healing process. Once the inflammation has gone, scar tissues and deposits from the swelling will remain, leaving a stiff joint. *Yogasana* assist in restoring function to an injured area by increasing flexibility and strength.

4.1.3. YogaSense™ Effectiveness

YogaSense™'s core principle of maintaining optimal alignment makes yoga effective for orthopedic injuries. In yoga, the body's muscles and soft tissues are stretched and strengthened while maintaining alignment. Gradually, the body's structures come into place with the strength and flexibility to maintain their alignment. There are treatments where the patient can be adjusted manually, and sometimes this is necessary. But, if possible it is better for the person to work to achieve the changes. Through a yoga practice, the changes will be more lasting and more apt to be adapted as part of daily living. The classic example is the person with back pain. They come in and someone does the treatment to them and the back feels better. But, generally the root cause of back pain is poor alignment of the vertebrae and imbalance of muscles of the back. If the patient works through the yoga poses aligning the spine, strengthening and stretching to rebalance the back muscles, the recovery will happen organically. Mindfulness, which is an integral part of yoga, will help the patient be successful in maintaining good posture and body mechanics.

4.2. Spinal alignment and pathology

4.2.1. Abnormal posture and alignment of the spine

Forward Head: A forward head posture is when the head is forward of the middle of the shoulder joint (acromion).

Kyphosis: Kyphosis is an increased curvature of the thoracic spine. Lack of core strength allows gravity to round the back into a kyphotic posture.

Lordorsis: Lordosis is an increased inward curving of the lower back and is a contributing factor to lower back pain. Weak abdominal muscles allow the pelvis to tip forward out of a neutral spine into a lumbar lordosis.

4.2.2. Pathologies of the spine

Herniated Disc: A herniated disc occurs when the disc between the vertebrae presses out from between the two vertebrae. Neurological symptoms appear as the disc presses on the nerve roots coming from the spine. The disc can herniate to the side, anteriorly or posteriorly. It is common for the disc to herniate posteriorly with a forward bending lifting injury. The disc may herniate anteriorly in yoga teachers or dancers doing a backbend movement. Medical management is recommended for a herniated disc to determine the location and severity of a herniated disc and the best course of treatment.

Spinal Degeneration and Stenosis: As we age, the disc between the vertebrae loses its jelly center, the fibrous tissues encapsulating the disc lose their elasticity and the surrounding ligaments that help keep our vertebrae in alignment become stiff. The result is the narrowing of the canals where the nerves exit. Pressure on the nerves causes symptoms of an aching back that may worsen with exercise, especially spinal extension.

Spondylolithesis: Spondylolithesis is when a vertebrae slips off from the vertebrae above. Most often spondylolithesis is seen in the lumbar vertebrae. A more serious location is when it occurs in the neck. Clearance from the medical profession is needed before participating in physical yoga. This is not to be confused with spondylosis, a degenerative arthritis of the vertebrae or spondylitis, an inflammation of the vertebrae.

Sacroiliac Joint (SIJ) Dysfunction: The sacroiliac joint (SIJ) is located where the pelvis and sacrum join together. The bones are held together with ligaments. Because of the irregular surfaces of the joint and the fact that the weight of the upper body is displaced to the lower body through this joint, the joint is vulnerable to injury. Those with more flexibility tend to be at greater risk of injury. Forward bends that involve twisting tend to irritate the SIJ.

Additional Pathologies affecting the spine include tumors, tuberculosis of the spine, or congenital deformities and other spinal diseases.

4.2.3. Yoga intention

Align and lengthen the spine to improve conduction of the nerves.

4.2.4. Key problems and recommended *yogasana*

Problem	Recommended *yogasana*
Kyphosis: Will have tighter anterior chest such as in the pectoralis and will have overstretched and weakened thoracic spinal extensors	Chest Opener – to stretch the anterior chest *Balasana* with extended arms, Standing Wall Stretch and *Adho Mukha Svanasana* – to lengthen the spine and reduce the thoracic curvature. Airplane and sphinx – strengthen the spinal extensors
Lordosis: Will have weakened abdominals. Hip flexors that attach to the lumbar spine are tight, thus pulling on the lower back. The long head of the hamstrings that attach to the ischial tuberosity will pull on the back	**Core Strengthening Routine** **Lower Back Exercise Routine** – to rebalance muscles of back
Poor body awareness	Verbal cues during yoga practice Kyphosis: Lift chest up Rounded Shoulders: Pull shoulders back and relax downward Forward Head: Tuck chin and lengthen the back of the neck

Problem	Recommended *yogasana*
Herniated Disc	Initially medical management to determine course of action. Post Herniation: Core Strengthening Sequence and posture awareness.
Spinal Stenosis	Limit extension in *yogasana*. Focus on lengthening the spine to open spaces between vertebrae.
Spondylolithesis	Clearance from medical professionals recommended before starting yoga. Core Strengthening Sequence Weight-bearing on the spine: head and shoulder stands are contraindicated.
Sacroiliac Joint (SIJ) Dysfunction	Avoid forward bends in sitting and avoid forwards bend with rotation. Do not go to end of range of motion in *yogasana* to avoid further stretching of the SIJ.

4.2.5. Safety and special commentary

When there is poor posture, the abnormal spinal alignment may interfere with nerve conduction through the spine. Onset of neurological symptoms, which include pain, weakness, sensation changes, bowel and bladder dysfunction, needs to be addressed by the medical profession as they may mean more serious pathologies of the spine. Back pain that worsens with exercise is a sign of more serious spinal disorders.

Involvement of bowel and bladder function needs immediate medical attention.

4.3. Scoliosis

4.3.1. Description and pathology

Scoliosis is lateral curvature of the spine. The curvature may be functional or structural. Functional scoliosis is when the curve can be reversed. The cause of the scoliosis may come from another part of the body, such as with a leg length discrepancy. Structural scoliosis can occur at any age. It may be due to defects in the vertebrae from birth or may develop idiopathically (with no known cause). It often shows up in children or adolescents during a growth spurt.

Scoliosis is named based on the location and the type of curve. The curve is either a "C" or "S" shape. An example of a common "S" curve is the right thoracic left lumbar curve. When a curve reaches a 40 degree angle, bracing and/or surgery may be indicated. Once the curve becomes significant, worsening of the curve will continue due to natural aging process and the pull of gravity over time. Intervention is necessary to prevent the curve from squeezing the lungs and heart as the ribs rotate and collapse with the lateral bending and rotation of the vertebrae. Compression of the vertebrae may interfere with nerve conduction in the spine, leading to leg weakness. Back pain and fatigue are common.

4.3.2. Presentation

Presentation includes uneven shoulder height, rib hump (noticeable upon a forward bend to 90 degrees) and uneven height of pelvis. In the front, breast may be uneven and protruding on the concave side.

4.3.3. Yoga intention

Yoga for the lengthening of the spine, de-rotation of the spine and strengthening the core to maintain the lengthened state.

4.3.4. Key problems and recommended *yogasana*

Problem	Recommended *yogasana*
Lateral bending in spine	Lengthening of spine with lateral bend to opposite side. *Tadasana* with lateral bending. *Trikonasana* with focus on lengthening.
Rotation of spine - rotation is forward to front of chest on the concave side and rotation is posterior on the convex side of the curve (creating the rib hump)	De-rotation of the spine. Spinal Twist - away from side of rib hump. *Pavritta Trikonasana* with focus on lengthening the spine.
Compression of the spine	Lengthening of spine in *yogasana*. Standing Wall stretch. *Adho Mukha Svanasana*: make marks on the mat to align self.

4.3.5 Safety and special commentary

For someone who has had a rod implanted in the spine, there is no mobility of the spine where the rod is located. Care should be taken not to create excessive mobility above and below the rod. Poses are practiced to both sides with the intention of achieving symmetry to the left and right.

4.4. Osteoporosis

4.4.1. Description and pathology

Osteoporosis is the condition where the loss of bone density creates fragile bones, which are then prone to fractures. The diagnosis is determined by Bone Mineral Density (BMD). The normal level is a T score of 1. When the BMD's T score is 2.5 or greater, osteoporosis is present. In osteopenia, the T score is between 1 and 2.5.

Osteoporosis is most common in post-menopausal women, but may occur at any age. Peak bone mass is reached around age 30. Up to that point, bone formation is greater than the bone re-absorption rate. The fastest rate of bone loss occurs in women in the first few years after menopause. Other risk factors contributing to bone loss include excess of alcohol, smoking, diet lacking in calcium and vitamin D, inactivity and long-term use of medication such as steroids.

4.4.2. Presentation

Osteoporosis often results in the rounding of the thoracic spine and collapsing of the vertebrae. Compression fractures of the vertebrae result in loss of height and pain in the back. Pain and fear of further fractures can lead to depression, reduction of physical activities and loss of independence in activities in daily living (ADLs).

4.4.3 Yoga intention
Maintain good posture and take actions to strengthen the bones.

4.4.4. Key problems and recommended *yogasana*

Problem	Recommended *yogasana*
At risk for fractures	**Supported Balancing Sequence** - guard against falls.
Kyphosis: deformity of the spine	**Chest Opening** *Yogasana*
Decreased bone density	**Strengthening Sequence** with weight-bearing *yogasana*. Diet rich in Calcium and Vitamin D.
Mental and emotional: depression and fear of fractures	Pranayama Meditation
Pain from fractures and compression of spine	**Restorative Yoga** **Guided relaxation**

4.4.5. Safety and special commentary

Forward bends create increased pressure in the lumbar vertebrae. Be sure to bend from the hips and keep the spine straight.

4.5. Arthritis

4.5.1. Description and Pathology

Rheumatoid arthritis: Rheumatoid arthritis (RA) is an inflammation that attacks the synovial linings of the joints. RA tends to affect the smaller joints. Joints become warm, painful and swollen during periods of exacerbation. Over time, the inflammation destroys the joint tissues. A common deformity of RA is the drifting of the fingers.

Osteoarthritis: Also known as degenerative joint disease, osteoarthritis occurs when the cartilage of the joints begins to wear. Without the protective covering on the joints, weight-bearing and movement is painful.

4.5.2. Presentation

Rheumatoid arthritis: characterized by swollen smaller joints, for example, the wrists and hands. A common deformity from RA is the ulnar drift of the wrists and hands, which impairs hand strength. Full weight-bearing on involved joints is not recommended.

Osteoarthritis: sufferers commonly experience stiffness with movement. Stiffness increases over time, especially with lack of movement. Larger weight-bearing joints are typically involved. Jumping in and out of poses is not recommended.

4.5.3. Yoga Intention
Gently lubricate the joints in non-stressful yoga.

4.5.4. Key problems and recommended *yogasana*

Problem	Recommended *yogasana*
<u>RA:</u> deformities of small joints. Period of Inflammation.	Breathing exercises and meditation recommended during inflammation period.
<u>OA:</u> progressive degeneration of larger weight-bearing joints.	Yoga postures in lying or positions of non-weight bearing recommended. **Pawanmuktasana** – gentle rotation of the joints improves circulation and reduces stiffness without stress to joints.

4.5.5. Safety and special commentary

During periods of inflammation, avoid weight bearing or stress to the joints. Less is better.

4.6. Lower Back

4.6.1. Description and pathology

Back pain is a leading cause of work related disability. Common risk factors include sedentary lifestyle, being overweight, a job that requires longs periods of sitting or a job that requires repeated or heavy lifting. The spine brings the weight of our upper body down through to the pelvis. Abnormal alignment of the pelvic bowl and lumbar vertebrae is seen with lumbar lordosis.

The key concepts in management of low back pain is restoring optimal alignment of the spine and pelvis, strengthening the core to maintain this alignment and to stretch any structures that may be pulling the spine out of alignment.

Sciatica: The spinal nerve roots that make up the sciatic nerve exit the spine from the L4, L5, S1,S2, S3 vertebrae and combine to make the largest and longest nerve in the body. The sciatic nerve runs from the low back, through the buttock and down the back of the leg. When compression and injury occurs to this nerve it is called sciatica. Sciatica may be caused by a herniated disc, spinal stenosis, spondylithesis or muscle spasm. Symptoms of sciatica may be pain in the back or anywhere down the leg to the foot. Changes in sensation and muscle strength may be present. In general, symptoms that include weakness and sensation changes to the leg and foot are more serious and require medical management.

4.6.2. Presentation

Lower back pain presents differently depending on the severity and etiology of the pain. The onset can be sudden as seen with a trauma or lifting injury, or the onset may be gradual as with degeneration of the spine. Symptoms vary from an ache in the back such as with sacroiliac joint dysfunction or may radiate down the leg as with sciatica. Neurological involvement is an indication of a more serious problem.

4.6.3. Yoga intention
Strengthening of the core with focus on neutral alignment of the lower back.

4.6.4. Key problems and recommended *yogasana*

Problem	Recommended *yogasana*
Spinal alignment	**Spinal Alignment Exercise** **Posture Awareness Exercise**
Abdominals	**Core Strengthening Sequence**
Back Extensors	*Bhujangasana*

Problem	Recommended *yogasana*
Stretching of Hip Flexors - these muscles attach to the lumbar spine and often pull on the back.	**Hip-to-knee Sequence**
Stretching of Hamstrings – these muscles attach to the posterior pelvis, which when tight, pull the pelvis and the spine out of alignment.	*Supta Padangusthanasana* (using the strap)
Tight lower back muscles	Double knees to chest– this opens the lower back

4.6.5. Safety and special commentary

In cases where there is onset of weakness in the extremities, numbness, tingling and/or bowel and bladder changes, a physician should be contacted.

Bowel and bladder symptoms should be treated as a medical emergency.

4.7. Neck

4.7.1. Description and pathology

Neck pain is a common complaint. In general, muscle spasms in the neck muscles are due to poor posture and work habits or lifestyle that results in neck pain. We may sleep in a crooked neck position, talk on the phone using the shoulder and ear to hold the phone, or sit at the computer with the shoulders tensed. Yoga that focuses on posture, core stability and relaxing muscle tension is excellent for improving this kind of neck pain.

More serious causes of neck pain include disc herniation, cervical stenosis and spondylolithesis. Whiplash, a common injury of the neck with a car accident or other trauma, may result in strain and tears to the

337

ligaments and muscles of the neck. Immediate X-rays to rule out fractures are recommended with all traumas to the neck.

4.7.2. Presentation

Less serious neck pain may be interpreted as a general feeling of stiffness and muscle aches. More serious symptoms may include pain radiating down the arm, numbness and tingling in the fingers, and weakness in the arm. These symptoms require medical assessment.

4.7.3. Yoga Intention

Yoga to reduce stress and tension in the neck area.

4.7.4. Key problems and recommended *yogasana*

Problem	Recommended *yogasana*
Tension in the neck muscles	**Restorative Yoga** Long deep breathing to relax muscles and to reduce stress.
Pain and stiffness in neck	**Pawanmuktasana**: gentle upper body.
Posture of neck may be tipped to side, or forward head posture, or other abnormal postures	**Posture Awareness Sequence** **Core Strengthening Sequence**

4.7.5. Safety and special commentary

For persons with neck pain due to trauma who wish to start yoga, it is imperative that he or she be cleared by a medical professional to rule out fractures prior to commencing classes.

Worsening symptoms that include pain down the arm, numbness or loss of strength should be investigated by a medical professional to rule out serious pathologies.

Weight bearing on the head and neck is not recommended.

4.8. Upper Extremities

4.8.1. Abnormal alignment of the upper extremities

Dysfunctional Scapula Humeral Movement: For every 15 degrees of shoulder abduction, 10 degrees is from the humerus in the shoulder joint and 5 degrees is from the scapula. This means that in extended *tadasana*, raising the arms requires rotation of the scapula combined with the humeral head externally rotating to tuck under the coracoacromion arch (Cailliet, 1977). Dysfunction is when this coordinated scapula and shoulder movement is not occurring.

Rounded Back and Forward Shoulder Posture: This posture prevents the external rotation needed for fully lifting the shoulder.

Hyperextension of the Elbow: In hyper-mobility, the elbow joint may hyperextend. In weight-bearing, the muscles are not doing the work bearing the weight but lock instead, using the bones. This is illustrated in *section 4.10*.

4.8.2. Common pathologies and injuries

Rotator Cuff: Tearing of the rotator or SITS muscles of the shoulder.

Frozen Shoulder: Capsule ligaments around shoulder tighten and limit movement of the shoulder.

Tennis Elbow: Inflammation of the lateral tendons of the elbow. The tendons are attachments for the muscles of the forearm that provide the muscle action for wrist extension.

Carpal Tunnel: Considered a repetitive use syndrome where the median nerve that crosses the wrist is being compressed. Weight-bearing on the wrist may further aggravate the existing carpal tunnel symptom.

Arthritis of the hand: This creates weakness, pain and deformities in the hand.

4.8.3. Yoga intention

Restore *strength and flexibility needed for functional use of the arms and hands in daily living.*

4.8.4. Key Problems and recommended *yogasana*

Problem	Recommended *yogasana*
Rotator Cuff	Open the shoulders and progress to strengthening poses for the shoulders. Standing poses in which arms extend against gravity are gentle strengtheners. *Chaturanga Dandasana* is not recommended if there is a rotator cuff injury. This pose requires good alignment and sufficient strength to maintain the alignment or injury is likely to result.
Frozen Shoulder	**Shoulder Opening Sequence** Supine *Tadasana* (using strap)
Tennis Elbow	Strengthen the forearm and wrist with standing *Virabhadrasana II*. Avoid weight-bearing arm balance poses until resolved.
Carpal Tunnel	Modify amount of weight-bearing – try use of a wedge.
Arthritis of the hand	Avoid weight-bearing on hands or reduce amount of weight.

4.9. Lower Extremities

4.9.1. Abnormal alignment of the lower extremities

Hips:
- **Anteversion** is the placement of the femoral head anterior to the acetabulum, creating a structural limitation of external rotation of the hips. This can result in difficulty with sitting in easy pose.
- **Retroversion** is the positioning of the femoral head posterior to the acetabulum creating limitation in internal rotation of the hips. This can result in difficulty with *virasana*.

Knees:
- **Genu Recurvaturm** is hyperextension of the knee. This is illustrated in *section 4.10*.
- **Genu Valgus** is knock knees.
- **Genu Varus** is also known as "bow legged".
- **Tibial Torsion** medial rotation of the patella.

Feet:
- **Pes Planus** is flat feet.

4.9.2. Common pathologies and injuries

Hip:
- Total hip replacement.
- Arthritis, bursitis and tendonitis of hip.

Knees:
- Total knee replacement.
- Meniscus and ligament tears.

Feet/Ankles:
- Stiffness in the ankles and toes.
- Weakness in the small muscles of the ankles often leads to instability at the joint.
- Neurological involvement leads to abnormal tone where the anterior tibialis overpowers the peroneals and pulls the foot into inversion.

4.9.3. Yoga intention

To restore strength and flexibility needed to support the body in functional movements.

4.9.4. Key Problems and recommended *yogasana*

Problem	Recommended *yogasana*
Hip replacement	Limited hip range – especially hip flexion and rotation. Extreme range runs risk of dislocating the hip. Poses such as *kapotanasana* which combines an extreme range at the hip plus body weight on the joint are contraindicated.
Anteversion of femoral head: limited external rotation of hips	In *padmasana* or other sitting poses, use blankets to raise height of pelvis and allow knees to be lower than the hips.
Hip arthritis, bursitis and tendonitis	Practice non weight-bearing yoga when hip is painful
Knees – replacement and other knee injuries	Extreme range and weight-bearing such as a squat are not recommended (avoid hips going lower than the knees). Standing poses that emphasize alignment such as *utkatasana* are a good strengthener for the knee.
Feet	**Foot Care Routine** Maintain good range of motion of toes and ankles. Flexibility and strength in the feet are needed for good balance and normal gait.

4.9.5 Safety and special commentary

Post-surgical and post-joint replacement practitioners need the surgeon to provide medical clearance and information regarding limitations and any contraindications before beginning a yoga program.

4.10. Hyperextended joints

Care should be taken throughout *yogasana* practice to ensure that these joints are not locked, but straight, soft and slightly bent if necessary, so that injuries from hyperextension do not occur.

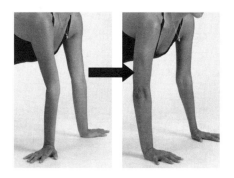

Elbows: turning the eyes of the elbows to look at each other.

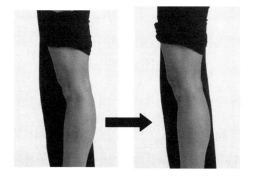

Knees: keeping the kneecaps soft so that the legs are straight with bones aligned to prevent bowing of the calves.

References

Cailliet, R (1977). *Shoulder Pain*. USA, F.A. Davis Co.

Book Three

YOGASENSE™:
Roadmap
Selected Routines and Exercises

YOGASENSE™ Master Sequence,
Selected Routines & Exercises
in DVD format
Details at the back of this book and from www.sunyoga.com

The YogaSense™ Roadmap

THE FUNDAMENTALS

1. Bandha (*p. 225*)

2. Pranayama (*p. 238*)

3. Chanting (*p. 243*)

4. Yoga eye exercise (*p. 256)*

5. Meditation (*p. 261*)

6. Sun breath (*p. 349*)

7. Pelvic floor routine (*p.364*)

8. Foot care routine (*p. 366)*

9. Pawanmuktasana sequence (*p. 367*)

10. Guided relaxation (*p.368*)

11. Tantra Yoga (*p.369*)

THE PHILOSOPHY

Book 1 *sections 7.3 and 8.9*

YOGASENSE™

YOGASENSE™ MASTER SEQUENCE DVD

Available from www.sunyoga.com

SPECIAL ISSUES

1. Brain organizing & grounding meditation (*p.350*)

2. Vestibular rebalancing exercise (*p. 351*)

3. Posture awareness exercise (*p. 352*)

4. Balance sequence (*p. 353*)

5. Spinal alignment exercise (*p. 355*)

6. Core strengthening exercise (*p. 357*)

7. Supported strengthening sequence (*p. 359*)

8. Wheelchair / chair yoga (*p. 360*)

9. Hip & hamstring opening exercise (*p. 361*)

10. Shoulder opening sequence (*p. 362*)

11. Lower back routine (*p. 363*)

12. Restorative Yoga (*p. 365*)

13. Gastrointestinal (GI) exercise (*p. 367*)

SUN BREATH SEQUENCE

Eka 1: Breath Awareness

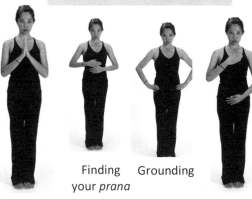

Namaskar

Finding your *prana*

Grounding

Aligning body with breath

Dve 2: Breath and coordinated movement

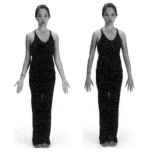

Inhale- palms facing forward
Exhale- palms facing backwards
(12 cycles)

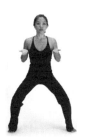

Inhale – lift palms and arms upward
Exhale- strong grounding motion with hands
(12 cycles)

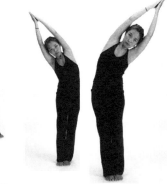

Energizing with your breath!

Trini 3: Nourishing

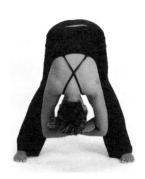

Chatvari 4: Chest Opening 1

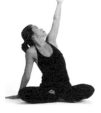

INHALE

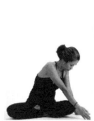

EXHALE

Panca 5: Chest Opening 2

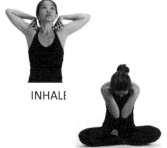

INHALE

EXHALE

BRAIN ORGANIZING & GROUNDING MEDITATION

Benefit	Body Part	Yoga
Brain balancing	Respiratory System	Balancing *Pranayama*: *nadi sodhana* (*Page 239*)
Balance and grounding	Crossed midline with deep pressure	*Garudasana*
Balancing left and right Brain	Coordinated cross-lateral movements	Windmill Yoga March
Centering and calming	Mind focus	Meditation (*Book 1: section 8.6*)

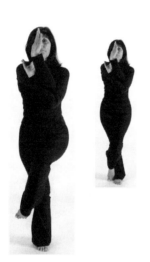

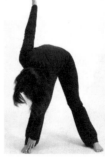

YOGA MARCH

(right)
Reciprocal movement pattern is achieved with repeated simultaneous lifting of the opposite arm and leg. This imitates the mature crawling of a baby and plays an important role in achieving bilateral coordination.

GARUDASANA

(above, main picture)
Deep pressure is applied while crossing midline at the forearms and thighs, calming the nervous system.

(above, inset)
Modification: keep the focus on being steady. If you have a balance problem keep the toe of the crossed leg on the floor.

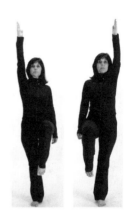

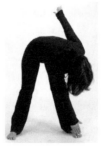

WINDMILL

(above)
The repeated movement of crossing midline helps to integrate the left and right brain.

VESTIBULAR REBALANCING EXERCISE

Benefit	Body Part/Movement	Posture
Vestibular system within the inner ear is retrained.

Episodes of dizziness and vertigo reduced. | Head lateral bend and rotation | *Trikonasana* |
	Head flexion/extension	Cat/Cow
	Head down with rotation	Thread the needle
	Head rotation with lateral bend	Windmill
	Head inversion	*Adho Mukha Svanasana*

Uttanasana |

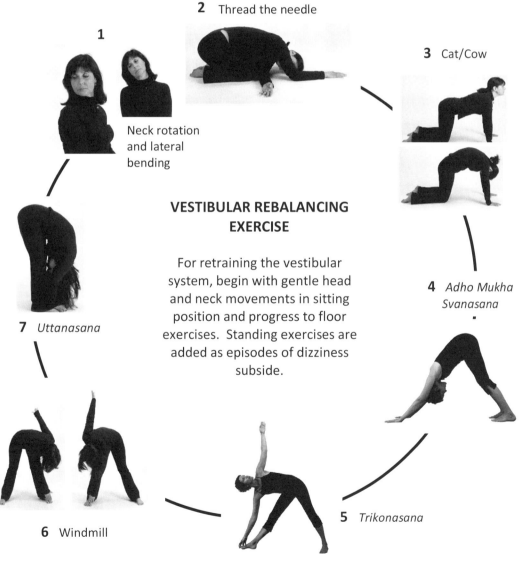

1

Neck rotation and lateral bending

2 Thread the needle

3 Cat/Cow

4 *Adho Mukha Svanasana*

5 *Trikonasana*

6 Windmill

7 *Uttanasana*

VESTIBULAR REBALANCING EXERCISE

For retraining the vestibular system, begin with gentle head and neck movements in sitting position and progress to floor exercises. Standing exercises are added as episodes of dizziness subside.

POSTURE AWARENESS EXERCISE

For posture awareness, bring your focus inwards. Visualize and realign your body starting with the feet, moving up through the body to the head.

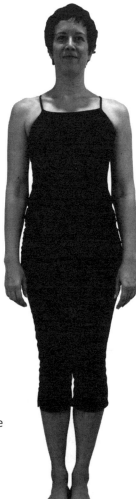

5

- Shoulders are pulled back but relaxed. The back of the neck is long in a slightly chin-tucked position.
- The arms are relaxed to the side.

4

The chest is lifted on each inhalation as the feet are grounded with each exhalation.

3

Thighs are lifted, hips are over the knees and ankle. The pelvis is in neutral position.

2

The knees are positioned over the ankles. Care is taken so as not to hyperextend the knee.

1

- Feet grounded, heels touching if possible. Otherwise, for stability, keep feet hip-width apart.
- Feet pressed downwards on the floor weight-bearing evenly on both feet.
- Weight is distributed evenly across the ball of the foot and the heel.
- Toes are spread out and the arch of the feet lifted.

BALANCE SEQUENCE

Balance awareness exercise

Close the eyes in *tadansana* to feel the inner balance. Extend the arms and move gently into side bending to challenge the balance.

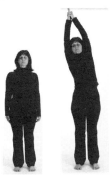

Pre-standing balance exercise

Before moving into standing balance poses start in the hands and knees position to learn to engage the core while lifting one arm or one leg. After you have learned to use your core, progress to simultaneous lifting of the opposite arm and leg.

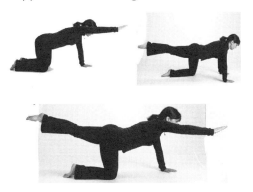

Static balance exercise

In single leg standing poses engage the core and keep the eye gaze steady. Use a chair for support or a toe on the floor until you are steady in single leg standing. For a challenge turn the head to the side as you maintain your balance.

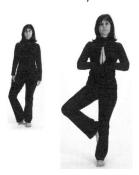

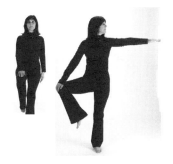

BALANCE SEQUENCE

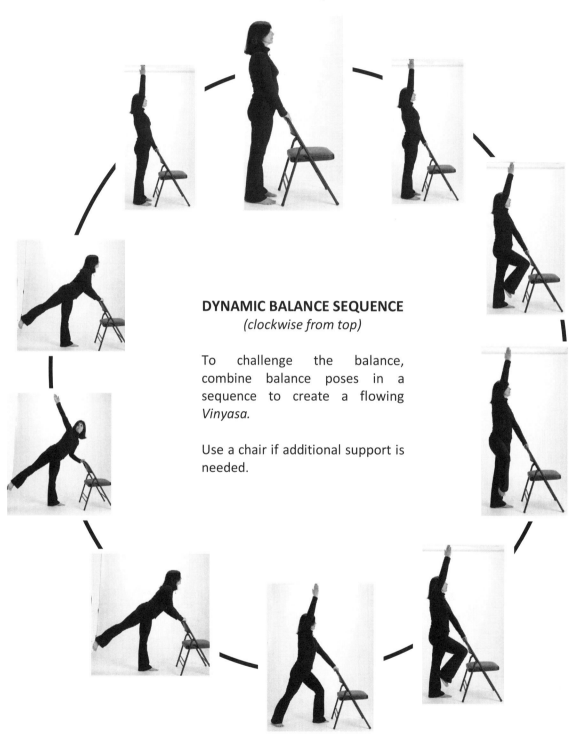

DYNAMIC BALANCE SEQUENCE
(clockwise from top)

To challenge the balance, combine balance poses in a sequence to create a flowing *Vinyasa.*

Use a chair if additional support is needed.

SPINAL ALIGNMENT EXERCISE

Lengthening the spine

- Follow the cues for postural awareness – engage core, lift chest, shoulder blades pulled back and lengthen the back of the neck.
- Ground the tailbone as you lengthen the spine upward.

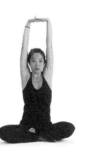

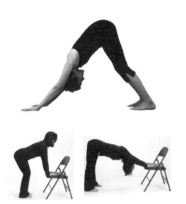

- *Adho mukha svanasana* lengthens the spine using gravity.
- To focus on spinal lengthening, bend the knees slightly to release the pull of the hamstrings on the back.
- Use a chair or wall as a gentle modification.

- *Balasana* opens the lower back and reverses the thoracic flexion (or kyphosis).
- Ground the tailbone as you stretch the arms forward.

Strengthening the spine

Plank and *adho mukha svanasana*: Moving between these two poses works the back extensors and abdominal while keeping the spine straight and lengthened.

Exhale

Inhale

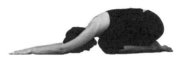

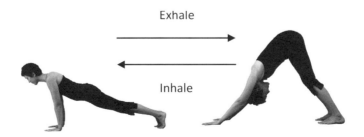

SPINAL ALIGNMENT EXERCISE

De-rotation of the spine

In scoliosis there is lateral bending of the spine and rotation of the vertebrae. Be sure to anchor in the tailbone and lengthen the spine as you rotate the trunk in the de-rotation yoga poses.

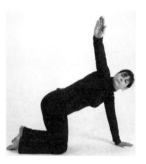

From hands and knees position lift one arm to rotate the spine. Try to make the rotation to the left and right symmetrical.

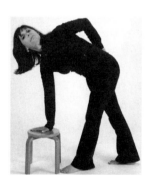

Revolved triangle is an example of a pose in which the spine de-rotates along the entire spine from the tailbone to the head.

Resting the arm on the back allows you to focus on the spine.

Opening the side of the body

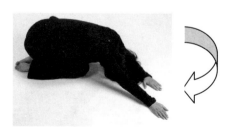

Balasana Arm Walk: From *balasana,* walk the hands over toward the convex side of the curve. This will open and lengthen the concave side of the spine.

CORE STRENGTHENING EXERCISE

Core awareness

To protect our back in our daily lives and during our yoga practice, engaging the core to maintain a neutral spine or neutral pelvis is essential. The pelvis is in a neutral position and the spine with the natural lumbar curvature when the pubic bone and anterior superior iliac spine are in the same plane.

Place the heel of the hand on the hip bone and the fingers pointing toward the pubic bone, creating a triangle. Neutral is the point in which the pelvic bowl will neither be tipped forward (anterior tilt with arching back) or tipped back (posterior tilt with flattened low back).

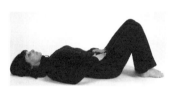

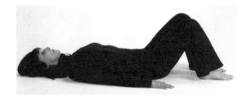

Practice long deep breathing while maintaining a neutral spine. Imagine in your mind, walking while maintaining the pelvic bowl upright, neither tipped forward or back.

Abdominal control with movement

To gain spinal stability, practice movement of the leg while maintaining a neutral pelvis.

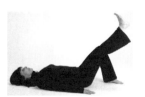

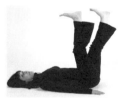

Leg Raises   Leg Circles   Leg Walk

CORE STRENGTHENING EXERCISE

Challenge and apply

Strengthen the Abdominals

Strengthen the Back Extensors

Modification for tight hamstrings or weak core

Core Strengthening

1. Reduces back fatigue

2. Reduces back pain

3. Improves breathing

4. Gives stability for moving

5. Helps maintain a straight spine

6. Protects internal organs

7. This is the container that holds the internal pressure for the breath and bowel movements.

Strengthen the pelvic floor muscles

Do pelvic floor exercises and apply *moolabandha* during *yogasana*

SUPPORTED STRENGTHENING SEQUENCE

Strengthening in motion

Using weight-bearing and gravity, this mini *vinyasa* builds strength throughout the range of motion.

Strengthen the arms by maintaining them up throughout the sequence

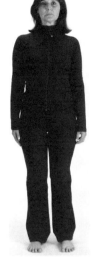

1

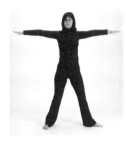

9

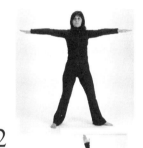

2

3

Standing poses are excellent for strengthening the body.

Engage the core throughout to build core strength.

8

4

7

6

5

Legs are strengthened by working in the wide stance.

The thighs are engaged throughout the sequence.

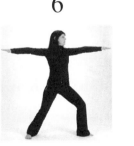

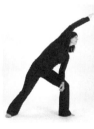

Ankles are strengthened by lifting up the arches and pressing down to engage the whole foot.

SUPPORTED STRENGTHENING SEQUENCE

Modified *Surya Namaskar*

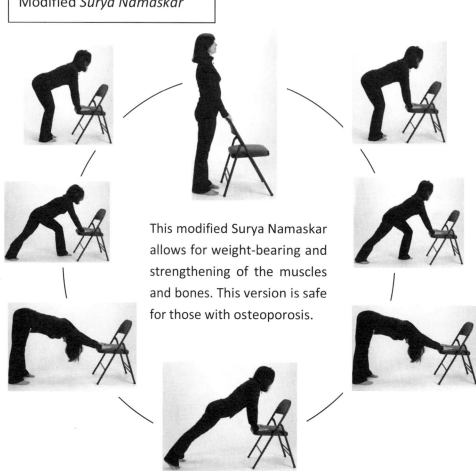

This modified Surya Namaskar allows for weight-bearing and strengthening of the muscles and bones. This version is safe for those with osteoporosis.

WHEELCHAIR / CHAIR YOGA

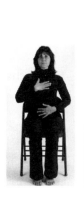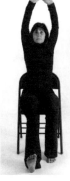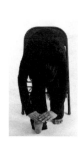

Many poses can be modified for the sitting position. Don't let the chair define your yoga.

HIP AND HAMSTRING OPENING EXERCISE

Assisted leg stretching with the strap

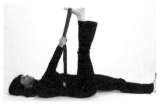 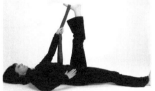 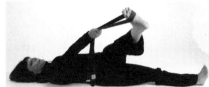

Stretching the leg straight upwards with a strap around the ball of the foot in *supta padagusthasana,* use your exhalation to release tightness.

Keeping the pelvis grounded to the floor, move the leg out to the side to stretch the hip adductors.

Allow the leg to cross over the midline to release tightness in the tensor fascia latae and the hip adductors.

Engage the core throughout the sequence to protect the back and stabilize the lumbar spine in neutral. Those with back issues or weakness of the core should practice the sequence with the opposite knee bent.

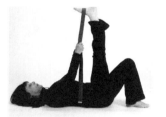

Additional stretches for the hip

 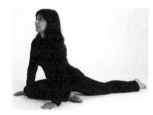 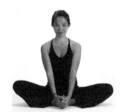

External rotators

External rotator on bent knee side; hip flexors on extended leg side

Hip adductor stretch with external rotation

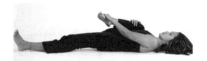 **Iliopsoas stretch:** hip flexors are stretched on the extended leg.

SHOULDER OPENING EXERCISE

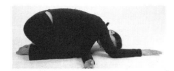

Mobilizing

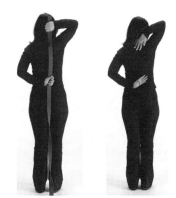

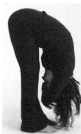

In Thread the Needle, the body weight gently brings the shoulder into horizontal adduction, stretching the deltoids and triceps.

Using the strap to open the shoulder – lower arm into internal rotation and the upper arm into external rotation

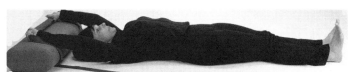

In *uttanasana* (*left*) and in lying *tadasana* (*above*), gravity is used to assist in opening the shoulders. The arms are supported on a bolster or cradled to allow the muscles to be stretched to relax in this pose.

Strengthening

Moderate challenge is created by working and stretching at end range.

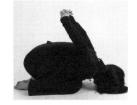

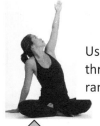

Using gravity through the range

Working against gravity and using the body weight, shoulder exercises can be graded to meet the individual's needs.

Gentle strengthening using self-assist.

Most challenging is moving in and out of poses while holding the body weight.

START

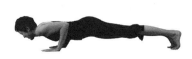

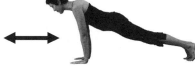

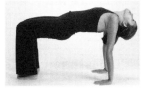

LOWER BACK ROUTINE

Pathway for a healthy back

Realign the spine: stretch hamstrings, hip flexors and back extensors that pull the spine out of alignment.

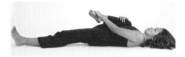
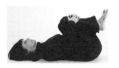
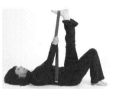
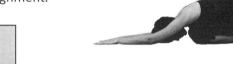

Core strengthening: build core awareness and core strength to maintain spinal stability in neutral spine. Refer to the **Core Strengthening Routine**.

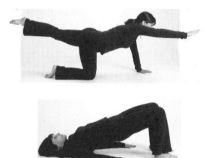
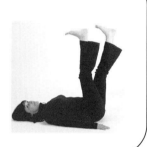

Functional stabilization: learn to maintain good postural alignment throughout the *yogasana* practice.

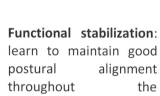
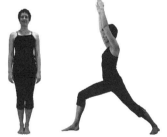
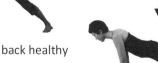

Good posture helps keep the back healthy

PELVIC FLOOR ROUTINE

Pelvic floor awareness

In yoga, the pelvic floor is part of applying the root lock or *moolabandha*. Refer to *Book 1, section 7.5.2.*

1. Begin in knee bent position. Breathe in and out. Begin to draw the breath in as if breathing in from the pelvic floor and release with the exhale.

2. Breathe in and tighten pelvic floor, hold tight and release the breath, then release the pelvic floor muscles. Learn to separate the breath from the pelvic floor.

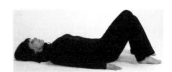

3. Lengthen the time with the pelvic floor muscles tightened to 10 breaths. Inhale deeply on the 10th breath and tighten the pelvic floor as much as possible. Exhale, then release the pelvic floor muscles.

> Pelvic floor exercises reduce incontinence, bring connection to first *chakra* and improve postural control.

Challenge and apply the *moolabandha*

1. Stand in Goddess pose (*below, left*). Breathe in and pull up pelvic floor. Hold for 3 breaths. Exhale and release pelvic floor muscles.

2. Repeat standing in Star pose *(below, middle)*. Tighten the pelvic floor and hold for 3 breaths

3. Repeat: stand in *tadasana* with arms raised (*below, right*). Tighten the pelvic floor and hold for 3 breaths.

4. Practice this routine during daily activities such as standing in the grocery line and sitting at your desk.

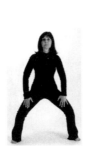 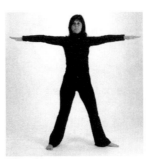 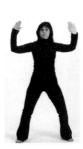

RESTORATIVE YOGA

Renewing your energy

In restoratives the body is supported for total relaxation. Focus on long deep breathing.

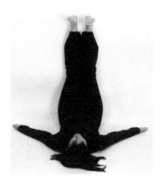

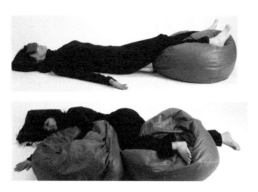

Benefit		Position
Reducing edema to legs, increase venous return to heart.	**Whole body calming of the nervous system:** Increase Parasympathetic System Decrease Sympathetic System	Legs up wall
Good for back pain or pregnancy		Sideline
Relaxation position to reduce pressure at low back.		Supported bent knee

Opening the chest with restoratives

Benefit	Body Part	Restorative
Expand rib and open shoulder: gentle stretching with gravity.	Intercostals of ribs Pectoralis muscles	Mat roll along spine
Reduce kyphosis – opening space for lungs.	Thoracic Spine	Mat roll perpendicular to spine

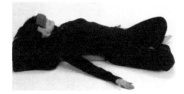

Placing a rolled mat along the spine perpendicular or vertically creates a gentle back bend and chest opener.

FOOT CARE ROUTINE

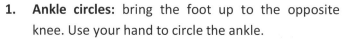

Mobilizing the foot

This is a gentle way of increasing circulation, flexibility and awareness to the feet. Start with these exercises before moving on to opening the ankles.

1. **Ankle circles:** bring the foot up to the opposite knee. Use your hand to circle the ankle.
2. **Toe bend**: use your hand to extend and bend the toes.
3. **Toe separation**: use your fingers to go between the toes, squeeze the fingers with the toes and relax.
4. **Toe pulls**: circle and pull each toe.

Opening the ankles

Having good balance includes having adequate flexibility in the ankles and toes. Those with decreased circulation or decreased strength of the feet will find that the ankles and toes become stiff. Practice long deep breathing while in this pose. If this is too painful, go back to the routine for mobilizing the foot.

1. *Balasana*: Ankles in extension. Surprisingly, some will find the stretch across the anterior foot painful. In this case, use a yoga mat or towel rolled under ankles.

2. *Vajrasana*: Sitting with toes flexed improves flexibility in stiff toes and stretches the sole of the foot. This can be painful for some so use blocks to support part of your body weight and reduce the weight bearing on the toes as needed.

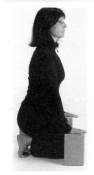

PAWANMUKTASANA SEQUENCE

Gentle lubricating of joints

Pawanmuktasana is an ancient yoga routine that gently rotates, flexes and bends the joints of the body. Starting with the toes, it moves up the body sequentially. The gentle movements lubricate all the joints of the body.

1. Toe – bend and extend
2. Ankle – flex and extend, circles
3. Knee – flex and extend
4. Hips – circles
5. Hands – open and close
6. Wrist – circles
7. Elbow – flex and extend
8. Shoulder – circles
9. Neck - turning side to side, side bend and gently nodding head.

GASTROINTESTINAL (GI) SEQUENCE

These *yogasana* reduce gas and increase the parasympathetic system which aids in digestion.

Twists are done to both directions, starting to the left.

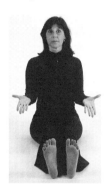

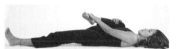

In *apanasana*, start with bending the right knee toward the right shoulder to press against the ascending colon. Follow with the left knee to the chest to stimulate the descending colon.

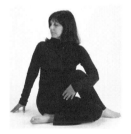

This series of yoga poses is relaxing, massaging the internal organs to aid digestion and elimination.

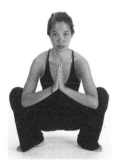

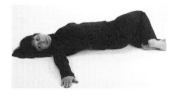

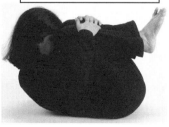

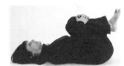

Keep your head to the floor in the double-knees-to-chest if you have neck issues.

GUIDED RELAXATION

Guided Relaxation is used to promote healing from within.

Preparing: Get comfortable in a quiet place. Clear your space so that your arms and legs are not touching anything.

Positioning: Close your eyes or use an eye pillow. Arms are positioned 6-12 inches out at side with palms up. The legs are 12-18 inches apart with the legs and feet rolled outward. Cover yourself with a blanket. Your neck should be in neutral alignment. Use a small pillow if needed.

Alternate positions: 1. Legs may be supported in the bent knee position. This is a good position if you have back problems
2. Lie on the side if lying on back is uncomfortable or if pregnant
3. Sit or lean on a desk if you cannot lie down

Instructions: Focus on the breath. Inhale, sending the breath to each body part and relax on the exhale. Start with the feet and work up the body ending at the head. Be sure to relax the jaw and tongue.
Feel the body surrender to the gravity. Maintain your focus on the breath and let go of any thoughts that may arise during your relaxation. Send the breath to a particular body part that needs healing energy.

Time: 5-20 minutes.

When: Relaxation is done at the end of yoga asana practice. It can also be practiced during the day if feeling tired or stressed.

Purpose: Promotes healing and nurtures the body and mind. Awaken rejuvenated.

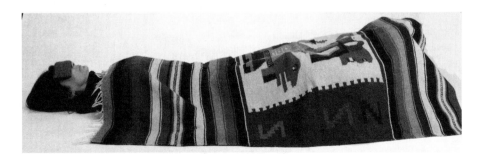

TANTRA YOGA

Union (*yoga*) and completion (*tantra*) through exploration, touch and pure love. Touch between two adults does not necessarily have to be sexual all the time. We all have the ability to heal with our hands, and it is through touching with pure intent and loving heart that we can bring healing, love, joy and completion to our partner. Tantra Yoga is about coming together through exploring and playing with each other.

Beginning your journey:

Set your intention. Your intention is to explore, to give and to heal, not sexual gratification. Therefore, in this beginning session, there will be no penetrative sex and no orgasm for either party.

Your first touch is Namaskar. Firmly lay your hands on your partner's body (shoulders are a good place) and hold that position. Tune in to your partner's breathing rhythm. Let your nostrils be filled with your partner's scent. Allow your hands to be the conduit for your body temperatures. Stay in this position until you feel your two bodies are equilibrated: same heat, same breath, same intention. Be totally absorbed.

Then slowly but confidently move your hands and lay them on another part of your partner's body. Get acquainted with the landscape and contours. Grow in your confidence.

Begin your exploration. Encourage your partner to vocalize: "That feels good", "Move lower", "Do that again", etc.

As you progress, you may wish to touch your partner with other parts of your body or your tongue. Give expression to the love in you. Grow as you heal. This is Tantra Yoga.

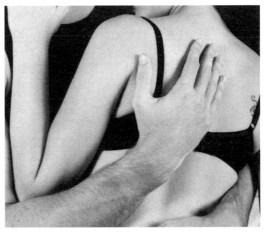

Tantra Yoga- Yoga for Lovers
by Jacqueline Koay
Sun Yoga (January 2010)
www.sunyoga.com

About Sun Yoga:

Sun Yoga is a global, not-for-profit organization dedicated to creating a more peaceful and fairer world through yoga. Founded in 2001 by Jacqueline Koay, Sun Yoga grew from small weekly classes taught out of Friendship House in Southsea, Hampshire (Jacqueline's hometown) into a global family of over 450 teachers. Today, Sun Yoga runs teacher training programs, workshops and classes in Europe, Asia and the United States.

Profits from Sun Yoga have been channeled into supporting projects benefiting children and the needy globally, eschewing its Founder's vision of creating a better world through yoga. Sun Yoga also provides opportunities for people from all walks of life to find a more meaningful, balanced and yogic way of life.

For more information, please email hello@sunyoga.com or visit www.sunyoga.com.

About Yogabilitation and YogaSense™ Therapy

Yogabilitation Physical Therapy Center is located in downtown Fairfield, Connecticut and offers a holistic approach to Physical Therapy for children and adults with medical, neurological and orthopedic concerns. **YogaSense™ Therapy,** developed by Theodora Barenholtz, is a blend of traditional physical therapy techniques with yogic teachings. Yogic techniques of breathwork, meditation, and postures are integrated in this highly effective therapy for motor, language, and social development as well as medical needs.

For information on YogaSense™ workshops, please email yogabilitation@aol.com or visit www.yogabilitation.com.

Sun Yoga's Teacher Training Programs:

Sun Yoga is a Yoga Alliance USA Registered School

Registered Yoga Teacher at 200 Hours (RYT200)

Beginning with the Foundation modules, students will then progress to take modules on Hatha, Kundalini, Contemporary and Children's Yoga. This modular program ensures that students are provided with a strong foundation (Techniques, Anatomy, Physiology, Philosophy, Ethics, Lifestyle and Teaching Methodology) as well as exposure to other key schools of yoga. Hands-on Practicum (assisting and teaching as trainee teachers) will ensure that the skills required to make a good and competent yoga teacher are finely honed.

Yoga Therapy (RYT500)

For students who have already achieved the basic 200 Hours qualification, this course is both heavily academic and hands-on. As a student, you will study the Foundation modules consisting of Yoga & Medical Science, Anatomy, Physiology and Ayurveda before undertaking the two main branches of Yoga Therapy, namely the Children's Yoga Therapy and Adults Yoga Therapy modules. You will also be working (under supervision) with real clients to give you the experience and exposure of working as a Yoga Therapist.

Other courses and workshops:
Sun Yoga Kids Teacher Training Program
Special Needs Yoga
Yoga in Schools
Prenatal Yoga

For more information, please visit www.sunyoga.com or www.yogasense.info.

Yogic Tools from Sun Yoga:

YogaSense™ Master Sequence, Exercises and Routines DVD.

Instructional DVD featuring the photographs used in this book in full color.

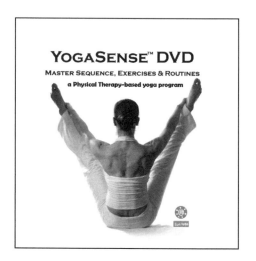

As an adjunct to this book, the YogaSense™ DVD contains all the materials presented here and much more. It further furnishes the exercises and routines presented in this book with clear and beautiful dialogue. The YogaSense™ DVD is a suitable practice accompaniment for all levels. **US$20**

Teaching Aid:
Yogasana flash cards

Invaluable tool for the new teacher

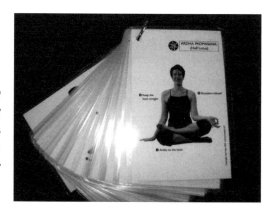

54 large color cards of common *yogasana* and Surya Namaskar illustrating the key points of each posture. Each *yogasana* is clearly photographed and annotated with the three / four key points, useful for dialoguing and self-practice. (14cm x 9cm) **US$35**

Live Patanjali! Yoga Wisdom for Everyday Living
(300 pages, printed on recycled paper)

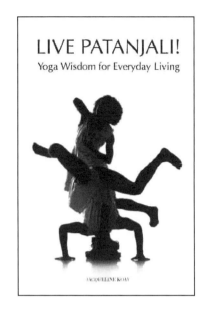

A simple-to-read discourse on the Yoga Sutra of Sri Patanjali, this book by Jacqueline Koay, Founder of Sun Yoga, has been serialized in Yoga magazine UK and widely reviewed. Written in plain English (with Sanskrit where relevant), Live Patanjali is based on the author's rich life and is redolent with humor and common sense. **US$20**

Simply Yogic.
Food for the Mind, Body & Soul
A simple, informational and relevant 100 page book on the yogic diet

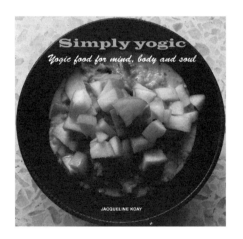

Written by Jacqueline Koay, whose first cookbook, *The Kundalini Yoga Cookbook*, was a finalist in the Gourmand World Cookbook Awards 2006 and is now published in three languages, this second cookbook from the author takes a deeper, more academic look into the subject and presents a collection of simple-to-prepare, delicious yogic food. **US$15**

Popular Yoga Mantra CD
(31 minutes)

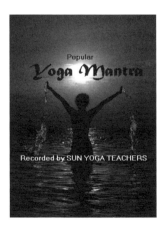

Recorded by Sun Yoga Teachers, this CD contains the popular mantra of the yoga tradition, in particular, Kundalini Yoga, including *Aad Guray Namay, Adi Shakti* and *Ramadasa*. Also included are the Gayatri Mantra and *Asatoma,* and instrumental tracks suitable for meditation. **US$10**

Fun With Sun Yoga. Yoga Cards and Booklet for Children's Yoga
An award-winning bestseller!

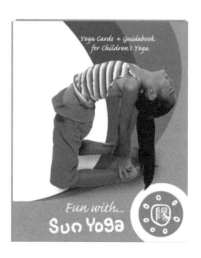

The prestigious Gold Award Winner of the Mom's Choice Awards 2009, this pack provides hours of yogic fun for the child. It also provides innovative class ideas for the teacher of children's yoga. The booklet contains information of the *yogasana* with suggestions on how to enrich each *yogasana* as well as games ideas.
US$20

Groovy Creatures Yoga DVD

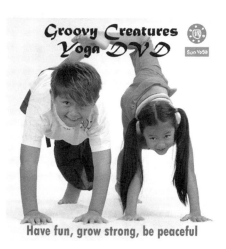

The Groovy Creatures are fun and original animals and plants created at Sun Yoga to deliver a physical therapy-based children's yoga program, and covers the following developmental areas: Brain balancing, Core strengthening, Whole-body strengthening & stretching, Balance and Positive Affirmation. This DVD is both fun and effective as a yoga therapy tool.
US$20

Children's Yoga Music CD
Fun yoga songs to get children moving as well as meditating.

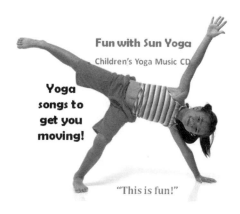

The songs borrow from classics such as 'I'm a Little Teapot' but with yogic themes. They are an ideal accompaniment to **Fun With Sun Yoga. Yoga Cards and Booklet for Children's Yoga.**
US$10

Peaceful Warrior Handbook

*A workbook for children and their parents
and teachers*
www.peacefulwarriorhandbook.com

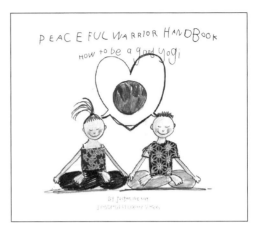

How to be a good yogi? Taking the abstractness out of the *yama* and *niyama*, this beautifully illustrated book gives the aspiring yogin/yogini a step-by-step guide to being a peaceful warrior. The heart-warming illustrations make this 32 page book a wonderful gift or a lovely activity to share with a child. (Color, 21cm x 17cm)
US$10

This book is available at quantity discounts.

Special purchase

The complete yogic toolkit containing all of the above is available at US$128, representing a saving of 20%!

Shipping, handling and applicable tax additional

Acknowledgements

Jacqueline and Teddi would like to thank:

Our teachers over the years who have contributed to our knowledge
Joanna Kraft and Rhonda Manware for being such lovely models
Teng Swee Ai and Tony Wong for accuracy (the mistakes are all ours!)
Katya Akermann and Adam Wilkinson for keeping us on track
and
Jan Barenholtz for feeding us when we were too busy to eat and for his
unending support and patience throughout this project.

With lots of love to our children, Nicky, Kit, Katerina, Jack and Georgina
(Jacqueline's) and Daniel and David (Teddi's).

SAT NAM